Environmental Health Hazards
and
Social Justice

Environmental Health Hazards
and
Social Justice

Geographical Perspectives on Race and Class Disparities

Florence Margai

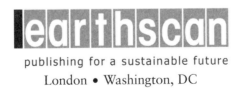

publishing for a sustainable future

London • Washington, DC

First published in 2010 by Earthscan

Earthscan Ltd, Dunstan House, 14a St Cross Street, London EC1N 8XA, UK
Earthscan LLC, 1616 P Street, NW, Washington, DC 20036, USA
Earthscan publishes in association with the International Institute for Environment and Development

For more information on Earthscan publications, see www.earthscan.co.uk or write to earthinfo@earthscan.co.uk

ISBN: 978-1-84407-824-0 hardback
ISBN: 978-1-84407-825-7 paperback

Typeset by OKS Prepress
Cover design by Susanne Harris

A catalogue record for this book is available from the British Library.

Library of Congress Cataloging-in-Publication Data

Margai, Florence M.
  Environmental health hazards and social justice : geographical perspectives on race and class disparities / Florence Margai.
      p. cm.
  Includes bibliographical references and index.
  ISBN 978-1-84407-824-0 (hardback) — ISBN 978-1-84407-825-7 (pbk.) 1. Environmental health—Social aspects. 2. Medical geography—Social aspects. 3. Health and race—Environmental aspects. 4. Poor—Health and hygiene—Environmental aspects. I. Title.
  RA566.M26 2010
  362.1—dc22   2010026789

Contents

Part III Social and Economic Factors in Population Health Disparities

List of Figures and Tables

Figures

Tables

Acknowledgements

This book is a culmination of years of teaching, conducting research and service in the field of geography and environmental health disparities. Its successful completion was contingent on the support received from many colleagues and students in my home institution and beyond. I am particularly grateful to my colleagues in the Department of Geography at Binghamton for providing the rich institutional environment for me to explore and write about these issues. Some of the ideas presented in this book were first explored in the classroom with my students, and/or funded research projects with preliminary findings presented in articles and presentations at conferences such as the Race, Ethnicity and Place Conference that was initiated in Binghamton in 2000. With valuable input from many individuals, in particular John Frazier and Eugene Tettey-Fio, and several of my colleagues in US institutions and beyond, I was able to develop these ideas further for presentation in this book.

I would also like to thank the residents of the communities in which I worked and gathered data for some of the case studies presented in this book. Through research and activism I will continue to bring attention to their challenges, and forever remain a strong advocate for improving their health and overall well-being.

My sincere thanks are offered to Tim Hardwick, the Commissioning Editor for Earthscan for his encouragement and patience during the writing of this book, and the rest of the publishing staff for the book production tasks. I am also indebted to my colleagues in Binghamton, and the anonymous reviewers for providing detailed comments and suggestions which helped to strengthen the various chapters of book.

Finally, my deepest gratitude goes to my entire family, most of all William, Luba and Konya for their patience, love and support over the years.

Preface

In an increasingly globalized world, the linkages between social and environmental injustices are becoming inherently complex with undeniable outcomes in the distribution of risks and disparities in population health. Evidence from both developed and developing countries suggests a multilevel and multifactorial basis of these disparities, with similarities in the core drivers of these hazards, but differential population vulnerabilities across the regions. Moving from one country to another, one finds many examples of environmental health challenges facing various segments of the population particularly those residing in low-income, working-class and minority communities. Disparities abound in different spatial contexts, from local to global, and in varied forms including the uneven distribution of clean air and water, nutritious foods, healthy neighbourhoods, access to quality and affordable health services, and all of life's other enhancing resources.

Examining the uneven distribution of these hazards and the differential impacts on human health is part of the broader mission of social justice, and therein lies one of the primary aims of this book. The text seeks to critically explore the geographic distribution of these hazards with emphasis on the interactions between social and environmental risk factors, the historical and current sources of these problems, and their collective impact on human health. Following a discussion of the foundational themes and concepts in Part I, the book examines the environmental aspects of health disparities in Part II and the social and economic aspects in Part III. This integrative approach is unparalleled in the literature and is best accomplished by framing the discourse within the discipline of geography.

Using geographic perspectives, the book offers a comprehensive overview of the conceptual frameworks, operational definitions and methodologies that are useful for addressing population health disparities. Several of the ideas and analytical strategies are based on the author's experiences garnered during the last two decades of research, teaching and service in the field of geography and environmental health. The chapters also reflect the increasing recognition of geography and spatial epidemiology in environmental and public health assessment. In particular, geographic perspectives and techniques are now firmly entrenched in all studies of population health disparities, the goal being to use these placed-based approaches to explore the human–environmental associations and outcomes of public health. Both academics and public health professionals now recognize the important role that geographic principles, geographic information systems (GIS), spatial epidemiology and geostatistics play in disease risk estimation, and detection and mapping of disease hotspots within communities. These approaches are useful not only for the geo-targeting of at-risk populations but also leveraging limited resources in needy and underserved areas.

In acknowledging the growing importance of these approaches, and in particular the need to educate a new breed of environmental health analysts with a social justice mindset, this book is purposely designed to introduce readers to these geographic perspectives. Using statistical data, charts and maps for different world regions, the geographic distribution of environmental health hazards are illustrated, along with the primary risk sources, the varying patterns of exposure among population subgroups, and the disproportionate health outcomes. The association between disease causing agents in the physical environment, and the socio-economic, cultural, behavioural and institutional factors that produce disparate patterns of disease and disability among various segments of the population are examined.

Another objective of the book is to expand the discussion of population health disparities to include a broader characterization of environmental diseases. The debate on this issue currently focuses on chronic, degenerational diseases such as diabetes, hypertension or infectious diseases such as HIV/AIDS. By extending the dialogue to problems such as lead toxicity, respiratory diseases, water-related disparities, food insecurity and environmentally induced cancers, we hope to more fully document the scope of health disparities.

On the issue of environmental injustice, the discourse is also heavily tilted toward the plight of marginalized communities within the United States and Europe, and often omits the comprehensive analysis and mapping of conditions facing vulnerable populations in low-income countries. This book offers a more balanced approach by drawing examples from regions in both the global North and South, particularly those groups that are most impacted in selected African countries. In using these case studies, we hope to draw attention to the emerging geographies of global environmental injustice and environmental health risks in the developing countries.

Finally, this book is written primarily for upper level undergraduate students and first year graduate students in a number of interrelated disciplines: medical geography, public health, environmental health, other population health fields in the social sciences (such as medical sociology and medical anthropology), and environmental studies. Students in more specialized programmes such as the various centres established for the study of health disparities, as well as professionals in health care and health policy institutions will also benefit greatly from reading the book. Overall, the notable features of the book include:

- Theoretical frameworks, operational definitions, and analytical methods for measuring and mapping important concepts and indicators of population health disparities. Various terminologies and concepts that are tackled in the text include environmental diseases, health disparity, health equity, race, ethnicity, class, social justice, measurable dimensions of segregation, and access to health services.

- Descriptions of relevant data sources for analysing environmental hazards, exposure and health outcome measures. Noteworthy here is the valuable information provided on the relevant sources, and methods for processing and mapping demographic and health data for developing countries.
- Overview of the primary statistical and geospatial methodologies used for mapping and visualization of health measures.
- Discussion of the social and economic aspects of health disparities particularly race, ethnicity and class status.
- Discussion of the environmental aspects of health disparities including major risk sources such as global climate change, emerging infectious diseases, toxic chemicals, waterborne hazards and food insecurity.
- Case studies drawn from local, regional and global contexts that explore these issues in depth, illustrating both the theory and practice of uncovering the root causes of these problems, and the similarities and differences across world regions.
- Using maps, charts and other visual illustrations to portray health disparities at different spatial scales including the hotspots that deserve immediate attention.
- Illustrating the effectiveness of a place-centred approach in the study of health disparities for assessing the spatial extent of these problems and supporting efforts to achieve environmental, social and health equity.

List of Acronyms and Abbreviations

AAPA	American Association of Physical Anthropology
AAPI	Asian Americans and Pacific Islanders
ADME	absorption, distribution, metabolism and elimination
AFB	African-born (blacks)
AIAN	American Indians and Alaskan Natives
AIDS	acquired immunodeficiency syndrome
AIRS	Aerometric Information Retrieval System
AR	attributable risk
ATSDR	Agency for Toxic Substances and Disease Registry
AU	African Union
BLL	blood lead level
BMI	body mass index
BRFSS	Behavioral Risk Factor Surveillance System
BSE	bovine spongiform encephalopathy
CAM	complementary and alternative therapies
CDC	Centers for Disease Control
CERI	Comprehensive Environmental Risk Index
CFC	chlorofluorocarbon
CHI	chronic health index
CHIPRA	Children Health Insurance Reauthorization Act
DALY	disease-adjusted life year
DDE	dichlorodiphenyldichloroethylene
DDT	dichlorodiphenyltrichloroethane
DHS	Demographic and Health Surveys
DTM	demographic transition model
DYCAST	Dynamic Continuous-Area Space–Time
EBD	environmental burden of disease
EC	environmental classism
EE	environmental equity
EJ	environmental justice
ENSO	El Niño Southern Oscillation
EPCRA	Emergency Planning and Community Right-to-Know Act
ER	environmental racism
ERIDs	emerging and re-emerging infectious diseases

ERNS   Emergency Release and Notification System
ERT   environmental risk transition
ES   exposure surveillance
ESDA   exploratory spatial data analysis
ETM   epidemiological transition model
EU   European Union
FFR   fast food restaurant
GBD   global burden of disease
GCM   general circulation model
GIS   geographic information systems
GO   Getis-Ord (statistic)
GPS   global positioning systems
GWR   geographical weighted regression
HadCM3   Hadley Centre Coupled Model
HCFC   hydrochlorofluorocarbon
HDI   Human Development Index
HepB   hepatitis B
HIV   human immunodeficiency virus
HOD   health outcome database
HSA   Health Service Area
HSPA   Health Service Professional Shortage Area
IDP   internally displaced person
IDW   inverse distance weighting
IHS   Indian Health Service
IMR   infant mortality rate
IOM   International Organization of Migration
IPCC   Intergovernmental Panel on Climate Change
IRS   indoor residual spraying
JMP   Joint Monitoring Programme (for Water Supply and Sanitation)
LBW   low birth weight
LISA   local indicators of spatial association
LULU   locally unwanted land use
MAUP   modifiable areal unit problem
MDG   Millennium Development Goal
MEA   multilateral environmental agreement
MRI   magnetic resonance imaging
MSA   metropolitan statistical area
MSM   male to male sexual contact
MUA   Medically Underserved Area
NAFTA   North American Free Trade Agreement
NATA   National Air Toxics Assessment
NBDPN   National Birth Defects Prevention Network
NCD   non-communicable disease
NCDB   neighbourhood change database
NCEH   National Center for Environmental Health
NCHS   National Center for Health Statistics
NHANES   National Health and Nutrition Examination Survey

NHIS	National Health Interview Survey
NIABY	not in anyone's back yard
NIH	National Institutes of Health
NIMBY	not in my back yard
NRC	National Research Council
NTC	National Toxics Campaign
NVSS	National Vital Statistics System
NYDOT	New York State Department of Transportation
OAU	Organization of African Unity
OBGYNs	obstetricians/gynaecologists
OECD	Organisation for Economic Co-operation and Development
OK	ordinary kriging
OMB	US Office of Management and Budget
OR	odds ratio
OSHA	Occupational Safety and Health Administration
PAH	polycyclic aromatic hydrocarbon
PAR	population attributable risk
PBDE	polybrominated diphenyl ether
PBT	persistence, bioaccumulation and toxicity
PCB	polychlorinated biphenyl
PCP	primary care provider
PFC	perfluorinated chemical
PIRG	Public Research and Interest Group
PMI	Presidential Malaria Initiative
POP	persistent organic pollutant
PSR	pressure–state–response framework
RDBMS	Relational Database Management System
REACH	Racial and Ethnic Approaches to Community Health
RR	relative risk of the disease
RS	remote sensing
SARs	Severe Acute Respiratory syndrome
SCCP	short-chain chlorinated paraffin
SCHIP	State Children's Health Insurance Program
SCP	specialized care provider
SDWIS	Safe Drinking Water Information System
SEER	Surveillance, Epidemiology and End Results Program
SES	socio-economic status
SMR	standardized mortality ratio
SPSS	Statistical Package for the Social Sciences
STIS	Space and Time Intelligence Software
TCEI	Toxic Concentration Equity Index
TCM	traditional Chinese medicine
TDDI	Toxic Demographic Difference Index
TDQI	Toxic Demographic Quotient Index
TEI	Toxic Equity Index
TESS	Toxic Exposure Surveillance System
TRI	Toxic Release Inventory System

TSDF	treatment, storage and disposal facilities
μg/dl	micrograms per decilitre
UNDAC	United Nations Disaster Assessment and Coordination
UNDP	United Nations Development Programme
UNICEF	United Nations Children's Fund
UNITAR	United Nations Institute for Training and Research
UNOSAT	United Nations Operational Satellite Applications Programme
USB	United States born blacks
USDA	United States Department of Agriculture
USEPA	United States Environmental Protection Agency
USGAO	United States Government Accountability Office
VOC	volatile organic compound
WHO	World Health Organization
WNv	West Nile virus
WPM	water point mapping
YLD	years lived with disabilities
YLL	years lost

PART I

THEMES AND CONCEPTS

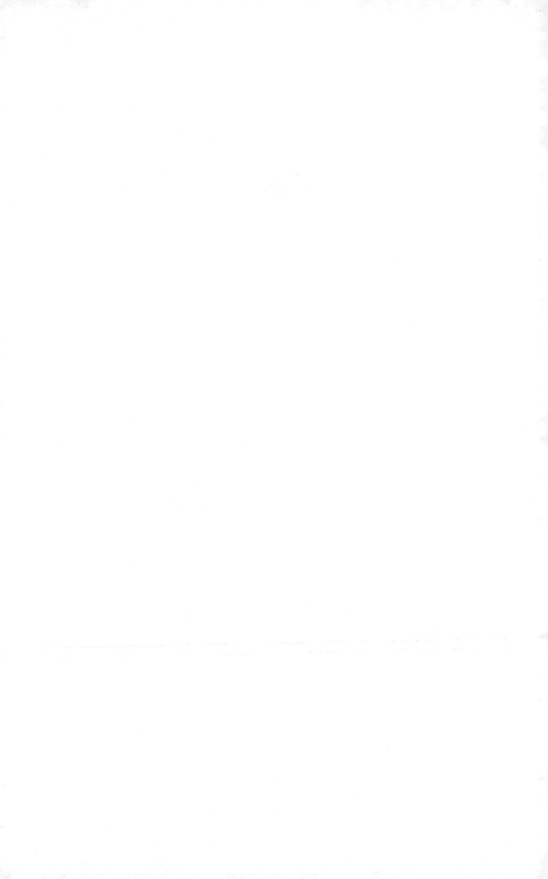

1
Geographic Foundations of Environmental Health Hazards: The Need for a Place-based Perspective

Introduction

As the 21st century unfolds, there are growing concerns that this new era is being marked, and perhaps permanently tainted, by an unusual set of geopolitical events, together with a series of economic, demographic and environmental challenges with profound implications for global health. During the course of this first decade alone, we have witnessed unprecedented levels of human agony and suffering caused by earthquakes, tsunamis, hurricanes, floods and other natural disasters, along with intentional acts of terrorism, civil wars and regional conflicts, all resulting in a significant number of deaths and disabilities. We have also witnessed the rapid integration of national economies into a new and increasingly unstable global economy, the emergence and dominance of multinational corporations, the convergence of global agricultural systems, food processing and distributional networks, changes in the structure and composition of labour markets, the rapid urbanization and large-scale movements of people within and across world regions. Not surprisingly, these events have been accompanied by an even greater transformation of the global and local environments, introducing a whole new set of environmental health hazards while exacerbating others.

Environmental health hazards are spatially differentiated with marked differences from place to place. Throughout the world, in developed economies, transitional and emerging economies one encounters evidence of racial, ethnic and class-based disparities in environmental exposure and health outcomes. The poor and underrepresented groups are too often the ones to bear the brunt of environmental hazards, the most likely to develop health complications from these exposures, and yet the least likely to gain access to beneficial health services that would detect and treat these problems. Knowledge of the environmental exposure risks, distributional patterns and their effects on population health requires a geographic perspective coupled with a social justice mindset to better understand the root causes, the situational contexts in which they occur and the disparities they produce among different population groups. This book offers these perspectives along with a discussion of the geographic tools and methodologies that are used to evaluate the distributional patterns of these hazards. Emphasis is placed on the environmental hazards and locational inequities that produce adverse health outcomes among disadvantaged population groups around the world. Key terminologies such as health disparities, health inequities and the various conceptualizations of race, ethnicity and social class are critically reviewed to draw out the inconsistencies in meaning, and interpretations across time and in varied contexts. The methodological challenges that arise in the use of these theoretical constructs to document population health disparities are discussed.

The text is applications-oriented, illustrating the combined use of demographic, health and environmental data, and geographic approaches to uncover the causes, contextual factors and processes that produce the contaminated environments. To illustrate the international scope of these issues, case studies are drawn from research conducted mostly in the United States and Africa, along with a review of related studies in Europe, Asia and South America. This comparative approach allows readers to gain a better understanding of the global distribution of these environmental hazards, their manifestation at different spatial scales, and the health inequities they produce among people in both developed and developing countries. In this first chapter, we shall examine the general characteristics of environmental hazards, noting the common risk sources, and potential health outcomes. This will be followed by an overview of the four traditions of geographic inquiry, highlighting the need for a place-based (or spatial) perspective in evaluating environmental health issues. The chapter concludes with a synopsis of the remaining chapters of the book.

Overview of environmental health hazards

Environmental health hazards are broadly defined in this text as the complete realm of disease causing agents, pathogens, events and processes in the external environment that threaten the health and well-being of people in their homes, neighbourhoods, communities and other surroundings. This definition calls further for the clarification of the term *environment*, as used in environmental health research. By environment, we are referring to all of the external circumstances and conditions that influence population health. Though many authors have offered their own interpretations in the literature (see, for example, Last, 1987; Moeller, 1992; Eyles, 1997; Briggs, 2000; Merrill, 2008), a more comprehensive characterization of the environment draws upon at least four frameworks that acknowledge the distinction between (i) the inner and outer environment of the human body; (ii) the personal versus ambient environment of individuals; (iii) solid, liquid and gaseous environments; and (iv) the biological, chemical, physical/mechanical and psychosocial environments. The latter is the most commonly used characterization in the study of environmental health hazards, and will be formally adopted in this book. This framework calls for a complete evaluation of the multiple risk sources of environmental diseases in our external surroundings: the biological, chemical and physical/mechanical factors as well as the psychological and socio-cultural factors. The latter may not always be readily observable but nonetheless have significant impacts on population health. Biological agents include the various forms of bacteria, viruses, parasites, fungi, spores and other pathogens that may be found in the air, food and water, some that are transmissible directly from person to person, or indirectly through animals or insects. Chemical agents consist of air pollutants such as sulphur dioxide or carbon monoxide gas, heavy metals such as lead and mercury, synthetic compounds such as dichlorodi-phenyltrichloroethane (DDT), polychlorinated biphenyl (PCB), and the many types of additives, pesticides, household cleaning agents and other hazardous materials. Physical/mechanical agents of disease originate from sick buildings, as well as excessive noise, heat or cold, and various forms of radiation in our surroundings.

Using the above classification of the environment, a summary of the most prevalent global environmental health hazards is provided in Table 1.1. The sources of origin and associated health risks are also provided. Though some of these hazards originate from natural sources, it is evident from the table that human activities now play a dominant role in transforming environments, introducing contaminants and/or triggering the state of events or processes that account for the emerging health hazards. For example, global atmospheric hazards such as ozone depletion, global warming and their attendant health problems observed in recent decades are triggered by anthropogenic activities. Noteworthy also are the residential, occupational and social environments of individuals that contribute further to environmental exposures and poor health outcomes.

As part of the discourse in this book, we shall map out the distribution of these hazards at different geographic scales – globally, regionally and locally – but more importantly examine the social injustices and disparities that are produced among individuals of different racial, ethnic and socio-economic backgrounds. In both developing and developed countries, income inequalities, residential segregation and isolation in contaminated environments, food insecurity, and limited access to life-enhancing resources all serve as key drivers of environmental exposure and ill health. Low-income, minority or working-class populations are often the most likely to bear the brunt of these disparities, which over the course of their lifetimes result in negative health outcomes. The illustration of these problems, globally and locally using geographic tools and perspectives will help draw out the commonalities across spatial scales while at the same time identifying the hotspots where prompt interventions are needed to correct the inequities. For those who are unfamiliar with geography, a brief overview of the discipline, the primary traditions and contributions to environmental health research is provided below.

Table 1.1 *Examples of environmental health hazards and associated health risks*

Category	Examples of hazards	Health risks
Natural hazards	Volcanic activity	Includes effects of direct injury by volcanic debris, lava, etc.; inhalation of gas, dust and indirect effects of famine, etc.
	Earthquakes	Direct injury from effects of earth tremors (e.g. building collapse), and indirect effects (e.g. flooding, tsunamis, epidemics and famine)
	Flooding/storms	Direct effects of drowning and injury by floods/storms, and indirect effects of water contamination
	Drought	Primary health effects due to lack of potable water and famine
	Hurricanes/wind	Direct effects of injury (e.g. collapsing buildings) but may also include longer term effects of contamination/loss of water supplies
	Soil erosion	Famine and poor diet due to effects of desertification on food supply
Atmospheric hazards	Outdoor air pollution	Wide range of respiratory, pulmonary and cardiovascular illnesses and cancers
	Greenhouse gases / global warming	Through indirect effects of hurricanes/flooding/ drought
	Ozone depletion	Increases exposure to UV radiation resulting in risks of skin cancer, cataracts and compromised immune systems
Waterborne hazards	Surface water pollution	Primarily diarrhoeal and gastrointestinal illnesses, but may also include chemical poisoning
	Drinking water contamination	Gastrointestinal and urinary diseases; rarely chemical poisoning
Food-borne hazards	Biological contamination	Bacterial agents cause wide range of diseases of the digestive system
	Chemical contamination	Food additives, pesticides such as DDT, hormone supplements and antibiotic residues cause a range of diseases including effects on digestive/urinary systems
	Food deserts	Limited access to nutritious food
Vector-borne hazards	Water related	Infectious and parasitic diseases
	Animal related	Infectious and parasitic diseases
Domestic/ residential hazards	Tobacco smoke / indoor air pollution	Wide range of respiratory and cardiovascular illnesses and cancers
	Lead-based paint	Lead poisoning with effects on nervous, cognitive and developmental systems
	Household chemicals / synthetic compounds	Adverse health effects from cumulative exposures to synthetic compounds such as phthalates, PFCs,and PBDEs. Accidents – physical injury and poisonings, suicide through use of chemicals, drugs and instruments

Table 1.1 (*continued*)

Category	Examples of hazards	Health risks
Occupational hazards	Industrial pollutants	Wide range of respiratory, pulmonary and cardiovascular illnesses and cancers; chemical poisoning
	Occupational accidents	Acute physical injury (e.g. by fire, explosions, accidents with equipment and chronic injuries (e.g. repetitive strain, back pain, etc.)
Infrastructural hazards	Hazardous accidents	Primarily acute physical injury (e.g. by fire, explosions) or chemical poisoning with respiratory effects
	Illegal dumps / abandoned waste sites, contaminated land	Many diseases including cancer clusters, and impacts on the digestive/urinary systems
Social conflicts	War	Almost all forms of health effects
	Terrorism	Acute physical injury (e.g. by fire, explosions) or chemical poisoning with respiratory effects
	Domestic violence	Physical injury; stress-related illnesses

Source: Modified after Briggs, 2000

The importance of geography in environmental health research

Geography is an integrative scientific discipline that examines the interactions and linkages between the natural environments and human societies, and how those interactions produce distinctive landscapes, spatial patterns, processes and outcomes. The discipline is particularly well suited for environmental health research because it offers a blend of natural science and social science paradigms that are crucial to understanding the environments in which we live, our adaptation and activities in those environments and how those interactions impact our health. As Parvis (2002) once wrote, environmental health professionals can benefit from geographic knowledge in several areas including the ability to read and produce maps, learn about atmospheric, hydrological and other geochemical cycles, learn the fundamentals of renewable and non-renewable energy sources, the physical limitations of our environment including the constraints of water and food resources, the use of chemicals in industry and agriculture, and global hazards such as ozone depletion, global warming and health impacts. The discipline also offers the ability to learn about different population groups in our local communities and around the world, the languages they speak, their religious practices, diet, customs and behavioural practices that contribute to ill health, as well as knowledge about the distribution of health-related services.

Geographic research is guided by a strong theoretical foundation that enables the spatial analysis of human–environmental problems. The discipline relies on cutting edge tools and technological methods such as computer cartography, geographic information systems (GIS), geomatics, statistics and remote sensing to compile and analyse spatially and temporally referenced data, and the underlying processes and factors that are responsible for the observable patterns. Contrary to popular myths of geography as a rote-based discipline, geographic research is applied with a focus on problem solving to address the real challenges facing people in their local communities and around the world. Issues of food access, air pollution, water quality and access, housing availability, environmental justice and poor health are matters that affect the lives of many around the world for which we need solutions.

The integrative nature of the discipline of geography is best seen in Figure 1.1 where one notices several subspecialties with a strong overlap with other disciplines in the natural and social sciences. Among these, medical geography is prominently featured with its cognate field in medicine and public health. The study of environmental health hazards and disease outcomes is deeply rooted in this subspecialty as will be evident in most of the chapters presented in this book.

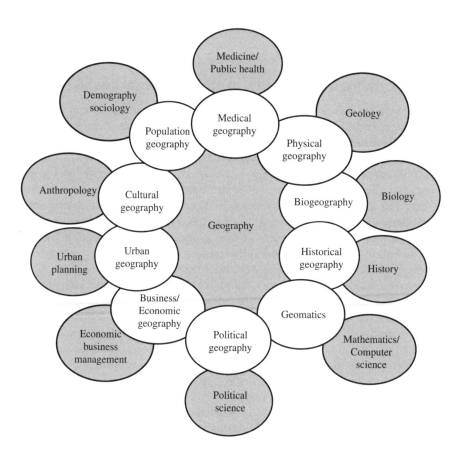

Figure 1.1 *The integrative nature of geography*

Geographic traditions

In a seminal piece first presented by William Pattison in 1964, he outlined four main traditions that guide geographic inquiry: the Earth Science tradition, the Culture–Environment tradition, the Area Studies tradition and the Spatial tradition. Within the context of environmental health, all of these four traditions serve as important rallying points for studying environmental hazards and disparities. The *Earth Science* tradition, the oldest of the four traditions, examines the underlying processes and factors that produce a detailed structure of our physical environment. A study of environmental hazards does require knowledge of these processes and the various elements that constitute the natural environment such as landforms, rocks, soils, climate, air quality, water and mineral resources. Knowledge of the distributional patterns of these elements and various ecosystems allows for a better understanding of the pathways and sources of exposure to disease agents and pathogens.

The *Culture–Environment* tradition emphasizes the interactions between people and the physical environments they occupy. This geographic tradition is centred on demographic patterns and trends, cultural diversity, social and political structures and the adaptive behaviours in different physical environments that produce distinctive cultural realms and landscapes. In environmental health research, this tradition provides valuable information for identifying anthropogenic activities that contribute most to major environmental health hazards such as climate change, and human vulnerability to such hazards. Migration, fertility and mortality rates, epidemiological transitions, institutional frameworks, social networks and settlement geographies provide further insights into the source areas of diseases, and global diffusion patterns.

The Area Studies, or *Regional Science* tradition, permits the subdivision of the world into homogeneous units, or regions, based on one or more properties such as the physical or cultural attributes, or the functional interrelationships between the places that constitute the region. Those regions that share common properties such as soil types, climate, religion, language or the same political jurisdiction are known as formal regions. An excellent example of the use of formal regions in environmental health can be drawn from the study of biomes, which reflect large regional groupings or communities of plants and animals around the world with distributional patterns that correlate strongly with the climatic regimes, altitude and latitudinal location of those areas. Knowledge of these biomes is useful in developing globalized patterns of disease systems, or environmental disease regions based on vectors such as ticks, mosquitoes and flies. This approach also provides a useful context for evaluating other health hazards that are linked directly to conditions in the natural environment (Meade and Earickson, 2000).

A second group of regions are functional regions which serve as useful frameworks in health-related studies. Such regions are defined by the interactions between places such as migration networks, commuting patterns, service areas and communication networks. For example, health care providers might be interested in the delineation of functional health regions to determine the spatial extent of their service area and how far patients are willing to travel to utilize these services. They might also be interested in examining the contributory role of functional regions and related nodes in the diffusion of diseases, or provision of services. In the United States, Health Service Areas (HSAs) are functional regions consisting of either individual counties or groups of contiguous counties that are relatively self-sufficient in terms of provision of health services. There are currently 824 such areas with clusters ranging anywhere from 2 to 20 counties. Two other examples of functional health regions are the Health Service Professional Shortage Areas (HSPAs) and Medically Underserved Areas (MUAs), consisting of areas where there are shortages in health professionals or service delivery, or which may have at-risk populations based on poverty levels, demographics and the prevalence of certain health conditions. The geographic delineation of these functional regions assists in the reallocation of health resources to minimize health disparities.

The fourth geographic tradition is based on the Spatial or *Locational Analysis*. As the name implies, this tradition stresses the importance of a spatial or place-based understanding of human–environmental interactions and the use of geographic technologies for mapping and analysing these processes and related outcomes. Environmental health geographers have utilized these tools effectively to study the spatio-temporal dynamics of diseases, produce disease maps, identify hotspots for health intervention and illustrate the inequitable distribution of hazards and health outcomes by race, ethnicity, income and other demographic parameters. These tools provide a great deal of information about the natural and built environments of different population groups around the world, their demographic attributes, level of social organization, institutional frameworks, political and economic relationships and the kinds of activities and behaviours in those environments that create or heighten the occurrence of environmental hazards. Analysing and mapping the geographical patterns and impacts of those hazards, the overlap between their occurrence and different racial and socio-economic groups has provided valuable insights for health surveillance and intervention.

Overall, the four traditions presented above offer a glimpse of the diverse range of topics and issues that are covered within geography, and the kinds of technological tools at our disposal for addressing these societal challenges. A question that many people often ask is *Why turn to geography to study environmental health and social justice?* The answer to this is most evident in the exhaustive list of studies conducted in recent decades demonstrating the need for a place-based perspective in addressing these concerns. Throughout this book, we shall draw upon the findings of these studies; however, for now, it is important to recognize several scholars who have been the strongest advocates of a geographically centred approach (Kearns, 1993; Briggs, 2000; Fitzpatrick and LaGory, 2000; Parvis, 2002; Hess et al, 2008). Below, we present a few examples offered as rationale for using geographic perspectives in studying environmental health disparities:

1   Environmental health hazards are not uniformly distributed across space; rather, they vary from place to place as a result of the natural processes that

occur in those environments and the human activities that transform those environments.

2   The countries, regions, communities and, more specifically, the neigh-bourhoods in which people live, and the physical, chemical, biological, psychological and social attributes of those environments influence their life chances, their access to resources and opportunities, and their overall risk of exposure to environmental hazards. Therefore, *place* matters in studying health disparities.

3   The increasing convergence of space, time and the integration of the global economies is apparent around the world. These activities and processes are readily visible in the transformation of natural environments, global trade, communication networks, labour markets, human mobility and disease emergence and re-emergence. Geographic principles and approaches are therefore needed to model these processes, specifically the dynamics and spatio-temporal patterns of emergent health hazards, and develop early-warning systems that reflect the threat levels within and across geographic territories.

4   The health outcomes of environmental health hazards are geographically expressed due to the confluence of the processes noted above as well as social injustices engendered through social stratification and group marginalization, institutional policies and practices. From a problem-solving perspective, many of the steps that are needed to redress the population-based disparities would have to be prioritized and targeted at specific locations. Geographic tools and methodologies enable the identification of areas or hotspots where the risks would be greatest, thus enabling the effective use of limited resources.

Organization of the book

The book is divided into three parts. Part I is foundational, emphasizing the important themes and concepts of environmental health, measurement, data collection and portrayal using geographic methodologies. Including Chapter 1, there are five chapters in this section. Chapter 2 examines the nature of environmental diseases followed by a presentation of the disease classification system including basic concepts such as disease incidence and prevalence. In Chapter 3, we grapple with the definition of health disparities, distinguishing between the concept and the notion of health inequity and social justice. The chapter also examines the theoretical foundations of health inequity. Drawing from the work of several scholars, a theoretical framework is presented that examines the interactive role of biology, geographic origin and the cultural, economic, political and legal factors in influencing the environment and health of individuals. Chapter 4 discusses the significance of race, ethnicity and class in evaluating health disparities. We examine the differences between race and ethnicity and the need for collecting health data on these population attributes. The overlap between race and class, and the need for separate analyses of these variables is discussed. Finally, Chapter 5 examines the different sources of health data, and the methods that are used to validate and portray health disparities at different geographical scales. An overview of relevant statistical methods and GIS will be provided. This chapter also introduces students to the use of geostatistical approaches in detecting environmental disease clusters and disparities.

Part 2 of this book focuses on the environmental aspects of health disparities. The chapters included in this section showcase several applications that address environmental health problems in various world regions with case studies drawn from the United States and Africa, and reported findings from other world regions. Seven chapters are included in this section. Chapter 6 examines the key sources of global climate change and other environmental disturbances, and the anticipated impacts on population health. The geographical differentiation of these impacts and varying patterns of population vulnerability are discussed. Further discussion of the health impacts of climate change is provided in Chapter 7, with emphasis on emerging and re-emerging health risks. In this chapter, the spatial (landscape) epidemiology approach is introduced using examples drawn from research conducted on the West Nile virus in the United States, and malaria in Sierra Leone. In Chapter 8, we examine the widespread production and use of toxic chemicals, including the major pathways and routes of human exposure. Then, using DDT and lead toxicity as examples, the adverse health effects of these toxic substances are discussed. The chapter ends with an illustration of the analytical approaches that are used to evaluate group health disparities based on their exposure to these chemicals. In Chapter 9, the focus is on the history of environmental justice in the United States with emphasis on the inequitable distribution of hazardous facilities in low-income and minority communities. The global geographies of environmental injustice and health consequences are explored in Chapter 10. A case study is presented using GIS to evaluate the health risks associated with the illegal dumping of hazardous wastes along the coast of Abidjan, Ivory Coast. Water- and sanitation-related health disparities are examined in Chapter 11. The chapter takes on a key concept, *access*, with dimensions that are measurable across various countries around the world. Efforts to provide universal coverage in water supply and quality are also discussed in this chapter. Chapter 12 addresses the increasing concerns about food contamination, food justice and food insecurity as well as the emergence of food deserts in the developed world. Using examples from Burkina Faso and the United States, a cross-cultural analysis of the issues and different health outcomes is presented.

The third part of the book contains four chapters that examine the social attributes and economic factors that produce population health disparities. Using the United States as an example of pluralistic society, Chapter 13 examines the settlement geography, residential segregation patterns and changing demographic profiles of the racial and ethnic minority groups and the unique health concerns confronting these groups. Chapter 14 examines the increasing population flows and movements within and between countries and the likely impact on emergent diseases in the destination areas. Using a recent US dataset, a comparative analysis of black immigrant health relative to their native-born counterparts is presented. Chapter 15 focuses on the various dimensions of health care in terms of geographic access, affordability and utilization among different population groups. The types of health resources are discussed along with the emerging trends in medical pluralism. In examining health affordability, we use geospatial analytical methods to identify the geographic hotspots and socio-economic profile of the uninsured in America. We then conclude in Chapter 16 with a discussion of key strategies that require the collective contributions of the public, governments, researchers and health professionals alike to undertake programmes that are geared towards health parity.

References

Briggs, D. J. (2000) 'Environmental health hazard mapping for Africa', WHO-AFRO, Harare, Zimbabwe, pp1–140, www.afro.who.int/des/pdf/healthhazard.pdf, accessed 2 December 2008

Eyles, J. (1997) 'Environmental health research: Setting an agenda by spinning our wheels or climbing the mountain?', *Health and Place*, vol 3, no 1, pp1–13

Fitzpatrick, K. and LaGory, M. (2000) *Unhealthy Places: The Ecology of Risk in the Urban Landscapes*, Routledge, New York

Hess, J. J., Malilay, J. N. and Parkinson, A. J. (2008) 'Climate change: The importance of place', *American Journal of Preventive Medicine*, vol 35, no 5, pp468–478

Kearns, R. A. (1993) 'Place and health', *Professional Geographer*, vol 45, no 2, pp139–147

Last, J. (1987) *Public Health and Human Ecology*, Appleton and Lang, East Norwalk, CN

Meade, M. S. and Earickson, R. J. (2000) *Medical Geography*, 2nd Edition, The Guilford Press, New York

Merrill, R. M. (2008) *Environmental Epidemiology: Principles and Methods*, Jones and Barlett, Sudbury, MA

Moeller, D. W. (1992) *Environmental Health*, Harvard University Press, Cambridge, MA

Parvis, L. E. (2002) 'The significance of geography in environmental health, or what geography can do for the environmental health profession', *Journal of Environmental Health*, vol 64, no 6, pp42 and 57

Pattison, W. D. (1964) 'The four traditions of geography', *The Journal of Geography*, vol 63, pp211–216

2
Environmental Health and Disease Indicators: Valuation Measures, Transition Frameworks and Burden of Disease Estimates

Introduction

Consistent with the definition of environmental health hazards presented earlier in Chapter 1, environmental diseases are the health effects of exposure to external agents and conditions in the environment. The study of the distribution of these health impacts is empirically grounded allowing experts in both the natural and social sciences to study the potential associations and putative risk factors of exposure and health. Spatial epidemiology, a subspecialty in geography, involves the compilation, analysis and visualization of the disease indicators across geographical space and time. It is very closely related to the broader field of epidemiology which involves the descriptive and analytical study of the distribution and determinants of the diseases in populations. Both fields depend greatly on health measures that quantify the disease patterns.

The primary goal in this chapter is to introduce these basic measures and indicators, and discuss their use in environmental health assessment. We start with a review of the issues surrounding the evaluation of health in general, the classification of diseases, and then proceed to describe the indicators that are commonly used to assess disease risks across populations. A review of disease standardization methods will also be presented followed by a discussion of how these measures are incorporated into population transition frameworks and used to develop disease burden estimates for different world regions.

Key concepts in environmental health evaluation

Health

Though many people are likely to equate good health and wellness with the lack of disease, as early as the 1940s the World Health Organization (WHO) formally defined health as a 'state of complete physical, mental and social well being, and not merely the absence of disease and infirmity' (WHO, 1946). This definition was a deliberate attempt to shift emphasis away from the traditional evaluation of health in terms of disease pathology and physical abilities of individuals to a more positive characterization of health as a multidimensional and dynamic outcome of the interactions between individuals and their surroundings.

To date, the WHO's characterization of health remains under scrutiny for being too idealistic with lofty goals that are difficult to measure or attain particularly in low-income countries (McWhinney, 1987; Jadad and O'Grady, 2008). This definition remains largely unchanged, however, and offers certain properties that are useful in the evaluation of health. First, it offers a holistic and systems-based approach to health evaluation by analysing individual health as a complete system that is quantifiable along multiple axes: the physical, biological, mental, spiritual and social dimensions. Second, it offers an approach that values the contribution of both the internal and external environments in individual health assessment.

Expanded definitions of health describe individuals as being on a continuum rather a static state. Specifically, the health of an individual is viewed as dynamic, and continually fluctuates as one adapts to changing conditions and risks in the external environment. The noted distinction between the internal and external environments is also beneficial in environmental health assessment because it allows us to hone in on both the exogenous and endogenous aspects of health. Environmental health constitutes all of the physical, chemical and biological factors that are mostly external to the person, including the multiple risk sources and behaviours that are today reflected in the growing number of diseases. Of the 102 major global diseases reported by the WHO, 83 per cent are partly or entirely caused by exposures to environmental risk factors (Pruss-Ustun and Corvalan, 2006). Evaluating the risk sources of these diseases remains the primary task of environmental health analysts.

Disease

Unlike the concept of health, which is latent and somewhat elusive in meaning, a disease is considered to be a definite pathological process characterized by a set of signs and symptoms that impacts the well-being of an individual. The distinction between an environmental disease and other diseases, however, remains blurry in the literature with some authors offering more inclusive characterizations than others. For example, Moeller (2005) classifies any disease that is initiated, sustained or exacerbated by exposure to causative agents in our external environment as an environmental disease. Another approach is to classify diseases as either environmental if they are induced by exogenous influences of the environment, or genetic if they are based on endogenous influences associated with the internal constitution of the individual (Hutt and Burkitt, 1986). Consequently, all diseases that are not genetically based are deemed environmental diseases (Smith, 2001). Increasingly, however, the need for differentiation between these two causal influences may be unnecessary. Many health professionals now recognize that the role played by one's genetic predisposition in shaping the response to external

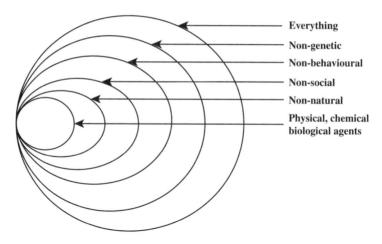

Everything

Non-genetic

Non-behavioural

Non-social

Non-natural

Physical, chemical
biological agents

Source: Adapted from Smith et al (1999)

Figure 2.1 *Different formulations of environmental risk factors of disease*

conditions may be more important than the dichotomy between the two classes of diseases. An excellent example is the case of Parkinson's disease, which is largely believed to be genetic but perhaps triggered by excessive exposure to environmental toxins such as pesticides. Further, Smith et al (1999) have argued for a more encompassing view of diseases noting

> *that genetic factors are actually also environmental, but merely on a different time scale. Thus, mutation, natural selection, and other mechanisms of evolution have changed the genetic composition of humanity according to environmental conditions existing in the past. In this context, ie, in which current genes are seen as the outcome of previous environments, all diseases are entirely environmental.* (p573)

Figure 2.1 shows the various formulations of environmental diseases, ranging from a narrow description that focuses on the physical, chemical and biological agents, to a definition that captures all disease agents and risk factors. We shall adopt the broader definition in this book.

Classification of environmental diseases

Environmental diseases may be distinguished further by their causative agents and modes of transmission. Globally, infectious diseases are the most prevalent diseases, accounting for 65 per cent of all human diseases, particularly in the developing countries. These diseases are caused by biological agents: bacteria, viruses, parasites, fungi, spores and other pathogens that are in the external environment. The animate and inanimate risk sources of these disease agents are known as *reservoirs*. They serve as the constant source of supply and provide the appropriate conditions for the pathogens to survive and multiply. Humans, for example, serve as reservoirs for diseases such as meningococcal meningitis, HIV/AIDS and tuberculosis. Infectious diseases that originate from wild and domestic animals, with pathogens transmitted directly from the animal reservoirs to humans, are known as *zoonotic* diseases. Examples include the West Nile virus, Lyme disease, rabies, Eastern Equine encephalitis and many more. Other disease agents may be circulated through non-living reservoirs such as contaminated soils and water sources. These include many of the bacterial and parasitic agents that cause gastrointestinal illnesses.

The transmission of biological pathogens occurs directly or indirectly though animate and inanimate objects. The process of *direct contact transmission* occurs when the disease is spread directly from an infected host to another without physical contact. This is common for contagious diseases that are spread through person to person contacts such as kissing, touching or sexual activity, or person to animal contacts, for example, animal bites. Inanimate objects also serve as disease transmission *vehicles*, as in the case of drinking from a contaminated glass of water, or using a dirt-ridden hand towel. Some of the world's most dangerous biological pathogens are also transmitted through *vectors*, live organisms such as mosquitoes and other arthropods that transmit diseases within and across animal species. Later in this text, we shall examine the environmental health challenges facing vulnerable populations as a result of vector-borne diseases such as malaria and the West Nile virus. There are increasing concerns about the increasing risks of transmission of these diseases and their expansion into new geographic territories as a result of global environmental degradation and climate change.

All other diseases originating from non-biological agents in the external environment are classified as the non-communicable diseases (NCDs). These diseases can be grouped into five categories based on their underlying etiology: (1) physical diseases; (2) chemical diseases; (3) developmental diseases; (4) neoplastic diseases; and (5) nutritional diseases. *Physical diseases* or injuries originate from sick buildings, hazardous occupations, vehicular accidents, violence in crime-ridden and war-torn environments, and exposure to repetitive activities, extreme temperatures, excessive noise and various forms of radiation in our surroundings (Moore, 1999). *Chemical diseases* are inherently more complex, resulting from exposure to environmental toxicants such as gaseous air pollutants, heavy metals such as lead and mercury, synthetic compounds, and the many types of additives, pesticides, household cleaning agents and other hazardous materials in our surroundings. Exposure to these chemicals interferes with the normal functioning of the human body resulting in a range of illnesses from asthmatic problems to lung diseases, cardiovascular diseases, endocrine and metabolic disorders, nervous system disorders and possibly also developmental and neoplastic diseases. *Developmental diseases* consist of various disorders that hinder the complete development of individuals to a point where their physical, emotional, cognitive or social functioning is below the norm expected for their age. The diseases originate from either endogenous influences, such as structural formation errors within the genes (or chromosomes), or exogenous conditions that are triggered by exposure to biological pathogens, chemicals or radioactive substances in the external environment. During stages of fetal development, maternal behavioural practices such as substance abuse, malnutrition and use of certain medications can also contribute to these kinds of disorders. These health events, however, may not just be limited to congenital anomalies, or infants. Development diseases can be pre- or post-natal with some cases of delayed outcomes that become evident well beyond the childhood years. *Neoplastic diseases* arise from the abnormal growth of body cells. These growths, often called tumours, may be benign (non-cancerous), or malignant (cancerous), endangering human lives as they grow outward to other parts of the body. Unfortunately, for many of these diseases, the underlying etiology is not well understood. Though some are genetically based, or the result of the aging process, many are believed to be the cause of external agents such as viruses, parasites, irradiation and exposure to toxic chemicals. Finally, *nutritional diseases* cover the range of illnesses that arise from overeating, malnutrition and poor dietary practices. The long-term effects of inadequate nutrition are most evident in marginalized and low-income societies where cases of stunting, wasting and vitamin deficiencies are prevalent, particularly among infants. In more affluent societies, nutritional disorders are manifested mostly in the form of overeating and poor food choices resulting in negative health outcomes such as obesity, diabetes and cardiovascular diseases.

Finally, from a spatial epidemiological perspective, the distinction between endemic, epidemic and pandemic diseases also becomes relevant in environmental health research, particularly when identifying the target areas for implementing disease surveillance and intervention programmes. *Endemic* diseases are usually present, year round, in a given geographic area. They are constantly present in the host community, with occasional spikes in incidence but generally remain within the expected level for that community. Examples include several kinds of transmissible diseases such as malaria, trypanosomiasis or schistosomiasis. Diseases may also be considered as *epidemics* when outbreaks occur or when they are introduced suddenly in a local community; or if they did exist year round in the community, their incidence increased beyond the expected level for the community. Examples such as cholera or the influenza epidemic are common but such designations may also apply to chronic or non-communicable diseases such as the recent declaration of an obesity epidemic in the United States. When epidemics spread globally, transcending national and continental boundaries, they are referred to as *pandemic* diseases. Examples include HIV/AIDs, SARS and, more recently, the H1N1 virus.

Measures of disease frequency and exposure risks in host communities

Defining, measuring and mapping environmental health indicators and disease outcomes are areas of increasing importance in global health as attention shifts towards the identification and control of environmental factors that influence human health. The process of uncovering these factors and evaluating the distributional patterns of the health-related outcomes is guided by a series of 'Who, What, Where and How' questions. As geographers, however, the initial point of inquiry is always place-centred: (i) *Where* do cases of the disease and health-related outcomes occur? (ii) Who is most affected by these outcomes? (iii) When are these health outcomes most likely to occur, and are there any discernible trends across space and time? (iv) What kinds of exposure agents and risk factors do vulnerable populations have in common? (v) How much risk is increased or attributable to exposure to these external agents? Addressing these questions requires the computation of relevant information on all health occurrences using a variety of indicators: incidence and prevalence rates, relative risk and attributable risk ratios, and summary measures of disease burden.

The analytical process begins with the collection and compilation of data on all cases of mortality, or deaths and related causes, and morbidity, or reported cases of disease and disabilities. Presented below is a basic set of epidemiological indicators that measure the frequency, magnitude or risk of occurrence of these health events.

Rates

Rates are the most commonly used measures for evaluating disease risks and comparing their occurrence across groups or regions. They are essentially proportions or fractions that relate the frequency of the health event to the size of the population at risk in a given area and within a defined time period. Depending on the nature and duration of the health event, one may decide to compute either the incidence rate or prevalence rate as described below:

Incidence rates: The incidence rate of a disease represents the rate at which new cases of the disease occur within the population during a specified time period. It is useful for measuring all types of health events, but more so for acute and communicable diseases. Computing the incidence rate requires some information regarding the total number of individuals that are susceptible to the disease, meaning the *population at risk* for the disease. Depending on the disease, this number could be a subset of the population, such as the elderly population, or it could be the entire population in the defined geographic area. Also relevant is the *time period* under investigation. Some diseases, particularly epidemics, are best monitored on a daily or weekly basis, whereas others, such as endemic diseases, may be best monitored using monthly or yearly data. One also requires information on the number of *new cases* diagnosed within the defined time period. With the available information, the incidence rate (I) is computed as follows:

$$I = \frac{Number\ of\ new\ cases\ in\ a\ specified\ period}{Number\ of\ people\ at\ risk\ during\ the\ specified\ period} \times K$$

where K is the multiplier used to express the derived measure either as a percentage form (by multiplying it by 100), or expressing it per 1000 people, and in other cases, per 100,000 people. The choice of K depends on the size of the at-risk population. When dealing with large population sizes, it is best to express the rate per 1000 or higher to avoid dealing with large fractions or decimals. For example, the crude death rate, a measure commonly used to compare mortality levels across countries, is expressed as a rate per 1000 people.

Prevalence rates: Disease prevalence rates are most effective for evaluating chronic illnesses or, in general, assessing the burden of disease in a defined geographic area. Unlike the incidence rates which focus on the new cases, the disease prevalence reflects the existing number of cases of the disease at a given time period. The prevalence rate (P) is computed as follows:

$$P = \frac{Number\ of\ people\ with\ the\ disease\ at\ a\ specified\ time\ period}{Number\ of\ people\ at\ risk\ at\ the\ specified\ time\ period} \times K$$

Since the measure focuses on both the new and existing cases in the population, the greater the time period under study, the greater the prevalence rate. Two related measures are the *point prevalence*, which provides the cases present at a very specific time (more like a snapshot of the disease burden), and the *period prevalence*, which measures the cases present over a given period, for example a year.

Ratios

Ratios, unlike disease rates, are measures of association that compare the risk of a health event under one set of criteria to the risk of the health event under another set of criteria. These criteria may depend on different geographic environments such as the presence or absence of exposure to a causative agent. Alternatively, the criteria might be based on a comparison of two or more population groups, or multiple time periods. For example, in a study of paediatric lead poisoning, the risk of elevated blood lead levels among children might be compared among those residing in homes built before the 1940s, versus children residing in newer residential structures. In another example, one might be interested in assessing the efficacy of a new vaccine during a clinical trial aimed at reducing the burden of malaria in a low-income community. This will require the comparison of the disease burden (prevalence) among subjects who are treated with the vaccine to the disease burden among those who are not vaccinated. In all of these instances, different measures of association can be calculated first by developing a contingency table, as shown below:

Table 2.1 *Contingency table used for estimating risk ratios*

Exposure or risk factor	Disease		
	Present	*Absent*	*Total*
Present	a	b	(a + b)
Absent	c	d	(c + d)
Total	(a + c)	(b + d)	(a + b + c + d)

Note: a represents the number of people with the disease in the exposed population group; b is the number of people without the disease in the exposed population group; c is the number of people with the disease in the unexposed group; and d is the number of people without the disease in the unexposed group.

Using the summarized information in the contingency table, the following measures could be obtained:

1 Risk of the disease among the exposed $(r_e) = \frac{a}{a+b}$
2 Risk of the disease among the unexposed $(r_u) = \frac{c}{c+d}$
3 Overall risk of the disease $(r) = \frac{a+c}{a+b+c+d}$
4 Attributable risk (AR) $= \frac{r_e - r_u}{r_e}$
5 Population attributable risk (PAR) $= \frac{r_e - r_u}{r}$
6 Relative risk of the disease (RR) $= \frac{a/a+b}{c/c+d}$
7 Odds ratio (OR) $= \frac{a/c}{b/d} = \frac{ad}{bc}$

The last two measures, RR and OR, are useful ratios for evaluating the association between an exposure agent and a disease outcome, or uncovering the benefits of a protective agent such as a treatment therapy. As shown above, the relative risk ratio (RR) compares the risk of a disease among the exposed population to the risk of the disease among the unexposed population. When RR is 1, there is no associative effect between the exposure agent and the disease outcome. When RR is greater than 1, it implies that the risk of the disease increases with exposure to the causative agent. When RR is lower than 1, it implies that the factor is protective, and therefore exposure lowers the risk of disease. A related measure of association is the odds ratio (OR) which compares the exposure risk among observed cases of the disease to the exposure risk among the non-cases (or healthy individuals). A computed OR that is two times or more higher among the cases than the non-cases implies a strong likelihood that an association exists between the causative agent and the disease.

Also noted above is the attributable risk (AR), a measure that is widely used in environmental risk assessment to determine the proportion of the disease burden that is attributable to an environmental agent. As shown in Figure 2.2,

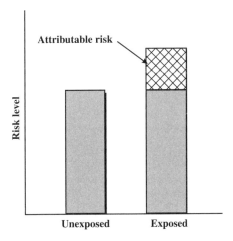

Figure 2.2 *Attributable risk*

AR assesses the excess risk of the disease among an exposed group. A related measure is the population attributed risk (PAR) which represents the risk of the disease in the entire population that can be attributed to exposure to the environmental health hazard. Both AR and PAR can be expressed as a percentage by multiplying the derived measures by 100. Although expressed as a percentage form, it is possible, when calculating multiple risks, for the attributable disease fractions to be less than 100 per cent and in some instances to exceed 100 per cent. The AR fractions are not necessarily additive and might result from the interactive or synergistic effects of multiple risk factors in the assessment of environmental health effects. Thus, an attributable risk in excess of 1, or 100 per cent, might be due to the interactive or synergistic effects of multiple risk factors that may heighten or dampen the contributory role of the others.

Table 2.2 provides examples of the mortality and morbidity indicators that are commonly used by health professionals (Checchi et al, 2007). All of the measures can be computed manually or through the use of statistical software packages that are readily available for data validation. These analytical tools allow for a more efficient examination of the data, and provide the appropriate tests of significance that confirm the degree of statistical confidence, and strength of the observed relationships. It is also important to note that some of

Table 2.2 *Examples of morbidity and mortality indicators*

Indicator	Basic formula	What it quantifies
Crude incidence rate	Number of health events due to any cause, in any age group/population at risk within a specified time period	Rate of occurrence of disease or death in the *general population.* Usually expressed per 1000, 10,000 or 100,000
Age-specific incidence rate	Number of health events in age group/population in age group at risk within a specified time period	Rate of occurrence of disease or death in a given *age group*
Group-specific incidence rate	Number of health events among members of a given subgroup/ population belonging to the group at risk within a specified time period	Rate of occurrence of disease or death in a given group. Usually calculated for vulnerable or disadvantaged population groups
Cause-specific incidence rate	Number of health events due to a given cause/population at risk within a specified time period	Rate of occurrence due to a certain cause in the general population
Case-fatality ratio	Deaths due to a given cause (disease)/total cases of a given disease	The likelihood of dying as a result of a given disease/ cause of ill health (lethality of a given disease)
Infant mortality ratio	Deaths among infants less than a year old/total live births within a specified time period	The probability of dying before age 1
Under-5 mortality ratio	Deaths among children under 5 years/total live births within a specified period	The probability of dying before age 5

Source: Modified after Checchi et al (2007)

these measures are *crude* measures based primarily on the aggregate population at risk. Others are more *specific* requiring the subdivision or stratification of the at-risk population into homogeneous groups based on the age structure, sex, race or other demographic attributes that are deemed to be relevant to the disease outcome under investigation. When analysing certain environmental diseases, the group specific rates are more informative than the crude measures.

Disease standardization

Standardization (adjustment) is a long-standing approach in epidemiological analysis that allows for the comparison of health indicators across different population groups or time periods, having controlled for confounding factors. In most applications, the disease rates are adjusted for the age structure of the population given the importance of the aging process in disease pathology, particularly for chronic illnesses. The process of age standardization is based on two approaches, direct and indirect, both geared towards the derivation of expected counts of disease in a study population.

Direct age-adjustment measures are preferable among health data analysts, and are widely reported by most governmental health agencies. The adjustment process employs either the *standard (reference) population*, a generalized demographic data provided by the WHO, or census statistics compiled for the region or country of interest. With the use of this reference information, the age-adjusted rate is calculated as a weighted average of the age-specific rates. The age-specific rates are calculated for each of the different age categories in the study population, and the weights that are applied are based on the population size in the corresponding age categories within the standard population. As reported in Table 2.3, the age-specific death rate (column 4) is generated by dividing the observed death count (column 3) by the number of individuals in each age category (column 2). Next, multiplying the age-specific death rate by the proportion of people in the same age group within the standard population (column 5) yields the expected death count for that age category (column 6). Finally, to obtain the direct age-adjusted rate, the expected counts are summed up and divided by the total population of the reference population. The results show that, when adjusting for the effects of age, the mortality rate for this

Table 2.3 *Computing age-adjusted death rates using direct standardization*

1 Age	2 Population	3 Deaths	4 Age-specific death rates	5 Standard population	6 Expected deaths
Under 1	1000	15	0.015	6000	90
1–14	3000	3	0.001	23,000	23
15–34	6000	6	0.001	41,000	41
35–54	13,000	52	0.004	30,000	120
55–64	7000	105	0.015	15,000	225
Over 64	20,000	1600	0.08	35,000	2800
All ages	50,000	1781	0.0356	150,000	3299

community is 22 deaths per 1000. This is in contrast to the crude death rate of 35.6 deaths per 1000. These results suggest overestimation of the crude death rate, a problem that would likely occur when evaluating diseases that are impacted by the aging process.

$$\text{Crude death rate} = \frac{1781}{50,000} * 1000 = 35.6$$

$$\text{Age-adjusted death rate} = \frac{3299}{150,000} * 1000 = 22.0$$

The direct standardization process illustrated above is best recommended for study areas with large populations in which the age-specific death rates are known and reliable. When evaluating health disparities, the derived measures are ideal for comparing health outcomes among different racial/ethnic groups, across different subregions, or multiple time periods.

A second approach is the indirect standardization method which works best for small study populations or situations where the observed cases of health events are rare with limited or no information on the age-specific death rates. In such cases, data on the age-specific rates of the standard population are utilized to generate the expected counts. As shown in Table 2.4, the third column has the age-specific rates for the standard population (*standard rates*). In each age category, the observed cases are then multiplied by the standard rate observed in each age category to produce the expected counts. These expected counts are then summed up across all age groups and then divided by the total observed counts to produce the standardized mortality ratio (SMR).

$$\text{SMR} = \frac{1781}{2032.5} = 0.876$$

As with other ratios computed in the previous section of this chapter, the SMR is a dimensionless indicator. An SMR that is greater than 1 implies that the mortality level is higher than expected, meaning that more deaths have occurred than anticipated in the community. If the SMR is less than 1, as in the observed case, it implies than when compared to the standard population, fewer deaths have occurred than anticipated. Unlike the age-adjusted death rate computed

Table 2.4 *Computing standardized mortality ratios using the indirect method*

1 Age	2 Population	3 Standard death rates	4 Expected deaths
Under 1	1000	0.02	20.0
1–14	3000	0.0005	1.5
15–34	6000	0.001	6.0
35–54	13,000	0.005	65.0
55–64	7000	0.02	140.0
Over 64	20,000	0.09	1800.0
All ages	50,000	17.4	2032.5

earlier, this ratio measure cannot be used for multi-group or interregional comparisons. However, it can be used to compare different disease outcomes within the same study population.

Using epidemiological measures in monitoring population health trends

Several of the measures presented so far in this chapter serve as useful indicators of health events in a community. These measures are reported regularly by governmental health agencies in several countries, and have been used consistently for intergroup and interregional comparisons. In this section, we shall examine the historical and recent applications of these measures in the development of population transition frameworks, and the more modern methods of health valuation using summary measures such as the global burden of disease (GBD) and the environmental burden of disease (EBD).

Population transition frameworks

For decades, many social scientists have investigated the causal linkages between economic development and the demographic, epidemiologic and environmental transformation of countries. Using historical evidence from mostly Western nations, a series of theoretical frameworks have been offered to explain and predict the likely course of events that would take place as countries transition from pre-industrialized to modernized societies. In particular, there are three population transition frameworks that rely on the basic measures of morbidity, fertility and mortality introduced earlier. These are the demographic, epidemiologic and environmental risk assessment frameworks (see Figure 2.3). Economic improvements, modernization and social change within countries are typically accompanied by changes in environmental conditions. These in turn produce modern risks, which along with the pre-existing traditional hazards compound the overall risks in these environments. Ongoing exposures to these environmental risks produce poor health outcomes that are manifested in the epidemiological transition. Increasing mortality and morbidity rates contribute to the demographic transition in these countries.

The oldest of these frameworks is the *demographic transition model* (DTM), which was first proposed in 1929 by Warren Thompson. The DTM proposes a transformation in the population structure of a country as it moves from an agro-based, non-industrialized economy to a highly industrialized, urbanized society. Drawing from the experience in Western Europe, the model uses the crude birth rates and crude death rates observed in these countries to develop four stages of demographic transition. This first stage, evident in most pre-industrial economies, is characterized by high birth rates and high death rates. Both rates fluctuate around 30 cases per 1000 persons, resulting in a high but stationary population growth pattern. In stage two, the death rates begin to decline as the economic circumstances begin to improve through industrial development accompanied by changes in agricultural practices, and improvements in health care, environmental health, sanitation and hygiene. The birth

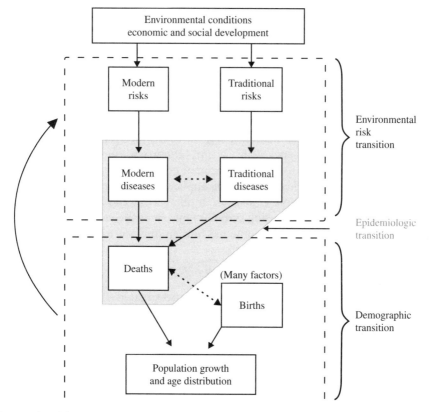

Source: Adapted from Smith and Ezzati (2005)

Figure 2.3 *Interrelationships between population transition frameworks: risk factors must change before morbidity and mortality patterns change*

rates, however, remain high, resulting in increasing population growth rates. The third stage is marked by declining birth rates, a process that could be triggered by factors such as rapid urbanization, societal modernization, late marriages and fewer children as a result of better educational and employment opportunities for women. Meanwhile, as death rates continue to decline, the overall growth rate of the population is reduced. In the fourth stage of the DTM, birth rates and death rates continue to decline to record low levels with observed rates below 10 cases per 1000 for both indicators. The overall population is likely to reach a low and stable rate, though in some countries birth rates are likely to fall even further below replacement levels. This has been identified as a possible fifth stage in which countries transition into a post-industrial economy dominated by service and knowledge-based activities. As with most theoretical frameworks, the dynamics and full applicability of the DTM are questionable, particularly in developing countries where in some cases the transition has been stalled by continuing high birth rates due to existing cultural norms and practices that differ significantly from the patterns previously observed in the Western nations.

A second transition framework that also employs several of the health indicators presented earlier is the *epidemiological transition model* (ETM). This theory examines the complex changes in morbidity and mortality patterns with the leading causes of death shifting over time from infectious diseases (denoted as traditional diseases in Figure 2.3) to chronic degenerative diseases. As in the case of the DTM, these epidemiological changes are the result of economic and technological developments as countries move from low-income, pre-industrialized economies to wealthy industrialized nations. The ETM, as originally proposed by Omran in 1971, identifies three major stages of the epidemiologic transition, all of which are guided by shifts in mortality patterns. The first stage is the Age of Pestilence and Famine, a phase associated with a high prevalence of infectious and parasitic diseases that take a heavy toll on the population. This is followed by an Age of Receding Pandemics in which mortality rates gradually decline, a stage that is no doubt consistent with stage two of the demographic transition. The third stage is the Age of Degenerative and Human-induced Diseases. As suggested by the WHO, this is the stage where morbidity rates overshadow mortality as indices of health. Chronic diseases associated with the aging process prevail in this stage, accompanied by diseases that are directly linked to environmental pollution such as hazardous accidents, lead exposure, ozone depletion and global warming. More recently, with global environmental change, some epidemiologists have noted that we might be re-entering the Age of Pandemics with the recent upsurge in infectious diseases such as SARs, H1N1 and their unprecedented rates of diffusion across the globe (Brilliant, 2009). The resistant strains of malaria parasites and tuberculosis also pose significant health risks at the global level.

The third transition framework, the *environmental risk transition* (ERT), builds upon the theoretical foundation established by the preceding models, the DTM and the ETM. Linking the health indicators to environmental hazards, the model suggests that there are discernible shifts in the character of environmental risks during the period of economic development in many countries around the world (see Figure 2.4). The ERT framework recognizes a three-phase transition in environmental risks that are first evident at the household level (also referred to as the brown level). With increasing economic development, these environmental risks gradually work their way to the community (grey) level, and then pan out to the global (green) level. The environmental risks at the household level are most evident in the poorest countries where residents grapple with issues of water supply and quality, waste disposal, hygiene and poor access to health care services. Infectious diseases prevail in these societies with mortality patterns consistent with stage 1 of the DTM and ETM. As countries become more developed and are able to tackle these problems a new set of environmental risks emerge. These new risks, though still impacting residents at the household level, are more likely to be manifested at the community level. Problems of urban air pollution, road traffic congestion and accidents, occupational hazards, lead pollution from households, industrial and transportation sources emerge as salient risk sources. Over time, these risks play out in more complex ways emerging at larger geographic scales with global implications. The environmental transition at this level is evident in global environmental hazards such as

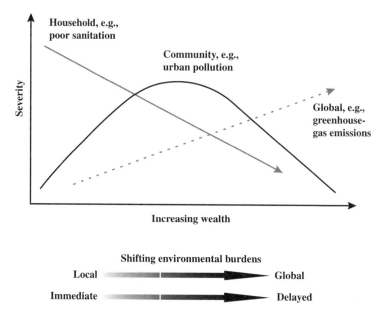

Source: Smith and Ezzati (2005)

Figure 2.4 *Environmental risk transition framework: household risks decline with increasing economic development, community risks rise and fall, while global risks increase throughout the development process*

climate change, stratospheric ozone depletion and land-use changes, accompanied by the emergence or re-emergence of pandemic diseases. Though the ERT framework was only recently introduced by Smith (2001), proponents contend, and rightly so, that environmental risks precede the epidemiologic transition and the demographic transition. The shifts in environmental risk factors occur before the disease outcomes and related demographic patterns emerge as predicted by the ETM and DTM. Some disease outcomes are likely to emerge quickly following the change in risk factors while others have longer latency periods resulting in slower changes in demographic or epidemiologic patterns.

Estimating global and environmental burden of disease

Since the 1990s, researchers have worked on the development of more comprehensive health measures that incorporate data on both mortality and morbidity outcomes. Among these, the most successful and now widely adopted measure is the disease-adjusted life year (DALY), an additive measure that combines the estimates of years lost (YLL) with the estimates of years lived with disabilities (YLD). The DALY is essentially a health gap measure that captures the difference between the ideal health status and the actual health status of individuals in a given country. The ideal health status is based on the notion that everyone regardless of regional location, race or income status is entitled to the same maximum life expectancy as their counterparts. Using the WHO world standard population as a reference, the maximum life expectancy is assessed at 80 years for males and 82.5 years for females. In computing the DALY,

YLL = number of deaths × standard life expectancy at age of death; and

$$YLD = I*DW*L$$

where I is the number of disability cases, L is the average duration of the disease and DW is a weight factor based on the perceived severity of the disease. This ranges from a scale of 0 (perfect health) to 1 (dead). For example, the untreated form of terminal-stage cancers are typically weighted as 0.81, whereas the untreated forms of other diseases are weighted much lower (asthma − 0.06; tuberculosis − 0.27; malaria − 0.20). The combination of the YLL and YLD produces the DALY measure which is expressed in time units or lost years of healthy life.

Following its initial development, the DALY has been quantified for major diseases and disease groups, as well as by age, sex, country and global subregions. Ezzati et al (2004) used this framework to assess the health impacts of 26 risk factors among 14 world subregions. The analysis focused on nutritional risk factors, sanitation and hygiene, substance abuse, physical inactivity, unsafe sexual activities, occupational hazards and environmental pollution. Overall, cardiovascular risk factors and tobacco use have contributed most to deaths at the global level. In terms of healthy years of life lost, underweight conditions, unsafe sex, blood pressure and tobacco and alcohol use are the leading risk factors. Subsequent analyses have provided insightful patterns of disease and disability risks at the global, regional and national levels.

A similar approach has been applied to derive a measure of the EBD. First introduced in 2003, this index measures the disease burden that is attributable to environmental risk factors. The EBD relies on an exposure-based methodology, with information gathered from three main sources: (i) the distribution of the risk factor exposure within the study population; (ii) the exposure–response relationship for the risk factor; and (iii) the DALYs lost to the disease associated with the risk factor. Analysts suggest that in the absence of the DALYs data, the disease incidence or mortality rates be substituted into the analysis.

The EBD has been applied in several studies to identify the attributable risk fractions of environmental hazards. Using the morbidity and mortality data to calculate the EBD, the results suggest that about 24 per cent of the number of years of healthy life lost is due to environmental risk factors. Similarly, among the deaths reported, roughly 23 per cent is attributed to these risk factors. Environmental attributable fractions of the diseases vary widely across geographic regions. In more recent applications of the EBD (2007), three indicators of environmental health are used to evaluate the DALYs across the subregions of the world. The first is based on diarrhoea, an indicator of access or lack thereof to clean water, sanitation and hygiene. The second is based on

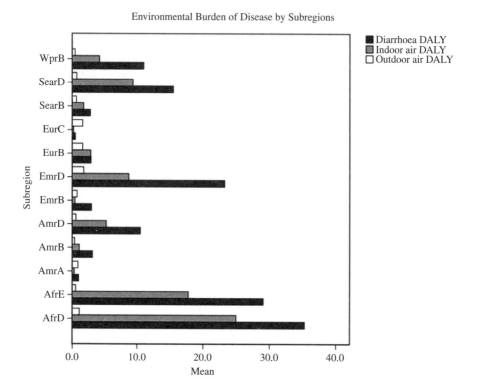

Figure 2.5 *Environmental DALYs across world regions*

indoor air pollution, and the third based on outdoor air pollution. The results show widespread disparities in the geographic distribution of the respective DALYs across the global subregions. Figure 2.5 summarizes the DALYs obtained across these regions. The highest DALYs are reported in African subregions D and E, followed closely by Eastern Mediterranean countries (such as Somalia, Sudan, Egypt, Pakistan and Afghanistan), and then the Southeast Asian countries.

Chapter summary

The basic epidemiological measures were introduced in this chapter along with an overview of the issues surrounding health valuation, and the classification of environmental diseases as diseases that are triggered or exacerbated by exposure to external agents. Different measures were presented for comparing morbidity and mortality trends within and across populations. We also explored how these measures are standardized to account for confounding factors such as age by comparing the observed outcomes to the expected from a reference population. Finally, the use of these indicators was further demonstrated through population transition frameworks and the development of summary measures such as the GBD, and the EBD estimates of population health.

References

Brilliant, L. (2009) 'The Age of Pandemics', *The Wall Street Journal*, 2 May, available at http://online.wsj.com/article/SB124121965740478983.html

Checchi, F., Gayer, M., Grais, R. F. and Mills, E. J. (2007) 'Public health in crisis-affected populations', *Humanitarian Practice Network*, vol 61, pp58

Ezzati, M., Rodgers, A. D., Lopez, A. D. and Murray, C. J. L. (eds) (2004) *Comparative Quantification of Health Risks: Global and regional burden of disease attributable to selected major risk factors*, World Health Organization, Geneva, Switzerland, available at www.who.int/publications/cra

Hutt, M. S. R. and Burkitt, D. P. (1986) *The Geography of Non-Infectious Disease*, Oxford University Press, New York

Jadad, A. R. and O'Grady, L. (2008) 'How should health be defined?', *BMJ*, vol 337, art 2900

McWhinney, I. R. (1987) 'Health and disease: Problems of definition', *CMAJ*, vol 136, no 8, p815

Moeller, D. W. (2005) *Environmental Health*, Harvard College, Boston

Moore, G. S. (1999) *Living with the Earth: Concepts in Environmental Health Science*, Lewis Publishers, London

Omran, A. R. (1971) 'The epidemiologic transition: A theory of the epidemiology of population change', *Milbank Memorial Fund Quarterly*, vol 29, pp509–538

Pruss-Ustun, A. and Corvalan, C. (2006) *Preventing Disease Through Healthy Environments: Towards an estimate of the environmental burden of disease*, World Health Organization, Geneva, Switzerland, available at www.who.int/quantifying_e-himpacts/publications/preventingdisease.pdf

Smith, K. R. (2001) 'Environment and health: Issues for the U.S. Administration', *Environment*, May, vol 43, no 4, pp34–38

Smith, K. R. and Ezzati, M. (2005) 'How environmental risks change with development: the epidemiologic and environmental risk transitions revisited', *Annual Review of Environmental Resources*, vol 30, pp291–333

Smith, K. R., Corvalan, C. F. and Kjellstrom, T. (1999) 'How much global ill health is attributable to environmental factors?', *Epidemiology*, vol 10, no 5, pp573–584

Thompson, W. S. (1929) 'Population', *American Journal of Sociology*, vol 34, no 6, pp959–975

WHO (1946) Preamble to the Constitution of the World Health Organization as adopted by the International Health Conference, New York, 19–22 June, signed 22 July by the representatives of 61 States (Official Records of the World Health Organization, no 2, p100) and entered into force 7 April 1948

3
Population Health Disparities and Social Injustices: Indicators and Spatial Patterns

Introduction

In a world where environmental hazards now play a major role in disease occurrence, environmental health indicators provide valuable markers for characterizing disease trends, delineating the spatial patterns, and comparing risks across regions. A few of these indicators were introduced earlier in Chapter 2, along with a discussion of their uses and applications in establishing population transition frameworks and evaluating disease burdens. This chapter goes a step further to examine these measures within the context of health disparities. The chapter begins with a clarification of the concepts and terminologies that are increasingly used in the literature to describe the differential health status of population groups. The growing disconnect between public awareness of these problems and their support for governmental intervention is also discussed along with research paradigms that seek to explain the underlying causes. In the last section, an overview of health disparities in the United States is presented, along with a recent national initiative to promote health parity and social justice.

The nature of health and social inequalities

The emerging literature on this topic is filled with several terms that describe the uneven patterns of morbidity and mortality, and the excess burden of ill health among underprivileged groups in many countries around the world. Concepts such as *health disparities, health inequalities, health inequities, social injustices* and related terminology are now commonly used to describe these differences in population health. The key to examining the differences, however, lies not only in knowing what these concepts are but also the contexts in which they are applied. For example, the first two terms, health disparities and health inequalities, are used frequently and interchangeably in the literature but differ in meaning and application. Specifically, the term *'health inequality'* is a generalized concept that describes the uneven distribution of morbidity and mortality outcomes within and between populations (Reidpath and Allotey, 2007). Though emphasis is often placed on the health outcomes, inequalities may exist in multiple health domains such as access to care, diagnosis, treatment, participation in clinical trials and self-reported health status.

The term, '*health disparity*' also acknowledges the existence of population health differences, but goes a step further to emphasize the underlying health disadvantage that one population group faces when compared to its counterpart population (Margai, 2006). This concept is particularly useful within the context of social justice, when comparing the burden of ill health among social groups that are underrepresented politically, and/or economically marginalized by virtue of their race, ethnicity or other social attributes. Health inequalities exist within and between populations at all spatial scales – between countries at the global level, and within populations in both developing and developed regions. At the global level, significant differences are apparent between the wealthy industrialized countries and the low-income economies when examining the prevalence of infectious diseases, nutritional health outcomes, life expectancies and overall mortality rates. One such measure with marked differences at the global level is the infant mortality rate (IMR) (Figure 3.1). A child born in a country in sub-Saharan Africa or southern Asia is roughly ten times more likely to die before the first birthday than a child born in Europe or North America, Japan or Australia. These disparities are further evident within the developing countries where group differences exist between the socio-economic groups and ethnic groups (Braveman and Tarimo, 2002).

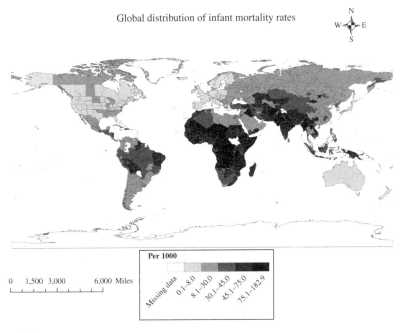

Source: CIESIN

Figure 3.1 *Global IMR*

The developed countries are not immune from such health disparities within their populations. They too have significant population differences in infant mortality and other negative health outcomes.

The Theory of Health Inequities

To a large extent, health disparities are inevitable as long as differences exist among various populations by geography, social status, income, race/ethnicity, culture, gender, age and other socio-demographic factors. Some authors have correctly noted that a situation can never arise in a country where the entire population has the same or equal health status (Low et al, 2003). This inevitability of population health inequalities, however, does not imply that such conditions are morally acceptable; and therein lies the difference between health disparities and health inequities. Specifically, the use of the term *health inequities* comes with a normative dimension that implies unfairness, injustice and a required response to address those disparities (Fabienne, 2001; Anand, 2002; Chang, 2002). Known as the Theory of Health Inequities, the principal claim is that uneven population health outcomes are (i) unjust; (ii) ethically and morally unacceptable; and (iii) steps must be taken to avoid and/or minimize these differences.

The various conceptualizations of this theory are all grounded within the underlying principles of justice and fairness. Whitehead (1990) for example described health inequities as population health differences that are unnecessary and avoidable, but in addition are considered to be unfair and unjust. Fabienne (2001) acknowledged that Whitehead's definition pointed in the right direction, but cautioned that a problem exists in determining precisely which of the inequalities in health outcomes are unjust or unfair. Payne-Sturges et al (2006) also discussed the ethical dimension of health inequities, noting that the moral obligation to correct such inequalities becomes even greater for disparities that are born out of environmental health hazards. Such outcomes, they noted, may be correctly described as *human-induced health inequalities*, since they are attributable mostly to anthropogenic activities. Environmental health disparities are also avoidable, and if and when they do occur, they should be corrected through human action and intervention.

The emphasis on *remediation* is apparent in the health inequities discourse. For example, the International Society for Equity in Health (2005) officially defined health inequities as the systematic and *potentially remediable* differences in one or more aspects of health across populations or population groups defined socially, economically, demographically or geographically. Margai (2003) too offered a three-pronged approach that highlights the need for response and remediation in the characterization of health inequities.

Framing the discourse within the context of morality and ethics also enables the recognition of the important links between *health inequity* and *social injustice*. The quest for environment and health equity is strongly linked to the overarching goals of social justice, an area that is broader and more encompassing in terms of the pursuit of fairness and justice. Building on the philosophical foundations of scholars such as Aristotle and Rawls, the moral significance of health as a basic human right principle is woven into the social justice principle as evident in major institutional declarations such as the United Nations Universal Declaration of Human Rights, the Millennium Development Goals, and the Healthy People 2010 initiative in the United States. This social justice principle is also apparent in the health disparities literature. For example, in writing about the approaches to health equity, Fabienne (2001) advocates an indirect approach that draws upon Rawl's theory of justice and fairness. The basic tenet is that social inequalities in health are unjust or unfair if they originate from a basic structure of society that is unjust. The author argues that the key to uncovering health inequalities lies in the basic structure of society. This social structure often reflects the various strata or positions that individuals find themselves in, with different expectations of life. The societal structure impacts the talents and abilities of individuals, and through the allocation of resources it impacts the opportunities and life's chances for those individuals. Societies with unjust structures impose undue disadvantages on those who are worse off or socially marginalized, and benefit those who are already better off in life (Fabienne, 2001). By uncovering these deep-seated injustices one may have a better shot at reducing health inequities and in so doing achieve social equity and justice.

Ruger (2004) also endorses the linkage between social justice and the moral significance of health but more in terms of human capability. The human capability perspective promotes the idea of giving individuals the opportunity to achieve good health and thus be free from escapable morbidity and preventable mortality (Ruger, 2004). As she describes it, the human capability view also has an element of human agency. Society is morally obligated to offer individuals a chance to pursue the lives that they value. The element of human agency occurs individually and collectively. As an individual, one should be free to make decisions about health habits, risks, lifestyle, priorities and treatment options. The collective agency plays out at the policy level with significant implications for health care delivery, resource allocation and decision making. Ruger suggests further that the capability view towards social justice of health (i) requires the prioritization of health and its determinants above all other social ends; (ii) ensures that health care is socially guaranteed; (iii) uses the democratic process to provide guidance and specifics on what types of health care should be guaranteed and to what level; and (iv) ensures that individuals are involved in the decision-making process (Ruger, 2004). It will be interesting to see how the balance between the individual and collective agency plays out in countries such as the United States that are currently grappling with the implementation of health care policies that strive toward health equity and affordability.

Another great example of the twin goals of health and social equity in the literature is offered by Levy and Sidel (2006). In their book, *Social Injustice and Public Health*, the authors provide examples of social injustices: wars and other forms of violence, global warming and other environmental hazards, corruption, erosion of civil liberties, restriction of scientific research, education and public discourse, and failure to provide essential health services to disadvantaged populations. Social injustices are described as violations of fundamental human rights that are often carried out in two ways: (i) the denial of socio-economic, socio-cultural, political and civil or human rights of specific groups based on their perceived status as inferior members of society; and

(ii) the implementation of policies and actions that adversely impact the societal conditions in which people can be healthy.

These perspectives underscore the varied contexts in which population health differences are formulated as: (i) health inequalities which merely refer to the observed differences; (ii) health disparities, which emphasize the disadvantages borne by some groups; and (iii) health inequities, which are linked to a broader mission of social justice. The latter encapsulate the differential health outcomes, the unethical concerns about these differences, and the need for societal intervention. In the next segment of this chapter, we shall explore these issues further, noting the trends in public understanding of the root causes of these disparities, and their support for governmental intervention.

The root causes of health disparities: Individual vs population-based frameworks

In the United States and around the world, public awareness of health disparities has increased significantly over the last decade. A recent study of the trends in the United States attributed this rise in public consciousness to the intense media coverage of the plight of low-income and minority groups particularly in the wake of disasters such as Hurricane Katrina in 2005 (Taylor-Clark et al, 2007). Trends at the global level also suggest a revival in public perception, a pattern that has been boosted by a new generation of studies that highlight the magnitude and nature of health problems facing underprivileged populations, and a greater concern for health system efficiency, sustainability and interest in equity (Gwatkin, 2000).

Unfortunately, even as awareness has increased, the general public has become less supportive of governmental interventions to address these health differences. Public support for governmental intervention has waned in part because, as revealed in a recent study, many people attribute health disparities to the personal limitations of individuals such as their failure to seek medical treatment, their failure to adhere to physician recommendations, or their inability to pay for health care services (Taylor-Clark et al, 2007). Sadly enough, these accounts are similar to historical accounts that blamed differential racial/ethnic health outcomes on traditional biomedical factors such as genetic susceptibility, racial/ethnic heritage, or the behavioural, nutritional and occupational characteristics of individuals.

Focusing on the personal attributes of individuals to account for health disparities is not only misleading, it also detracts from the more important task of uncovering the fundamental causes of these problems. Health disparities are not necessarily due to individual shortcomings, but the result of major root causes that exist at the population level. Efforts to understand and address these problems require an 'upstream', macro-scale or population-based perspective rather than an individual-based or micro-scale view. This approach becomes even more meaningful and apparent when examining the geographic distribution of disease outcomes, the group-related characteristics and socio-spatial experiences.

One of the key drivers of population health disparities is social privilege. In the literature, social privilege has been variously described in terms of wealth, power, prestige and perceived social standing of a dominant group over others in a given society. But as Braveman and Tarimo (2002) rightly pointed out in their study, social privilege is not unique to only a few societies:

> *In virtually every society in the world, social privilege varies among groups of people categorized not only by economic resources but also by gender, geographic location, by ethnic or religious differences, and by age; other dimensions can be important as well, but these are nearly universal, and they often interact with each other to make some groups, for example poor women in ethnic minority groups, particularly disadvantaged with respect to opportunities to be healthy.* (p1623)

The ripple effects of social privilege play out in all areas of society. They are most evident in the decision-making processes of various institutions and societal actions that impact the lives, both the biographies and geographies of underprivileged populations, confining them to neighbourhoods of social distress, deprivation and environmental degradation. Actions such as residential segregation, racial/ethnic discrimination, land-use and zoning regulations, and the siting of noxious facilities, all create unhealthy environments and poor living conditions that produce adverse health outcomes. These outcomes are most observable at the population levels and not at individual level. The investigation of the root causes of health disparities therefore requires an ecological perspective that is linked to group-related characteristics and experiences.

Ecological or population-based approaches to studying health disparities also involve the incorporation of risk factors that play out at multiple levels (Diez-Roux et al, 2000; Gee and Payne-Sturges, 2004). As shown in Figure 3.2, there are at least five levels at which these disparities can be evaluated either independently or simultaneously using techniques such as multilevel analysis. These include the family or household level, the cultural/ethnic group that the people identify with, their workplace or occupational environments, the neighbourhood and the larger community in which they reside.

Many research frameworks have been developed to account for these different layers of vulnerability and the relative contribution of the key determinants of disparities. One of the most recent conceptualizations identifies the primary causes of environmental health disparities (Gee and Payne-Sturges, 2004). Termed the exposure–disease–stress model, it differentiates between individual and community processes, noting that the latter are the most important determinants of poor health conditions. Community processes include neighbourhood attributes such as residential segregation, structural factors such as zoning policies, and tax incentives that lure polluting industries into the area. All of these factors contribute to individual stressors and long-term health disparities.

Another framework developed earlier focuses on race/ethnicity as a pivotal factor in the emergence of health disparities (Williams, 1997). Williams

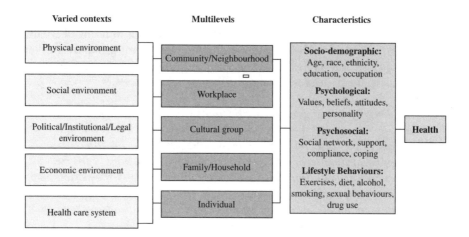

Figure 3.2 *Levels of health disparities*

identified several basic causes (culture, biology, geography, economic, political and legal structures) that impact the social and occupational status of the less privileged groups. These factors subsequently produce surface causes such as racial/ethnically segregated and socio-economically distressed neighbourhoods and poor health practices in those communities. Over time, these stressful conditions impact the human biological processes (such as the endocrine, neurological, immune systems) resulting in adverse health outcomes. Though Williams previously identified nativity and group origin as contributory factors, geographical factors such as housing, settlement patterns and poor environmental conditions also serve as determinants of health in low-income and minority neighbourhoods (Margai, 2006). The model as illustrated in

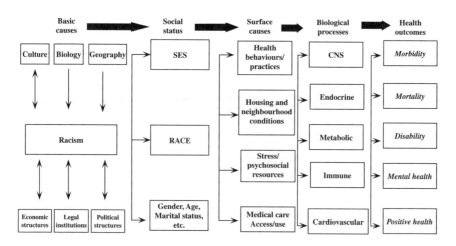

Figure 3.3 *Williams' theoretical framework for understanding the role of race in health*

Figure 3.3 is most applicable to the US context but can be easily replicated in other countries using the markers of social privilege and group marginalization in those countries.

Overview of health disparities in the United States

As noted earlier in this chapter, health inequalities exist at the global level between countries, and within populations at the national level regardless of the country being a wealthy industrialized nation or not. When it comes to documenting these disparities, the United States is perhaps one of the most widely researched countries because of its pluralistic and racially diverse composition, along with an unfortunate history of racially based policies and practices. Health inequalities are reported among many different segments of the population by race/ethnicity, national origin, gender, socio-economic status, language proficiency and geography (Liao et al, 2004; Kawachi et al, 2005). The most persistent and the most complex set of disparities, however, are those based on the racial/ethnic characteristics of the population (Carter-Pokras and Woo, 1999; Kingston and Nickens, 2000). The health of racial and ethnic minorities who already face major economic and social disadvantages is threatened by even greater challenges. When compared to the white majority, these groups, especially blacks, Latinos and Native Americans, face more chronic health conditions, greater risk factors, limited access to health care resources, linguistic barriers, and limited utilization of health-related services.

The disparities by race and ethnicity are pervasive and cut across all health events, including morbidity and mortality outcomes, functional limitations and disabilities, as well as self-rated health. When examining the various forms of disease, there are higher prevalence rates of chronic infectious diseases such as tuberculosis and HIV/AIDs, environmental diseases such as asthma, lead poisoning and pesticide exposures, developmental diseases such as learning disabilities and birth defects, neoplastic diseases such as liver and prostate cancer, and nutritional diseases such as hypertension and obesity. These disparities also cut across all life stages from infants, to adolescents, adults and elderly populations.

Racial and ethnic health disparities in the United States also have an element of place with the geographical clustering of these health events in areas that are clearly linked to the settlement geographies of these groups. The contrasts between rural versus urban areas, segregated and non-segregated communities, poor housing quality and environmental conditions in these areas have all contributed to the geographical differentiation of the observed health outcomes. The negative dimensions of health are best witnessed in the urbanized areas where groups such as African Americans tend to reside and are likely to pay an *'urban health penalty'* with excessively high rates of tuberculosis, sexually transmitted diseases, HIV/AIDS, asthma, homicides, infant mortality and other adverse health outcomes.

Summarized in Table 3.1 below are some of the race-specific morbidity and mortality rates observed among the groups. The information presented for the five major racial and ethnic groups, non-Hispanic whites, non-Hispanic blacks, Hispanic (Latino), Asian Americans and Pacific Islanders (AAPI) and American Indians and Alaskan Natives (AIAN), shows marked differences. For example, the infant mortality rate within the black population is more than twice the observed rate among whites, a pattern that is also consistent with the primary risk factor, low birth weights. Blacks also face the highest mortality rates of coronary heart disease, stroke and overall cancer deaths. When examining cause-specific rates for these cancer deaths, one finds that the death rates for lung and prostate cancers are also high among the black population. The female breast cancer death rates remain high among blacks despite evidence of lower disease incidence among them when compared to their white female counterparts. The reasons behind these disparities are very complex and are linked to societal, cultural and environmental risk factors that play out at the population subgroup level rather than just the individual level.

Along with some of the factors alluded to earlier in this chapter, health access and the utilization of the health services also matter. Evidence of this disparity is shown by the differential levels of health insurance availability among the groups in Table 3.1. The lack of health insurance often leads to late diagnosis and differential treatment approaches resulting in lower survival rates among the underprivileged groups.

Exposures to environmental contaminants also contribute significantly to the emergence of these health disparities. As shown in Table 3.2, the minority groups face a disproportionate burden of exposure to air pollutants resulting in a greater likelihood of respiratory diseases such as asthma, a problem that is linked to both indoor and outdoor pollutants. Hispanics and Asian-Americans face relatively high exposure levels to ozone, particulates and carbon monoxide, a pattern that could well be linked to their residential locations in the metropolitan areas in the East and West of the country. Blacks too are among the most susceptible populations to asthmatic conditions with death rates that are four times higher than the white or average national rates observed for all age categories.

The health indicators presented in Tables 3.1 and 3.2 provide a very useful barometer for comparing disease rates across social groups. To summarize the magnitude of the observed differences between the groups, the index of disparity can be computed using the following basic formula proposed by Pearcy and Keppel (2002):

$$Disp = \frac{\left(\sum |r_{(1-n)} - R|/n\right)}{R*100}$$

The disparity index is computed by taking the average of the absolute difference between the rates observed for the specific group (r) and the reference population group (R), divided by the rate of the reference group (R). To express the index as a percentage, the computed value is multiplied by 100.

As an example, the disparity index was calculated for infant mortality rates among blacks and whites. Using the white population as the reference group, the index was calculated for the black population across all counties in the United

Table 3.1 *Morbidity and mortality indicators among the US racial and ethnic groups*

Health indicators	US total	White	Black	Hispanic	Asian	American Indian
Infant mortality rate (2005, per 1000 live births)	6.9	5.8	13.6	5.6	4.9	8.1
Low birth weight <2500g (2005, per cent)	8.7	7.3	14.0	6.9	8.0	7.4
Coronary heart disease deaths (2005, age adjusted per 100,000)	154	153	198	125	87	102
Stroke deaths (2005, age adjusted per 100,000)	47	45	66	36	39	35
Prevalence of diabetes (2005, age adjusted per 1000)	57	49	89	77	–	118
HIV rate (2005, persons aged 13+ years)	11.8	5.6	43.5	16.4	2.0	4.4
Overall cancer deaths (2005, age adjusted per 100,000)	183.8	187.0	226.8	122.8	110.5	123.2
Lung cancer deaths (2005, age adjusted per 100,000)	52.6	55.5	59.6	22.4	25.7	34.1
Female breast cancer deaths (2005, age adjusted per 100,000)	24.1	24.0	33.5	15.0	12.2	15.2
Prostate cancer deaths (2005, age adjusted per 100,000)	24.5	22.4	54.7	18.5	10.4	17.6
Mental disorder (2003–2005, age adjusted rate)	21.1	21.7	22.9	12.6	8.2	18.8

Note: Data presented are for white non-Hispanic and black non-Hispanic populations. A dash denotes missing data.
Data Source: CDC Wonder DATA 2010; Centers for Disease Control and Prevention, Atlanta, GA.

Table 3.2 *Selective indicators of environmental risk factors and diseases among the US racial and ethnic groups*

Environmental health indicators	US total	White	Black	Hispanic	Asian	American Indian
Persons exposed to Ozone (2004, per cent)	39	33	43	59	66	23
Persons exposed to PM <10 mcg (2004, per cent)	10	7	6	28	22	13
Persons exposed to carbon monoxide (2004, per cent)	7	4	4	20	17	8
Paediatric lead poisoning						
Ever had asthma (2005, age adjusted per 100,000)	12.9	13.5	14.9	10.7	–	–
Deaths from asthma under 5 yrs (2005, per 1,000,000)	2.0	2.3	9.2	–	–	–
Deaths from asthma 5–25 yrs (2005, per 1,000,000)	2.4	1.1	8.0	–	–	–
Deaths from asthma 25–34 yrs (2005, per 1,000,000)	4.1	3.0	13.3	1.6	–	–
Deaths from asthma 34–64 yrs (2005, per 1,000,000)	12.7	9.9	37.7	7.7	5.3	–
Deaths from chronic obstructive pulmonary disease excluding asthma 45+ yrs (2005, per 1,000,000)	118.82.0	130.9	79.1	51.8	38.2	78.8

States. The derived values were then exported into ArcGIS 9.3 to illustrate the geographic differentiation across the country (Figure 3.4). The results provide evidence of a place-based pattern of racial disparities in infant mortality rates. Areas of extreme disparities appear along the Atlantic Seaboard, the Southeastern United States, and in selected counties on the West Coast.

Efforts are underway to reduce group inequities by funnelling health resources into high-risk communities. One such approach is the Racial and Ethnic Approaches to Community Health (REACH) programme implemented by the US Centers for Disease Control (CDC) in 1999. The key objective of this programme is to eliminate racial/ethnic health disparities through the use of community networks and participatory-based approaches that are implemented in various care-giving settings such as hospitals, clinics, schools and after-school programmes, and in the workplaces and neighbourhoods. Starting initially in about 40 racially diverse communities, the programme has identified the most persistent indicators of health disparities as the priority areas: infant mortality rates; breast and cervical cancer screening and management; cardiovascular diseases; diabetes; HIV/AIDS; adult immunizations; hepatitis B; tuberculosis; and asthma.

Since its inception, the changes in the targeted communities have been monitored and documented. Data collected so far suggest that the programme has been effective in reducing some of the health disparities particularly in the management of chronic conditions such as diabetes and cardiovascular diseases. For example, cholesterol screening rates have improved for Hispanics in all educational levels in REACH communities. Among African Americans in REACH communities, the screening rates for cholesterol have also increased and exceeded

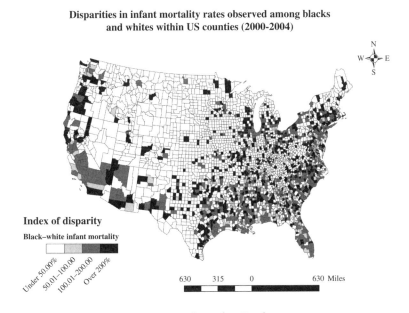

Figure 3.4 *Index of IMR disparity*

the national levels. Gaps in mammography rates between whites and blacks have also been sharply reduced in some of these communities. Similarly, improvements have been reported in the management of diabetes and related complications such as heart disease, stroke, blindness, renal failure and amputations (CDC, 2009).

Chapter summary

In all societies where people differ by race, ethnicity, place, income, age, gender and other dimensions, health inequalities and disparities are inevitable. The key to addressing these challenges, however, lies in acknowledging their existence as unjust, morally unacceptable and remediable. Addressing these inequities fulfils the broader mission of fairness and social justice within countries. In this chapter, we have examined the major concepts and terminologies as well as the existing frameworks that offer reasonable explanations for the root causes of health disparities and social injustices. As an example, we also chose the United States to discuss the primary indicators of health disparities among the racial and ethnic groups and the steps that are being taken to address these challenges. Given the measurable progress in the targeted communities so far, the government now plans to expand the successful strategies of the REACH programme into other communities across the nation. These efforts demonstrate that, while health differences are likely between population subgroups in any country, the observed differences can be minimized and even eliminated by the implementation of meaningful approaches that address the underlying causes of the disparities.

References

Anand, S. (2002) 'The concern for equity in health', *Journal of Epidemiology and Community Health*, vol 56, pp485–487

Braveman, P. and Tarimo, E. (2002) 'Social inequalities in health: Not only an issue for affluent countries', *Social Science and Medicine*, vol 54, no 11, pp1621–1635

Carter-Pokras, O. and Woo, V. (1999) 'Health profile of racial and ethnic minorities in the United States', *Ethnicity and Health*, vol 4, no 3, pp117–120

Centers for Disease Control (2009) 'REACH: Finding solutions to health disparities', available at www.cdc.gov/nccdphp/publications/AAG/pdf/reach_success.pdf, accessed 17 June 2009

Chang, W. C. (2002) 'The meaning and goals of equity in health', *Journal of Epidemiology and Community Health*, vol 56, pp488–491

Diez-Roux, A. V., Link, B. G. and Northridge, M. E. (2000) 'A multilevel analysis of income inequality and cardiovascular risk factors', *Social Science and Medicine*, vol 50, pp673–687

Fabienne, P. (2001) 'Health equity and social justice', *Journal of Applied Philosophy*, vol 18, no 2, pp159–170, reprinted in Anand, P. and Sen, A. (eds) (2004) *Public Health, Ethics, and Equity*, Oxford University Press, Oxford, pp93–106

Gee, G. C. and Payne-Sturges, D. C. (2004) 'Environmental health disparities: A framework integrating psychosocial and environmental concepts', *Environmental Health Perspectives*, vol 112, no 17, pp1645–1653

Gwatkin, D. R. (2000) 'Health inequalities and the health of the poor: What do we know? What can we do?', *Bulletin of the World Health Organization*, vol 78, no 1, pp3–18

International Society for Equity in Health (ISEqH) (2005) 'Working definitions', available at www.iseqh.org/en/workdef_en.htm, accessed 19 September 2008

Kawachi, I., Daniels, N. and Robinson, D. E. (2005) 'Health disparities by race and class: Why both matter', *Health Affairs*, vol 24, no 2, pp343–352

Kingston, R. S. and Nickens, H. W. (2000) 'Racial and ethnic difference in health: Recent trends, current patterns, future directions', *America Becoming: Racial Trends and Their Consequences*, volume 2, The National Academies Press, Washington, DC, www.nap.edu/openbook/0309068401/html/253.html, accessed 15 April 2009

Levy, B. S. and Sidel, V. W. (2006) *Social Injustice and Public Health*, Oxford University Press, Oxford

Liao, Y., Tucker, P., Okoro, C. A., Giles, W. H., Mokdad, A. H. and Harris, V. B. (2004) 'REACH 2010 Surveillance for health status in minority communities: United States, 2001–2002', *MMWR Surveillance Summaries*, 27 August, vol 2004/53, no SS06, pp1–36

Low, A., Ithindi, T. and Low, A. (2003) 'A step too far? Making health equity interventions in Namibia more sufficient', *International Journal of Equity in Health*, vol 2, no 5, pp7

Margai, F. M. (2003) 'Indicators of environmental inequities and threats to minority health in urban America', in Frazier, J., Margai, F. and Tettey-Fio, E. (eds) *Race and Place: Equity Issues in Urban America*, Westview Press, Boulder, CO, pp189–212.

Margai, F. M. (2006) 'Racial and ethnic disparities in health and health care: A geographical review', in Frazier, J. W. and Tettey-Fio, E. (eds) *Race, Ethnicity and Place in a Changing America*, Global Academic Publishing, Binghamton, NY

Payne-Sturges, D. C., Zenick, H., Wells, C. and Sanders, W. (2006) 'We cannot do it alone: Building a multi-systems approach for assessing and eliminating environmental health disparities', *Environmental Research*, vol 102, pp141–145

Pearcy, J. N. and Keppel, K. G. (2002) 'A summary measure of health disparity', *Public Health Reports*, vol 117, pp273–280

Reidpath, D. D. and Allotey, P. (2007) 'Measuring global health inequity', *International Journal for Equity in Health*, vol 6, no 16, pp1–7

Ruger, J. P. (2004) 'Health and social justice', *Lancet*, vol 364, pp1075–1080

Taylor-Clark, K. A., Mebane, F. E., SteelFisher, G. K. and Blendon, R. J. (2007) 'News of disparity: Content analysis of news coverage of African American healthcare inequalities in the USA, 1994–2004', *Social Science and Medicine*, vol 65, pp405–417

Whitehead, M. (1990) *Concepts and Principles of Equity and Health*, World Health Organization, Copenhagen, Available at www.euro.who.int/__data/assets/pdf_file/0010/74737/E89383.pdf

Whitehead, M. (1992) 'The concepts and principles of equity in health', *International Journal of Health Services*, vol 22, pp429–445

Williams, D. R. (1997) 'Race and health: Basic questions, emerging directions', *Annals of Epidemiology*, vol 7, no 5, pp322–333

4
Conceptualization and Measurement of Race, Ethnicity and Class

Introduction

Health disparities and social injustices cut across several levels of human categorization. Disparities exist by race, ethnicity, social class, religion, gender and other socially defined stratifications of the population. The most widely documented disparities, however, have been based on race, ethnicity and class differences and, as previously stated, recent research findings have renewed global attention on these issues as many governments now seek ways to redress the inequities. Unfortunately, many of the studies that monitor these efforts have been deterred by methodological challenges in the conceptualization and measurement of these three dimensions.

Race, ethnicity and class are conceptually fluid constructs whose meaning and interpretations have varied over time and across countries. Many observers have complained about the vagueness in the definition of these concepts and the inconsistent ways in which they are operationalized in current health research. Among these three concepts, race has been perhaps the most problematic, politically charged and divisive concept, forcing some authors to argue that emphasis be placed instead on ethnicity and class as the key drivers of health disparities (Harrison, 1995; Schwartz, 2001; Cooper et al, 2003). Other scholars have indicated that the ongoing problems and inconsistencies in measuring these concepts are likely to deter the replication of such studies, as well as hinder the overall progress in scientific research (Laws and Heckscher, 2002; Sankar et al, 2007). This chapter will discuss the problems surrounding the use of race, ethnicity and *socio-economic status* (SES) in health disparities research with emphasis on measurement and operationalization. We shall examine whether all three factors deserve equal treatment in the literature, and whether they should all be retained in the tracking of health disparities.

Transitions in the conceptualization of race

The inclusion of race in the assessment of health disparities remains a hotly debated topic in the literature. Part of the discourse is fuelled by the way in which race has been defined and conceptualized over the years, and the myriad ways in which those racial classifications have been incorporated into the institutional, legal and policy frameworks of many countries such as Japan, Brazil, South Africa, Australia and the United States. For some scholars, race is a conceptually unstable concept that no longer has a scientific basis for inclusion in the evaluation and measurement of health disparities (Harrison, 1995; Fullilove, 1998; Schwartz, 2001; Cooper et al, 2003). Yet, its societal impacts and health consequences are so real, and so persistent that it cannot be totally excluded from the analysis.

The concept and meaning of race has gone through several iterations over the years starting out first as a biological classification of human beings and then evolving into the present-day sociological construct. There are at least five different formulations of race in the scientific literature: (i) race as biology; (ii) race as social class; (iii) race as culture; (iv) race as ethnicity; and (v) race as a nation (Herman, 1996).

Race as biology is the oldest fabrication of race that has left a lasting impact on the ways in which society perceives and treats different population groups from around the world. As a biological construct, the concept of race was previously used to classify people into groups based on certain genetic and biological attributes that supposedly characterized these groups. The origins and most influential sources of these false classifications are traceable to natural scientists, who categorized human beings into distinct subspecies based on what they claimed to be innate biological differences and phenotypical attributes as manifested in skin colour, hair texture, blood composition and facial features. Notable among them were the French physician, Bernier (1625–1688), a French naturalist, Buffon (1707–1788), a German professor of medicine, Blumebach (1752–1840) and Linnaeus (1707–1778), a Swedish biologist and physician. Linnaeus, for example, proposed five classes of human species (Europeanus, Asiaticus, Africanus, Monstrosus and Americanus). Using a set of criteria that was initially based on geographic origin, and later skin colour and behavioural traits, he produced a ranking that strategically placed the Europeans at the top, and Africans at the bottom of the classification scheme. Subsequent classifications by others reinforced these ethnocentric ideas, later forming the basis and rationale for promulgating racist doctrines, and other global injustices that played out in the form of eugenics, the Holocaust and anti-Semitism, slavery, segregation and Jim Crow laws in the United States, apartheid in South Africa, and imperialism and colonialism in several world regions.

Racial classification based on inherent biological attributes has long since been debunked by natural and social scientists. In 1996, the American Association of Physical Anthropology (AAPA) put out a definitive statement that sought to eliminate these biases in scientific research noting that:

> *All humans living today belong to a single species*, Homo sapiens,
> *and share a common descent... Pure races in the sense of*

genetically homogenous populations do not exist in the human species today, nor is there any evidence that they have existed in the past. (AAPA, 1996, pp569–570)

The above statement is supported by scientific findings showing that globally, there is more genetic variation within racial groups than there is between different racial groups. Nearly 95 per cent of the observed genetic differences that exist are prevalent within the racial groups, and only about 5 per cent of the differences are between the groups. Further, a lot of intermixing has occurred between racial groups such that scientists can confidently claim today that there are no longer any pure genetic pools in the world. Recent results from the Human Genome Project confirm further that the human population has 99.9 per cent of its DNA in common (Lander et al, 2001).

Unfortunately, when discussing the characteristics of population groups, there is a still a tendency for many to focus on the visible physical characteristics of individuals like skin colour, hair texture or facial features. Scientific data, however, show that these phenotypical differences observed between the races are mostly adaptive features that are tied to the physical environments in which the groups reside. For example, the presence of darker skin colour in populations within tropical regions is largely a function of melanin production to protect against excess ultraviolet radiation in these regions. Thus, race as a biological construct is a conceptualization that has no scientific merit and should not be used for group classification in health disparities research.

It is important to reiterate, however, that despite the academic dismissal of race as a biology, the damage caused by this initial categorization of population groups has been persistent and nearly irreversible since the perceived differences in physical attributes, behaviour and cognitive abilities remain firmly ingrained and internalized in the public's psyche, and in the systemic structures (legal, institutional and policy frameworks). These perceptions have been translated today into the social construction of race, a subjective level of understanding that has been imposed and collectively accepted by people within and across various world regions. Previous cases of imposition include the definition of coloured people during the South African apartheid regime, and the classification of mixed races in the Pardo group in Brazil. Another example can be drawn from the previous classification of Italians and Irish as non-whites, but later as whites in the United States. This evolving colour line in the United States was once described by Thomas (2001) as follows:

The color line is not fixed but ripples through time, finding expression at distinct stages of our development as a nation. As the meaning of race has changed over time, its burdens and privileges have shifted among population groups. At one time in our history, for instance, the Irish and Italians were considered 'non-White', along with other immigrants who were not descendants of the early Anglo-Saxon Protestant settlers. (p1046)

Another example of group imposition and racial designation in the United States can be drawn from the iniquitous one-drop rule. This rule was applied primarily to people of African ancestry. Anyone with a trace of the African ancestry, regardless of skin complexion, was classified as black unless their racial background was proven otherwise by having an alternate non-white ancestry such as being Native American or Asian. This system was used to promote prejudice, racial discrimination and the disenfranchisement of African Americans during the Jim Crow era (1876 to 1965).

To better understand the nature of race and the societal consequences in America, it is best to describe the process of *racialization*, and in particular the historical formation of the white identity. A lot has been written on this in recent years, some from geographers who have examined the enduring impacts of this process on the American landscape (Frankenberg, 1993; Ignatiev, 1995; Hill, 1997; Kobayashi and Peake, 2000; Hoelscher, 2003). As Kobayashi and Peake (2000) describe it, racialization is one of the fundamental means of organizing society. It is the process through which racial groups are identified, assigned stereotypical attributes, and forced into specific living conditions that typically involve social and spatial segregation. Though much has been made of the racialization and evolution of blackness, Latina or Asian identities, too often the discussion of whiteness is downplayed or overlooked. Scholars like Kobayashi and Peake (2000) and Hoelscher (2003) argue, however, that deconstructing the process by which whiteness is enacted in the American society and the social, political and material consequences is a key step towards addressing societal inequities.

Whiteness is a social construction much like any of the other racial categories. It is also a conceptually fluid, and mobile construct that has a trend line and a geographical expression that is readily visible in the American landscape, particularly in the Deep South. Hoelscher (2003) argues that though the South is not unique in its struggle with racial injustices, it provided the main stage on which Americans played out the social construction of race (p662). Drawing on the work that was first presented by Frankenberg (1993), these authors identify at least three dimensions of whiteness. The first is the position of *structural advantage* that a white person has over others in society. The advantage, often referred to as '*white privilege*', is expressed in many forms and varied contexts in society such as greater access to jobs, housing, educational opportunities, upward mobility, higher earnings, better access to health care resources and better treatment in the legal system, health care system, and other public and private institutional settings.

A second dimension of whiteness has been characterized as a vantage point, or occupation of space, literally in terms of physical, psychological and social space. Kobayashi and Peake (2000) describe this dimension as a standpoint or place from which to look at oneself, others and society. It may also be described as a racial lens through which others are perceived and judged. Since the notion of whiteness is very rarely discussed, it remains under the radar, and is recognized implicitly as the norm, the standard, the reference point against which all other racial groups are compared. Evidence of this can be drawn from several of the instruments used to evaluate the anthropometric characteristics of people such as body weight, height, shape and other measures within the United States and around the world.

The third dimension of whiteness follows from the preceding connotations, in which whiteness is often associated with a standardized set of values, norms, attitudes, belief systems and behaviours that are perceived to be morally upright and acceptable to society. Collectively these three dimensions embody the distinctive attributes of whiteness which are deeply entrenched in the American society. Though many studies have focused primarily on the United States, these same processes and sociological constructions of racial identities take place in several other countries, especially in Europe, where race has played a role in the organization of society. As Hoelscher (2003) contends, whiteness is expressed in varied spatial contexts and scales, from nation-states, to regions, to cities, to neighbourhoods and factory floors (p662).

To summarize, the social construction of race remains a powerful undercurrent in most societies. In countries such as the United States, race is deeply woven into the societal fabric with impacts on all institutions, including the educational, legal, housing and health care systems. Race remains a proxy not only for ethnicity, but a proxy for culture, identity, class, social privilege and geographic space. The biological meaning of race may have been debunked by scientists as a complete fabrication, but its effects on society and on population health in particular remain real. Race as a social construct therefore deserves recognition and inclusion in health disparities research. The key question that needs to be addressed now is how best to capture an empirical measurement of this unstable concept in health research.

Improving the measurement and operationalization of race

The measurement of race in health disparities has been problematic because of the issues cited above, the incendiary nature of the concept, and the feelings of guilt, discomfort, prejudice and stereotyping that it conjures among people. In many countries around the world, race is not included in the data collection systems. In the United States, however, race is consistently measured in the census as well as in many health data collection systems. While these data systems serve as valuable sources for computing race-specific health measures and assessing health disparities in the country, some measurement problems have been uncovered that hinder the quality of the data (Laveist, 1994; Williams, 1999; Laws and Heckscher, 2002; Sohn et al, 2006). Two ways in which measurement errors creep into these data collection systems are through observer-recorded errors and self-recorded errors.

Observer errors arise in instances where the racial background of a subject is misrepresented because the interviewer or data recorder fails to ask the subject directly about his/her racial background due to the sensitivity of the topic. Instead, the observer records this racial information based on the subject's observable physical attributes. Such errors have been found to occur during the decennial censuses, in hospital admission records, patient discharge records, birth certificates, and in death certificates submitted by funeral homes (Laveist, 1994; Williams, 1999). Errors introduced by undercounting members of a racial group can propagate from data collection right through to the aggregation and computation of race-specific disease rates. These produce unreliable health records, resulting in the underestimation of racial disparities, particularly for non-African American minorities (Sohn et al, 2006).

The US Office of Management and Budget (OMB) revised the standards for the collection of data on race and ethnicity in an effort to correct the problems associated with observer records. These standards, which took effect in January 2003, suggested the use of self-identification as the mode for collecting data on race. The revision also included the ability for individuals to report multiple races. Self-recorded measures have been shown to be more reliable than observer records (Sohn et al, 2006); however, the likelihood of measurement errors still exists. Accounts of individuals self-identifying with other groups in order to take advantage of the perceived group benefits and privileges have been reported. Williams (1999), for example, detected this problem when evaluating the demographic trends of the American Indian population, describing it as follows:

> *Between 1960 and 1990, there was a six fold increase in the American Indian population. This dramatic growth of the population cannot be explained either by biological growth or international migration. It appears to reflect the change in self-definition, with more adults of mixed ancestry identifying themselves as American Indian.* (p128)

Similar accounts have been given of individuals concealing or reclaiming their racial background in the United States, Japan and elsewhere, as people opt for the racial categories that would be most advantageous in terms of the benefits of education, housing, employment, health care access and other privileges accorded to underrepresented minorities or the dominant majority groups in these countries (Sweet, 2005). Thus, the use of the self-identification method does not necessarily eliminate all measurement errors associated with the collection of race-based data.

Given the problems noted above, it is no surprise then that some scholars have called for alternate measures of group classification to evaluate health disparities. However, we should not be quick to dismiss this variable since it remains a vital component in the surveillance of health disparities. Specifically, within the causal framework of health disparities, race and racism are strong precursors of these poor health outcomes. The damaging health effects of race and racism have been presented not only by Williams, but also by several authors over the course of the last several years who argue that racism in particular is the neglected pathogenic factor in the study of health disparities (Winker, 2004; Smedley and Smedley, 2005). Carter-Pokras and Woo (1999) for example, in their study of the health profile of minorities noted that

> *racism transforms the social status of individuals such that SES indicators are no longer equal across the different racial groups. Racism restricts access to public education, health care, housing,*

> *recreational facilities and a host of services. Racial discrimination and racism can also induce psychological distress further compounding health disparities.* (p119)

Collecting and analysing data on race in health data systems enables the assessment of the negative health effects of racism and the tracking of progress towards the elimination of health disparities. Sondik (2000) discusses the importance of such data, particularly the data portraying trends in race-based measures. He rightfully notes that trend data provide valuable information on the changes that are taking place, identifying emerging health problems or improvements in various population groups, and more importantly assisting in the evaluation of the effectiveness of health intervention programmes. Findings from the analysis of such data are useful in setting goals, establishing priorities and policies geared toward health equity.

Making the case for keeping race in health data collection systems requires that steps be taken to better describe this construct, and minimize the errors or discrepancies associated with the measurement process. The OMB proposal to focus on self-reported measures is a step in the right direction. As Winker (2004) notes, 'individuals should self-designate race to ensure that the designation most closely matches what they believe reflects their personal and cultural background' (p1613). Brown (2007) and Williams (1999) also provide several good ideas relating to the self-identification, collection, and analysis of race-based data. These strategies require the development of culturally appropriate materials, the translation of questionnaires and data instruments for groups with limited English proficiency, the periodic monitoring and update of current measures, and the interpretation of research findings derived from studies that include racial data in their analyses. All studies that rely on race-based measures must justify the relevance of race in the study, discuss how the concept was measured and the limitations of the data, and identify the specific factors that link race to health. Sondik (2000) too proposes new research directions that focus on strengthening the methodological approaches such as conducting a cognitive test of race and ethnicity questions with multiple race respondents, identifying the best ways to bridge data collected under different measurement criteria, and evaluating the potential impact of technological changes such as the use of electronic health data records on the collection of race data within the various health data systems.

Ethnicity as an alternative classification scheme in health disparities research

Ethnicity has been suggested as a better classification scheme for tracking group differences in health. Some scholars have opted not to dismiss race entirely but to use the term race/ethnicity, an approach that we would also adopt in this book. This does not imply however that the two concepts are synonymous, though they overlap in some respects. Ethnicity is a broader conceptualization that is used to classify people into homogeneous groups based on a common heritage. Heritage is reflected in either a single or multiple set of attributes that people have in common such as their culture traits, language, religion, diet, beliefs, customs and behaviours, their ancestry or national origin, and sometimes the physically identifiable features associated with their race.

Like race, ethnicity involves the construction of sociological boundaries that are self-defined, or imposed by others; the notion of 'us' versus 'them'. These boundaries also change over time and space. For example, in both the United States and United Kingdom, changes in racial and ethnic categorizations have been made repeatedly in the decennial censuses to accommodate the demographic shifts in race and ethnicity, and the acceptable designations of various population groups.

Though advocated by many in health disparities research, the measurement and operationalization of ethnicity is not without its share of difficulties. Chaturvedi (2001) rightfully described ethnicity as a complex construct that encompasses both biological and environmental exposures of disease. This complexity comes with some strengths and weaknesses. Among the strengths, the ethnicity construct is broad and flexible enough to allow researchers to design a composite measure of exposure risks that could be refined later to match the precise research objectives. However, other observers view this conceptual flexibility as problematic, potentially giving rise to inconsistencies and the lack of consensus in group categorizations (Smith, 2000; Nazroo, 2003; Brown, 2007).

In health disparities research, ethnicity is particularly useful for inter-group comparisons to identify at-risk populations. Examples of this abound in the literature. For example, Kant and Graubard (2008) examined the ethnic differentials in the concentrations of selected nutritional biomarkers, in an effort to evaluate nutritional deficiencies and potential health risks. Again this strength can arguably be seen as a weakness because too often inter-group comparisons are based on measurement instruments that are derived from 'normal' values within European populations. For example, the instruments used by the World Health Organization to measure underweight or stunted children, or compute the body mass index (BMI) are based on standard reference values. This approach, some would argue, covertly endorses the ethnocentric views of health such that, when the measures taken from other populations deviate from these 'standardized' values, those populations are deemed abnormal and unhealthy.

Ethnicity is also a politically charged concept, and the basis of recent conflicts in several parts of the world. Examples include the ethnic cleansing in Rwanda and the Balkans, the persistent calls for self-determination and autonomy in Quebec, the North–South split in Italy and the rifts between the Belgian Walloon and Flemish populations. Group classifications based on ethnicity can therefore be as intense and divisive as racial classifications between groups.

Using ethnicity for group categorization has also led to overgeneralizations and the aggregation of groups that have very little in common. For example, in both the United States and the United Kingdom, there is a tendency to use designations such as 'Asians' or 'Blacks' when these groups consist of many subpopulations with differences in geographic origin, socio-cultural experiences, socio-economic status, health beliefs and behaviours. Ethnicity, like race, is therefore an imperfect candidate for health disparities research. The guidelines offered earlier for improving the data collection and interpretation of race-based measures also apply to the collection, analysis and interpretation of ethnic-related measures in health data systems.

Measurement and conceptualization of socio-economic status (SES)

Following the norm in the literature, the terms social class, social standing and socio-economic status (SES) are used interchangeably in this book though subtle differences do exist between them. The emphasis has been for the most part on SES, as an explanatory variable in health disparities and the degree to which it produces poor health outcomes. Many findings support the *social gradient* hypothesis which suggests the existence of SES differences in morbidity and mortality across various population groups. Specifically, lower SES has been shown to (i) reduce access to health care services and the quality of care received; (ii) limit the knowledge and opportunity to make healthy lifestyle choices and behaviours; (iii) heighten the risk of exposures to environmental hazards; (iv) increase exposure to material deprivation and stressful psychosocial environments over the life course of individuals (Lantz et al, 2001; Knesebeck et al, 2003; Margai, 2006).

SES has also been used as a control variable in many studies when examining the associative and predictive effects of other variables on health. For example, the age and sex differences within the population have been examined within the context of SES and health. When examining age, some studies have shown that SES differences in health persist and expand right up to the late middle age of individuals following which they decline as a result of selective mortality, social sector programmes that are geared toward the elderly and the dominance of biological effects over social determinants at the older ages (Herd, 2006).

SES has also been used as a proxy for race and ethnicity in some studies due to existing research findings that suggest a significant correlation between minority status and low SES of residents. In the United States, for example, minorities are over-represented within the low-income groups, and in the absence of data on income, researchers have opted for race as a proxy variable for income in their research. Some have argued, however, that the use of race as a proxy for SES is misguided and could potentially lead to the over-controlling of the causal effect of race on health (Kawachi et al, 2005). Others have voiced similar concerns noting that race and SES are two separate constructs, and race remains a significant determinant of health even after controlling for the SES of individuals (Williams, 1997; Carter-Pokras and Woo, 1999).

In the quest for reliable and comprehensive measures of SES, several indices have been developed over the years, some dating back as early as the 1960s. These include Duncan's 1961 Socioeconomic Index (SEI), Nam and Power's 1965 Occupation Status Scores (OSS), Hollingshead's 1971 Index of Social Prestige (ISP), Rossi et al's 1974 Household Prestige Score (HPS) and Treiman's 1975 Standard International Occupational Prestige Score (SIOPS). All of these measures have been based on one or more of the following three empirical indicators: income, education and occupation. More recently, some studies have added other indicators such as assets and home ownership to the mix (Knesebeck et al, 2003).

The popularity of SES as an explanatory, control or proxy measure in health disparities research, and the ongoing development of composite indices do not mean that the construct is free of controversy and debate. Like race and ethnicity, a series of theoretical and methodological problems have accompanied the conceptualization and measurement of this concept. Many scholars have commented on these issues, most notably Oakes and Rossi (2003) who, following a review of the SES literature, discovered a wide gap between studies that address 'SES measurement' and those that examine 'SES in health'. Describing this drawback in the literature as 'everyone putting the cart before the horse', they noted that so far, 'little work has focused on defining SES, operationalizing existing definitions, or evaluating the properties of the measures'(Oakes and Rossi, 2003, p771).

The two major problems associated with the current SES measures are the lack of consensus on the nominal definition of SES, and the absence of application of sound measurement theory to the construction of SES measures. To overcome these, Oakes and Rossi (2003) proposed a new composite measure, CAPSES, an acronym based on the words 'Capital' and 'Socioeconomic status'. In the CAPSES scale, which is rooted primarily in traditional social theory and psychometric techniques, SES is designed to measure the differential access to desired goods and resources. Using a systematic framework, individuals, families, households, neighbourhoods, countries or other socio-spatial entities may be grouped hierarchically based on their relative access to, and consumption of those goods and services to produce the SES characteristics.

In proposing the CAPSES scale, Oakes and Rossi (2003) accurately note that SES should be viewed not only as access to resources, but also as a function of three domains which uniquely place each individual, family or household within a given social structure. These three domains are the material capital, the human capital and the social capital:

$$SES = f(\text{material capital}, \text{human capital}, \text{social capital})$$

The material capital refers to tangible assets and endowments such as homes, cars, income earnings, savings, investments and stocks, inheritances and other items that are readily identifiable and measurable. Human capital tends to be a more latent component of the CAPSES measure. It includes the physical, mental or cognitive attributes of individuals such as their intelligence, motivation, drive and stamina, as well as the level of educational attainment, skills, abilities and knowledge base which may be acquired through the investment of time, money and labour. Having material and human capital is not sufficient, however. The third component in the CAPSES measure is social capital, a multidimensional construct that has been more widely researched than the other two domains in terms of the health impacts. Social capital can be viewed primarily as a collection of goodwill, fellowship, reciprocity, civic engagement and social trust that is shared by a network of individuals in a given neighbourhood or community (Bourdieu, 1985; Coleman, 1990; Portes, 1998). It offers significant benefits for the health of the individuals within the network. Collectively, the people within these networks work to promote group cohesion in their neighbourhoods and communities. Social capital not only promotes bonding among a homogeneous set of people, it also bridges the gaps among diverse racial and ethnic groups. Unlike the material and human capital reviewed earlier, social capital can be viewed as a renewable resource that is not depleted by use; rather it is strengthened further by use. Significant health and economic benefits exist in communities with a high social capital, including lower levels of infant mortality, lower welfare dependency, lower teenage pregnancy, employment opportunities, educational achievement and social mobility. There are also negative outcomes associated with social capital such as gang formation, organized crime or other networks that operate against societal interests (Oakes and Rossi, 2003).

The extent to which social capital influences health has been assessed at both the individual and the collective level. The CAPSES model suggests the use of multiple levels including the individual, family and household level, a perspective that is shared by others (Snelgrove et al, 2009). Some contend that the health benefits of social capital are best witnessed at the collective level (Lochner et al, 1999). Overall, as shown above, the efforts to operationalize this SES concept have entailed the inclusion of several empirical indicators.

Chapter summary

Race, ethnicity and SES are the three most commonly documented areas of health disparities in the United States and around the world. As research efforts continue to bring attention to these disparities, some key questions remain regarding the definition and operationalization of empirical measures and the potential errors introduced in the analytical process. The discussion in this chapter reveals that none of these concepts are immune from the theoretical and methodological problems. Though race is a politically charged concept, it should not be abandoned in favour of ethnicity and SES in health disparities research. Rather, the research focus must remain on the notion of race as a social construct, and steps must be taken to improve the calibration of this concept using self-reported data.

Ethnicity is also beset with problems that include the lack of consensus in definition, the likelihood of developing ethnocentric health measures, and the tendency to overgeneralize or aggregate dissimilar groups. The guidelines suggested earlier for improving race are also recommended for this concept. Finally, efforts to calibrate SES have also been met with some challenges; however, in relative terms, the most progress made so far has been in the operationalization of SES rather than race and ethnicity. Several scales have been proposed over the years, though some are not amenable to cross-cultural comparisons and appear to have limited functionality beyond the Westernized countries in which they were first designed. These SES scales focus mainly on income, educational and/or occupational attributes of individuals. The CAPSES model presented in the latter part of this chapter provides the first real attempt to overcome these challenges by offering a comprehensive framework that is based on well established analytical techniques. The inclusion of three components, material, human and social capital, provides a complete measure that is amenable to the evaluation of health disparities across multiple levels, spatial and temporal scales.

References

AAPA (American Association of Physical Anthropologists) (1996) 'Statement on the biological aspects of race', *American Journal of Physical Anthropology*, vol 1001, pp569–570, http://physanth.org/positions/race.html, accessed 28 May 2009

Bourdieu, P. (1985) 'The forms of capital', in Richardson, J. G. (ed) *Handbook of Theory and Research for the Sociology of Education*, Greenwood, New York

Brown, M. and The PLoS Medicine Editors (2007) 'Defining human differences in biomedicine', *PLoS Med*, vol 4, no 9, e288 doi:10.13721/journal.pmed.0040288

Carter-Pokras, O. and Woo, V. (1999) 'Health profile of racial and ethnic minorities in the United States', *Ethnicity and Health*, vol 43, no 3, pp117–120

Chaturvedi, N. (2001) 'Ethnicity as an epidemiological determinant: Crudely racist or crucially important?', *International Journal of Epidemiology*, vol 30, pp925–927

Coleman, J. S. (1990) *The Foundations of Social Theory*, Belknap Press, Cambridge, MA

Cooper, R. S., Kaufman, J. S. and Ward, R. (2003) 'Race and genomics', *New England Journal of Medicine*, vol 438, pp1166–1170

Frankenberg, R. (1993) 'Growing up white: Feminism, racism and the social geography of childhood', *Feminist Review*, vol 45, pp51–84

Fullilove, M. T. (1998) 'Comment: Abandoning "race" as a variable in public health surveillance: An idea whose time has come', *American Journal of Public Health*, vol 88, no 9, pp1297–1298

Harrison, F. V. (1995) 'The persistent power of "race" in the cultural and political economy of racism', *Annual Review of Anthropology*, vol 24, pp47–74

Herd, P. (2006) 'Do functional health inequalities decrease in old age?', *Research on Aging*, vol 28, no 3, pp375–392

Herman, A. A. (1996) 'Toward the conceptualization of race in epidemiologic research', *Ethnicity and Disease*, vol 6, pp7–20

Hill, M. (ed) (1997) *Whiteness: A Critical Reader*, New York University Press, New York

Hoelscher, S. (2003) 'Making place, making race: Performances of whiteness in the Jim Crow South', *Annals of the Association of American Geographers*, vol 93, no 3, pp657–686

Ignatiev, N. (1995) *How the Irish Became White*, Routledge, New York

Jackson, P. (1998) 'Constructions of "whiteness" in the geographical imagination', *Area*, vol 30, no 2, pp99–106

Kant, A. K. and Graubard, B. I. (2008) 'Ethnic and socioeconomic differences in variability in nutritional biomarkers', *American Journal of Clinical Nutrition*, vol 87, pp1464–1471

Kawachi, I., Daniels, N. and Robinson, D. E. (2005) 'Health disparities by race and class: Why both matter', *Health Affairs*, vol 24, no 2, pp343–352

Knesebeck, O. V. D., Luschen, G., Cockerham, W. C. and Siegrist, J. (2003) 'Socioeconomic status and health among the aged in the United States and Germany', *Social Science and Medicine*, vol 57, pp1643–1652

Kobayashi, A. and Peake, L. (2000) 'Racism out of place: Thoughts on whiteness and an antiracist geography in the new millennium', *Annals of the Association of American Geographers*, vol 90, no 2, pp392–403

Lander, E. S., Linton, L. M., Birren, B., et al (2001) 'Initial sequencing and analysis of the human genome', *Nature*, vol 409, pp860–921

Lantz, P. M., Lynch, J. W., House, J. S., Lepkowski, J. M., Mero, R. P., Musick, M. A. and Williams, D. R. (2001) 'Socio-economic disparities in health change in a longitudinal study of U.S. adults', *Social Science and Medicine*, vol 53, pp29–40

Laveist, T. A. (1994) 'Beyond dummy variables and sample selection: What health services researchers ought to know about race as a variable', *Health Services Research*, vol 29, no 1, pp1–16

Laws, M. B. and Heckscher, R. A. (2002) 'Racial and ethnic identification practices in public health data systems in New England', *Public Health Reports*, vol 117, no 1, pp50–61

Lochner, K., Kawachi, I. and Kennedy, B. P. (1999) 'Social capital: A guide to its measurement', *Health and Place*, vol 5, no 4, pp259–270

Margai, F. M. (2006) 'Racial and ethnic disparities in health and health care: A geographical review', in Frazier, J. W. and Tettey-Fio, E. (eds) *Race, Ethnicity and Place in a Changing America*, Global Academic Publishing, Binghamton, NY

Nazroo, J. Y. (2003) 'The structuring of ethnic equalities in health: Economic position, racial discrimination, and racism', *American Journal of Public Health*, vol 93, no 2, pp277–284

Oakes, J. M. and Rossi, P. H. (2003) 'The measurement of SES in health research: Current practice and steps toward a new approach', *Social Science and Medicine*, vol 56, pp769–784

Portes, A. (1998) 'Social capital: Its origins and applications in modern sociology', *Annual Review of Sociology*, vol 24, pp1–24

Sankar, P., Cho, M. K. and Mountain, J. (2007) 'Race and ethnicity in genetic research', *American Journal of Medical Genetics A*, vol 143, no 9, pp961–970

Schwartz, R. S. (2001) 'Racial profiling in medical research', *New England Journal of Medicine*, vol 344, pp1392–1393

Smedley, A. and Smedley, B. D. (2005) 'Race as biology, is fiction. Racism as a social problem is real', *American Psychologist*, vol 60, no 1, pp16–26

Smith, G. D. (2000) 'Learning to live with complexity: Ethnicity, socio-economic position and health in Britain and the United States', *American Journal of Public Health*, vol 90, no 11, pp1694–1698

Snelgrove, J., Hynek, P. and Stafford, M. (2009) 'A multilevel analysis of social capital and self-rated health: Evidence from the British Household Panel Survey', *Social Science and Medicine*, vol 68, pp1993–2001

Sohn, M., Zhang, H., Arnold, N., Stroupe, K., Taylor, B. C., Wilt, T. J. and Hynes, D. M. (2006) 'Transition to the new race/ethnicity data collection standards in the Department of Veteran Affairs', *Population Health Metrics*, vol 4, no 7, pp1–10

Sondik, E. J. (2000) 'Race/ethnicity and 2000 census: Implications for public health', *American Journal of Public Health*, vol 90, no 11, pp1709–1713

Sweet, F. (2005) *Legal History of the Color Line: The Rise and Triumph of the One-Drop Rule*, Backintyme Publishing, Palm Coast, FL

Thomas, S. B. (2001) 'The color line: Race matters in the elimination of health disparities', *American Journal of Public Health*, vol 91, no 7, pp1046–1048

Williams, D. R. (1997) 'Race and health: Basic questions, emerging directions', *AEP*, vol 7, no 5, pp322–333

Williams, D. R. (1999) 'The monitoring of racial/ethnic status in the USA: Data quality issues', *Ethnicity and Health*, vol 4, no 3, pp121–137

Winker, M. A. (2004) 'Measuring race and ethnicity: Why or how', *JAMA*, vol 292, pp1612–1614

5
Environmental Health Data Collection, Analysis and Visualization: An Overview of Geographic Methodologies

Introduction

During the last two decades, remarkable progress has been made in the development of geographic tools and spatial epidemiological approaches used to evaluate environmental health problems. Advances in cartography, geographic information systems (GIS), statistics and geostatistical modelling, remote sensing (RS), and global positioning systems (GPS) have enabled the timely acquisition and compilation of spatially referenced data on various health events, and the analysis, visualization and presentation of these events relative to socio-demographic and environmental risk factors. The use of these methodologies to address health problems has been part of a well established tradition in medical geography, dating as far back as the 1800s when maps were used in environmental and public health decision making and prioritization of preventive measures.

An often cited illustration of the beneficial uses of spatial epidemiology and other geographic approaches is the work of John Snow during the 1854 cholera epidemic in London. Plotting a dot density map of deaths from the disease, Snow was able to delineate the disease cluster, and later identify the contaminated water pump as the risk source of the disease (see Figure 5.1). This prompted the implementation of health intervention strategies that halted the spread of the disease and prevented the emergence of new outbreaks.

The methods used in spatial epidemiology have since flourished, expanding beyond dot density and choropleth mapping techniques to include highly sophisticated methods that allow for advanced ecological analyses of diseases, cluster detection using space and time algorithms, disease surveillance and risk assessment. As with all analytical tools, however, the success of these methods depends greatly on the availability of reliable data on the demographic characteristics of the population, the health events, the community and

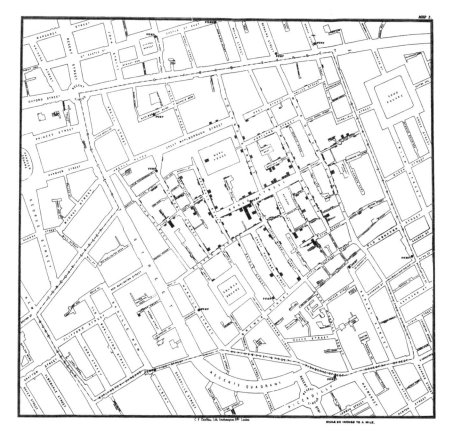

Figure 5.1 *John Snow's original dot density map*

neighbourhood contexts, and the putative risk factors. Some of the issues surrounding data measurement and quality were discussed in the previous chapter with specific reference to race, ethnicity and class. These constructs, however, cover only a small part of the comprehensive database required to establish linkages between exposures to environmental hazards and health disparities. Along with the demographic data, spatial data layers are required on the distribution of the hazardous events, the exposure sources and health outcomes in the population.

This chapter will first examine the sources and characteristics of the environmental health databases. Using examples drawn mostly from the United States, we shall explore the secondary sources of data on environmental hazards, exposure and health outcomes. The second part of the chapter will examine the spatial analytical methods that are commonly used to analyse and visually portray the distribution of these health problems. These techniques are discussed under four broad categories: disease mapping, ecological analysis, disease clustering and spatial prediction. The foundational elements of these approaches are presented along with the analytical pitfalls that accompany their use. More detailed applications of these methods will follow in the remaining book chapters, using case studies.

Environmental health surveillance systems and GIS databases

Environmental health analysts have come to rely on data garnered from public health surveillance systems for their research. These surveillance systems are designed to routinely collect environmental and health statistics, and disseminate the results to decision makers and other health professionals (Thacker et al, 1996). With recent advances in computer technology and greater recognition of the benefits of geospatial technologies, these systems are increasingly being set up within a GIS environment.

A GIS system is a comprehensive digital information management system that captures and stores data garnered from multiple sources. The GIS also enables the analysis, modelling and visualization of the derived information through the use of maps, charts and statistical tables. Central to the GIS are the spatially referenced data that are captured from both primary and secondary sources. Public health surveillance systems, cross-sectional health surveys, individual case-control studies, and cohort or longitudinal studies all serve as feeder lines of data into a GIS. Spatial data describing the location and characteristics of specific environmental hazards and other risk factors may also be generated using compatible geographic technologies. For example, the use of GPS units during field sampling and collection of water or soil quality measurements allows for easy integration of this information into the GIS. Remote sensing systems are used for the acquisition of aerial photographs and satellite imagery on land-use and land-cover characteristics. Digitizing tablets are used to obtain additional spatial data such as drainage and transportation networks, land-use patterns or administrative boundaries from pre-existing maps.

Within the GIS environment, the data may be grouped into two major types – the spatial databases and the attribute databases. Locational data in the form of geographic coordinates that describe the precise position of different features on the Earth's surface are captured in the spatial databases. These features could be presented either as points, lines or areas in the database. Point features represent the specific locations of health events or other geographic entities in space such as the location of schools, hospitals, factories, landfills or toxic release sites. Lines in the spatial databases represent linear features such as roads, rivers and other drainage systems, and political boundaries. The area features in the spatial databases are captured as polygons representing definable areas on the Earth's surface such as census blocks, tracts, counties, health administrative districts, countries and other spatial entities. Health districts, medically underserved areas or primary care services areas are all useful spatial scales at which data can be extracted and integrated into a GIS for mapping and visualization.

Also included in the GIS are the attribute databases which contain descriptive information regarding the points, lines and areas. For example, area polygons such as health districts may include the population size, the number of households, lung cancer incidences reported, median household income and the percentage of black, white, Asian or Latino populations. Attribute databases on points might include measurements taken from sampled water points or air quality monitoring stations. Similarly, information can be provided for each line in a spatial database and these quantitative or qualitative data serve as input into the data manipulation, analytical and visualization functions of the GIS.

Within the GIS environment, the success of the geospatial methods depends in part on the quality of the data acquired, the appropriate use of the data and the consideration of data limitations (Mather et al, 2004). To promote the analysis of different types of exposures and health outcomes, new guidelines have been put in place for establishing data infrastructures, metadata, and data exchange and coordination systems (Pew Commission Report, 2000). These guidelines encourage the use of the hazard–exposure–outcome axis proposed earlier by Thacker et al (1996). This framework specifies the process through which disease agents in the environment produce adverse health outcomes in human hosts (Figure 5.2).

When examining the health effects of environmental exposures within a GIS, environmental health analysts are encouraged to use this framework as a guide for integrating data from at least three data surveillance systems. Following is brief description of each data system, including examples of the compilation and management process within a GIS, and the inherent limitations.

Hazard databases

As shown in Figure 5.2, hazard surveillance systems are used to identify and track the conditions, activities and events that produce physical, chemical or biological disease agents in the environment, as well as the potential

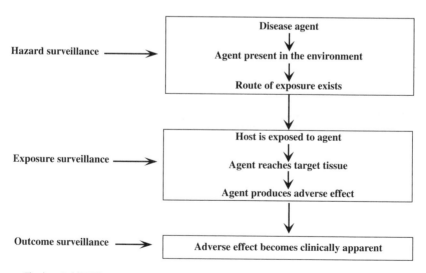

Source: Thacker et al (1996)

Figure 5.2 *Linkages between hazard, exposure and surveillance databases*

environmental pathways and routes of human exposure. Within the United States, there are several federal and state agencies responsible for collecting such information. One of the most successful systems is the Toxic Release Inventory System (TRI), a hazards surveillance database that is compiled annually and disseminated by the United States Environmental Protection Agency (USEPA). The system was set up in 1987, in response to the Emergency Planning and Community Right-to-Know Act (EPCRA). Through EPCRA, residents are informed about the dangers of chemical hazards that are generated, treated or stored in their communities. The TRI system compiles information on all waste management activities by industries and federal facilities. This information is then made accessible to the public through various information tools such as TRI Explorer that allow data queries to be performed by year, geographic location, type of industry, chemicals produced and the nature of disposal or other releases on-site or off-site.

Other useful data sources of environmental health hazards include the Aerometric Information Retrieval System (AIRS), the National Drinking Water Contaminant Occurrence Database and the Safe Drinking Water Information System (SDWIS). These databases provide valuable information for environmental health analysis in a GIS environment. However, they must be used with caution and effort must be made to validate the records through ground truthing. Experts warn against the timeliness of reporting data in some of the surveillance systems, the gaps in geographic coverage and the likelihood of sampling and measurement errors (Thacker et al, 1996; Mather et al, 2004). Notwithstanding these limitations, the surveillance systems remain valuable in environmental health studies, and have been used extensively to examine the spatial distribution of environmental toxicants in communities, and evaluate claims of environmental racism, inequities and associated health disparities.

Exposure databases

A second data source that is worthy of inclusion in an environmental health GIS is an exposure surveillance (ES) database that covers all of the relevant information regarding the hosts, or affected populations. ES systems capture all of the processes through which individuals are exposed to disease agents, together with biological markers that confirm the presence or absence of these agents within these populations. One example can be drawn from the National Health and Nutrition Examination Survey (NHANES) which is administered to a nationwide sample of adults and children in the United States. First implemented in 1971, this survey collects information on the health and nutritional status of the population for use in analysing the relationships between clinical, nutritional, behavioural and environmental risk. Environmental exposure data are also generated from biomarkers through a series of laboratory tests. The data have been useful for evaluating racial and ethnic health disparities such as obesity and paediatric lead poisoning.

Another example is the National Air Toxics Assessment (NATA) which provides an estimate of people's exposure to air toxics. The exposure estimates are derived from computer modelling of the atmospheric concentrations of toxic compounds using air toxics emissions estimates from different sources including cars, trucks, factories and waste incinerators. The assessment is useful in identifying large areas that present the greatest risks to the largest number of people. Using this database, geographers and other social scientists have documented the racial and ethnic disparities associated with these exposures and the respiratory and lifetime cancer risks (Morello-Frosch et al, 2001; Chakraborty, 2009).

Other examples of exposure surveillance databases include the Toxic Exposure Surveillance System (TESS), a national surveillance system implemented in 1985, to compile data on all human exposures reported to US poisoning control centres, and occupational exposure data compiled by the Occupational Safety and Health Administration (OSHA). As with most databases, there are certain challenges that accompany the use of these datasets. Specifically, exposure does not necessarily translate to negative health conditions. Even though the biological markers provide tangible evidence of hazard exposure, the level of toxicity within a person, and the potential health outcome depends on other factors such as the route of exposure, the frequency and duration of exposure, the age, genetic predisposition and behavioural characteristics of the host. The absence of this information during the analytical process may limit the functional utility of the data.

Health outcome databases

Health outcome databases (HODs) provide valuable information regarding the morbidity and mortality outcomes associated with exposures to disease agents in the environment. In Chapter 2, several of these environmental diseases were discussed along with the approaches used to compute the disease rates. Some of the databases that provide such information are probably the common and most widely used surveillance systems for environmental health analysis. Within the United States, there are many such systems at the national level, with most of them available through the National Center for Health Statistics (NCHS). Some databases are derived from nationwide surveys such as NHANES reviewed earlier, the National Health Interview Survey (NHIS), the National Hospital Discharge Data, National Vital Statistics System (NVSS), and the Behavioral Risk Factor Surveillance System (BRFSS).

Another federal agency that collects data on health outcomes is the Agency for Toxic Substances and Disease Registry (ATSDR). This agency manages data on toxic exposure outcomes such as the Hazardous Substances Emergency Events Surveillance Systems and the National Exposure Registry. Also worthy of consideration when building a comprehensive environmental health GIS is the Pesticide Exposure Surveillance database, the National Birth Defects Prevention Network (NBDPN), for birth defects surveillance, and the Surveillance, Epidemiology and End Results (SEER) Program, a primary source for cancer statistics. SEER is managed by the National Cancer Institute, an organization that oversees several state registries and guides the collection of data on cancer incidence, prevalence, survival and mortality from specific geographic areas. Representing about 26 per cent of the population nationally, the sampled population in SEER includes about 23 per cent blacks, 40 per cent Hispanics, 42 per cent American Indians and 53 per cent Asians. These registries routinely collect data on patient demographics, primary tumour site, tumour morphology and stage at diagnosis, first course of treatment, and follow-up for vital status.

In some of the HODs, such as the NHIS, usable data on various health events are presented at the individual level, along with their social, economic, behavioural and environmental risk factors. To maintain confidentiality, however, the residential addresses and related geographic information are often not disclosed, limiting the scale at which geospatial analysis of the data can be performed. Other limitations associated with these databases include the likelihood of errors from the misclassification or misdiagnosis of the disease, the changing diagnostic criteria, overgeneralization of health outcomes to the rest of the population, and the underreporting of certain conditions resulting in the incompleteness of the data (Mather et al, 2004).

Overall, along with data derived from primary sources, there are several sources of data for use in environmental health analysis. When building a comprehensive GIS for environmental health analysis, it is advisable to pool together an array of data layers that identify the environmental hazards, exposure characteristics and the related health outcomes. Data originating from public health surveillance systems are valuable sources for such analyses. The examples provided so far are drawn from the United States, but there are many examples of successful surveillance systems in other developed countries such as the UK, Australia and New Zealand. Efforts are also under way to establish and/or improve the systems in developing countries (Nsubuga et al, 2006). International efforts to institute global health data systems are slow due to inconsistencies in data definition, poor data quality, timeliness of reporting and the weak public health infrastructure in some countries. The World Health Organization (WHO), however, has established a few surveillance systems to monitor selected health events such as infectious diseases, and food-borne illnesses, and is now working toward the development of chronic disease surveillance systems. The data compiled in these systems are generated from a loose network of national public health agencies, non-governmental organizations, regional and country offices of other United Nations agencies, laboratory networks and many other health-related entities operating in these countries (Nsubuga et al, 2006). Though limited in scope, these databases are useful for the analysis of diseases such as malaria and HIV/AIDs, the detection of global hotspots and for disease forecasting.

Spatial statistical analysis and geo-visualization of health data

Spatial statistical analysis is one of the by-products of the quantitative revolution in geography that saw a paradigmatic shift from descriptive approaches to more analytical modes of inquiry in the discipline. Starting initially in the 1950s and then continuing through to the mid-1970s, many geography departments in Europe and the United States formally integrated advanced statistical courses into their curriculum to complement existing technical courses such as cartography, aerial photography and remote sensing. The advent of personal computer hardware, and later more powerful statistical and GIS software, spurred the development of new spatial techniques with wide ranging applications in the discipline. Recent improvements over traditional methods such as regression analysis now include the use of geographically weighted regression, empirical Bayesian methods, Poisson kriging, automated zoning methodology and multilevel modelling, to name a few.

One of the beneficiaries of these analytical developments is the field of public and environmental health where many researchers now routinely use GIS and spatial statistics to explore environment–disease associations. These studies are often conducted at small area levels (census blocks, tracts, wards) though there are also examples of individual case level analysis. Following is a description of the most common applications and the analytical challenges and barriers that arise when conducting these studies.

1. Disease mapping

Disease mapping involves the statistical analysis and visual representation of health data to identify the geographical patterns of disease and the potential association with putative risk factors. Maps are produced using either point features (as in point pattern analysis), line features (as in flow maps showing the diffusion of disease across places) or areal features (as in choropleth mapping to show the disease rates in a region).

Over the years, this cartographic process has been greatly enhanced by the use of GIS which enables the integration and analysis of large volumes of data. Using GIS, the analyst is able to capture, update, analyse and present this information with greater speed and precision. Data layers that reflect the demographic, economic or environmental characteristics of the study area are also mappable. Figure 5.3 shows the distribution of low birth weight babies in Erie County New York using the dot density approach (Margai, 2003). These health events are mapped alongside the demographic and economic risk factors. A manual classification scheme was used to map the distribution of the minorities, while the natural breaks classification scheme was used to map median household income levels. Also, using Pesticide Surveillance database, the environmental risk of pesticide applications is depicted using proportional symbols. Collectively these maps illustrate visually the relative associations between these risk factors and the poor reproductive health outcomes. Additional benefits of GIS include the ability to perform spatial queries to pinpoint the location of certain events or facilities, compute distances between places, create buffers around hazardous facilities and perform overlays to identify associations between two or more variables in the database.

The key to executing the various analytical functions is the Relational Database Management System (RDBMS) embedded in the GIS environment. This allows the analyst to explore potential relationships between multiple data layers, select elements according to some specified criteria, and analyse and map those elements with similar spatial characteristics.

Mapping the data within the GIS environment also requires logical reasoning and careful planning in order to produce meaningful maps. Maps may be presented as disease rates or standardized mortality or morbidity ratios as reviewed earlier in Chapter 2.

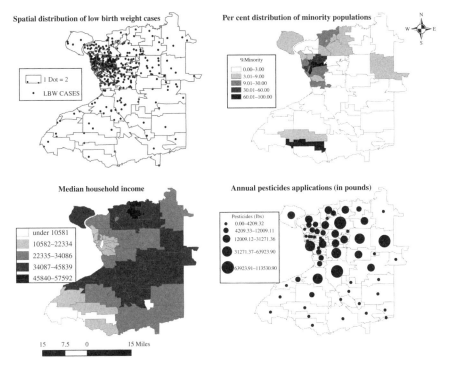

Data source: NYDOH; US Census, 2000; pesticide surveillance database

Figure 5.3 *Mapping patterns of low birth weight*

Data classification schemes

Most analysts start out by exploring the data using frequencies charts, and computing the statistical measures of centre (mean, median or mode), spread (standard deviation or variance), relative position (Z scores) and shape (skewness and kurtosis), as well as normality. These measures assist in the detection of any problems inherent in the data such as deviations from normality, the presence of missing values or statistical outliers that would potentially limit the application of more advanced spatial analytical techniques. Further, the preliminary statistical measures may assist the analyst in deciding how best to map the data.

Given the large volume of information on hand, continuous data are often categorized prior to mapping, using one of the following conventional classification schemes: (i) natural breaks (Jenks) based on the natural groupings inherent in the data; (ii) equal intervals; (iii) quantiles recommended for normally distributed data; and (iv) standard deviation to show the distribution of the features around the reported mean. Instead of using these default options within most GIS software packages, the analyst may decide to manually devise a classification scheme that is more suitable to the data and research objectives. In choosing the number of categories for mapping the data, it is also recommended that about four, and no more than eight categorical levels be used because of the difficulties in visually assimilating more than eight shades of colour or grey tones on a map (Olsen et al, 1996). Listed below are additional things to watch out for when creating the disease maps.

a. Modifiable areal unit problem Caution must be exercised in the selection of the spatial scale, or size of real units used for mapping. The analysis of the same dataset at different spatial scales often produces maps that convey different and sometimes contradictory results, a problem that is known as the *modifiable areal unit problem* in geography (Openshaw, 1984). If at all possible, it is advisable to map the data using the smallest geographic units, though this decision often depends on the availability of data at those finer scales.

b. Small numbers problem This is another problem to watch out for during the production of disease maps. The analysis of health events within small areas, such as census tracts or wards, introduces a problem in which the observed rates of the disease become unstable with larger variances. This commonly occurs in the study of rare diseases with small counts of the disease, or instances where the at-risk population within some of the spatial units is sparse within counts of 5000 people or less.

One way in which this problem can be handled is by masking the sparse data on the maps to minimize their visual effect. For example, in the cancer atlas produced by the NCI, rates based on small counts were reclassified as sparse data and hidden on the maps (Devesa et al, 1999). A more effective method is to use empirical Bayesian methods to produce smooth estimates of the disease risk. Smoothing is attained by shrinking the observed rates derived from the small populations towards the mean value obtained from the entire map (that is, the global mean) or a using a local mean obtained from the information contained in neighbouring units. Over-smoothing the data, however, may equally increase the likelihood of producing biased estimates, rendering the maps unusable with homogeneous surfaces that mask the true distribution of the disease risk (Beale et al, 2008).

c. Spatial autocorrelation When mapping disease rates, environmental health analysts must also be cognizant of the problem of spatial autocorrelation, the likelihood of obtaining a large degree of spatial dependence, or similar values among observations taken from nearby locations. This phenomenon is well recognized in geography, and perhaps best captured in Waldo Tobler's *First Law of Geography* which generally states that all places and their respective characteristics are related to one another; however, those places that are closer tend to be more related than those that are farther away.

Though problematic when using traditional statistical methods such as regression, spatial autocorrelation can actually be put into good use when analysing health data. Based on the autocorrelation of disease rates, several analytical tests have been developed to identify the hotspots and coldspots of disease. These also serve as the basis for spatial prediction of disease risks using inverse distance weighting, kriging and other geostatistical algorithms. These applications are discussed later in the chapter.

2. Ecological correlation analysis

Throughout the environmental health literature, one finds several examples of ecological correlation studies. Essentially, these are investigations that explore potential relationships between the environment and health using data averaged across spatial units. Instead of using individual-level data, these studies rely on data aggregated across small areal units using variables that measure disease risks (incidence or prevalence rates), and the socio-economic or environmental attributes such as the median household income, the average levels of ozone, the average soil lead levels, or the percentage of black, white or Asian populations residing in those spatial units. Lacking the measures that directly assess the linkages between the health effect and exposures to contaminants in the external environment of each individual in the study sample, ecological studies are limited by their inability to establish a direct causation between the environment and health. Studies based on ecological correlations are also criticized as misleading because the variability in the underlying individual data is lost by aggregation and computation of average rates. Another challenge comes with the interpretation of the results. Some studies are vulnerable to *ecological bias* by drawing inferences about the individual units based on analysis of the information at the aggregated level.

Overall, notwithstanding the potential pitfalls of the ecological approach, there are multiple benefits that can be derived from its use in geospatial analysis of health data (Elliot and Wartenberg, 2004). First, ecological studies take advantage of hazard, exposure and disease outcome databases that are routinely compiled and reported by state and federal agencies. Examples include the TRI, NATA and NHANES databases reviewed earlier. Individual-level data are not readily available for conducting such investigations due to privacy and confidentiality regulations. Further, the scales at which some of these secondary demographic and environmental health data are available often preclude researchers from working at finer spatial scales.

Another potential benefit is the ability to explore associations between variables and identify areas that require more detailed inquiries through individual-level observations and environmental monitoring. As such, these studies are considered to be valuable in exploratory spatial data analysis (ESDA), generating questions, research hypotheses and appropriate designs about disease causation.

Finally, from an analytical viewpoint, many of the challenges noted earlier in the disease mapping approach apply here as well, including: the need to explore the statistical distribution of the data; the choice of spatial scale at which to perform the analysis; and the concerns of spatial autocorrelation. To avoid misleading the public about possible causation between variables, correlation techniques should be used instead of regression analysis to evaluate the relationships. Traditional regression analysis is a stringent statistical technique that is susceptible to spatial data flaws such as spatial autocorrelation, spatial heterogeneity and heteroscedasticity, as well as multicollinearity between the variables. These data violations are likely to produce biased estimates that limit the use of the research results in public health decision making. If utilized, every effort must be taken to meet all of the statistical assumptions before proceeding with the analysis and to use the necessary diagnostic measures before and after the regression estimates are produced. The more recent introduction of statistical methods such as geographical weighted regression (GWR) represents major steps toward addressing these spatial data problems.

3. Detection of disease clusters

Due in part to intense media coverage and growing public anxiety over toxic environments, public health agencies are increasingly compelled to conduct disease cluster investigations. Previous investigations show that such studies cover various diseases such as birth defects, and many types of infectious diseases (Thun and Sinks, 2004). Today, however, these investigations tend to address health concerns that are linked to environmentally induced cancers originating from different exposure sources such as radiation from nuclear power plants and electromagnetic sources, pollution from landfills and contaminated water sources, exposure to pesticides, and specific chemicals such as benzene, trichloroethylene, dioxins and arsenic.

In the United States, there are reportedly over 1000 cancer clusters suspected around the country each year. Many investigations are triggered by public perception over an unusually high number of disease cases observed in a community. About 1300–1650 requests for cancer cluster investigations are received annually, averaging about four requests per day (Greenberg and Wartenberg, 1993). Often, these turn out to be perceived clusters that could not be scientifically validated. Perceived clusters also comprise a mix of unrelated health conditions among different population groups (and pets), making it difficult to establish a significant causal relationship with the suspected agent in the external environment. Of the 1000 or so investigations conducted each year, only about 15 per cent of these situations turn out to be true cancer clusters with specific health outcomes that are related to putative risk factors. These are only verifiable scientifically through a series of spatial and temporal analytical tests. Following below is an overview of the attributes of true disease clusters that lead to detailed etiological investigations.

Defining a true disease cluster

The National Center for Environmental Health (NCEH), in the United States, defines a true cluster as a situation in which the number of observed cases of the disease is greater than the expected number of cases that occurs in a group of people in a definable geographical area, and over a defined period of time. George Knox (1964), who derived one of the original statistical tests for cluster detection, offers a simpler definition, describing a disease cluster as an aggregation of health events in space and time. Aggregation in this context implies that the health events are of sufficient size and concentration that they are unlikely to have occurred by chance. Both definitions offer key features of true disease clusters. First, these are unusual health events with excess risks that are greater than expected, and unlikely to have occurred by chance. The evaluation of such events therefore requires statistical tools to show that the observed deviation from the norm is statistically significant.

A second characteristic of true disease clusters is that they occur within the definable boundaries of space, time or both. The aggregation of excess health events within a definable geographic area constitutes a *spatial disease cluster*. When the excess events occur in a definable time period, say having more cases of childhood leukaemia than expected within a five-year period, this is a *temporal disease cluster*. In situations where the excess disease cases are closer in space and time, meaning nearer cases occur at about the same time, than cases that are farther away, such instances reflect a *space–time interaction* in the emergence of the disease cluster.

The delineation of cluster boundaries, particularly in space, has been the subject of much debate because it is subject to bias. Specifically, without any clear or definitive guidelines, researchers or health analysts may engage in boundary tightening or shrinkage in order to validate the existence of a disease cluster, or vice versa. Also referred to as the *Texas Sharpshooter Syndrome* in the literature; this is analogous to the situation in which the sharpshooter first fires several gunshots into the barn door, and then draws the target around the bullet holes. By reducing the geographic boundary, the at-risk population within the delineated area will likely be smaller, resulting in a higher than usual estimated risk of the disease. This methodological bias should be avoided at all costs during a cluster investigation (Elliot and Wartenberg, 2004).

Spatial epidemiologists have examined these analytical challenges in the hopes of generating more robust cluster detection methods. So far, more than 100 analytical methods are currently available in a variety of software packages that are continually being upgraded to accommodate the needs of the health analysts. In this book, we shall rely mostly on ArcGIS, ClusterSeer and TerraSeer SPACESTAT programs to detect disease clusters. These packages offer GIS capabilities that allow for interactive data exploration, visualization, and statistical analyses using advanced techniques such as Poisson kriging and GWR. The SPACESTAT package also integrates several methods for detecting disease clusters as well as examining these patterns within the context of health disparities. We shall explore some of these applications later in the text.

When conducting cluster investigations, geographers are mostly interested in the spatial clusters, though several methods now exist for temporal and space–time patterns of disease risk. Spatially, the data collected for such analyses are based on individual occurrences or disease cases (point data) or they are based on aggregated disease rates within census tracts, wards, counties or other spatial units.

The methods available in the software packages noted above allow for the use of data collected on events, people, features or field measurements (Jacquez, 2008). Some studies have used events-based data typically coded as points or geographic coordinates that reflect the residential location of the patient. For example, Wheeler (2007) used individual case data to evaluate the spatial distribution and clustering of leukaemia incidence among children in Ohio. The data, covering a time period from 1996 to 2003, were garnered from the Ohio Cancer Incidence Surveillance System.

Cluster analysis can also be performed at the population level using aggregated information such as disease rates. Oyana and Margai (2007) examined the distribution and clustering of child lead poisoning cases in Chicago using disease rates measured across census blocks in Chicago, Illinois. Spatial clustering analysis may also be performed using field measurements such as soil lead levels measured within communities, or feature-based data using boundaries or polygons derived from field data (Jacquez, 2008). The cluster detection methods can also be classified according to the method of interest: global, local and focal:

a. Global clustering tests Global tests are designed to statistically assess whether there is evidence of significant clustering of disease without pinpointing the location of the clusters in the study area. The tests rely on the underlying spatial structure of the data, specifically spatial autocorrelation, to determine the significance and extent of clustering that exists. A commonly used measure is the Moran's *I* statistic which is calculated as:

$$I = \frac{n\sum_{i=1}^{n}\sum_{j=1}^{n}w_{ij}(y_i - \bar{y})((y_i - \bar{y}))}{\left(\sum_{i=1}^{n}(y_i - \bar{y})^2\right)\left(\sum_{i=1}^{n}\sum_{j=1}^{n}w_{ij}\right)}$$

where w_{ij} is the weight applied based on the spatial proximity between the data zones, y_i represents the attribute value and $\bar{y}$ its related mean, and n represents the total number of adjacent zones. The current GIS packages determine the degree of adjacency between the spatial units using one of three criteria: 'queen', 'rook' or 'bishop'. The queen criterion is the least restrictive, enabling the use of all common boundaries and vertices between the area polygons in the study area. The rook criterion on the other hand uses only the observations that share an edge rather than the corner or vertex between zones. The bishop is the most restrictive and very rarely used since it employs only the corners and vertices in calculating the degree of connectivity between adjacent zones.

The statistic derived from the analysis is called Moran's *I*, a weighted correlation coefficient that essentially describes the average degree of spatial dependency in the observed rate of the disease across the study region. As with all correlation coefficients, the absolute value of *r* reflects the strength of the observed relationship between adjacent data points. A positive *I* value represents positive spatial autocorrelation implying a clustering of spatial units with similar rates of disease. A negative *I* reflects a clustering of spatial units with dissimilar values, and a value of zero indicates no spatial autocorrelation. Moran's *I* is among the earliest global tests developed to detect spatial clusters. Others include the Joint Count Statistics for categorical data, and Geary's C statistic.

b. Local clustering tests In the mid-1990s, several local tests were developed as counterparts to the global tests. Instead of examining the phenomenon at the global level, the local tests are designed to depict the disease pattern around specific points in space. In doing so, the tests show the exact location of the disease clusters in a given study area. Examples include Kulldorf's Spatial Scan, and Getis and Ord's statistics. Another popular test is Anselin's (1995) LISA (local indicators of spatial association) statistic, a variant of the global Moran's I, which is computed for each spatial unit, as follows:

$$L_i = z_i \sum_{j=1}^{n} w_{ij}\, z_j$$

where z_i is the standardized disease rate in location i that is under investigation, and z_j represents the observed rates for neighbouring locations j, that share a common border with i. All values are standardized to have a mean of zero and a unit standard deviation (z scores). In addition to providing a global test, the LISA statistic and its associated significance test provide evidence of one of four patterns of the underlying spatial structure: a cluster of high values; a cluster of low values; evidence of high or low spatial outliers; or evidence of spatially random pattern that is not statistically significant. A negative LISA statistic indicates that there is negative local autocorrelation (spatial dissimilarity) and the likely presence of a spatial outlier where the individual units (i) have a lower (higher) disease rate than the average value of surrounding units. A positive LISA statistic indicates the presence of a cluster of low (or high) values within the adjacent spatial units. This test is available in ArcGIS and is useful for the detection of hotspots and coldspots in disease risk mapping.

Recently, Goovaerts and others, in their development of the SPACESTAT software, have modified the bivariate LISA statistic to enable the detection of disease clusters and disparities among any two racial/ethnic categories (Goovaerts et al, 2007). For example, to calculate the bivariate LISA at location i for disparity in lung cancer between white and black males, the revised statistics would be computed as follows:

$$L_{i,\,BM \times WM} = Z_{i,\,BM} \sum_{j} w_{ij} z_{j,\,WM}$$

where $z_{i,\,BM}$ is the standardized lung cancer mortality rate for black males at that location, $z_{j,\,WM}$ is the standardized rate observed for whites in location j adjacent to i. Therefore, the term $\sum_{j} w_{ij} z_{j,\,WM}$ represents the average white male lung cancer mortality for locations adjacent to i. A positive bivariate LISA statistic would imply that the observed lung cancer rate at neighbouring locations is similar for both racial groups, and a negative value would imply disparity between the groups. The computed statistic is accompanied by a test of significance.

Overall, the multiple tests available for cluster detection reflect the level of commitment on the part of geographers and spatial epidemiologists to develop appropriate techniques for describing the spatial distribution of diseases, identifying the hotspots, coldspots or anomalies of disease, and using the information to generate new research hypotheses or conduct more detailed etiological investigations. Some analytical challenges remain, however. Specifically, the effectiveness of these methods is dependent on how complex the disease etiologies are, including the length of the latency periods, the possibility of multiple exposures, genetic susceptibility and population mobility

(Kingsley et al, 2007). In tackling these challenges, the greatest need is for reliable, valid and complete data gathered at the finest geographic scale possible. Where necessary, it is important also to integrate the residential histories of individuals into the analysis in order to capture the multiple risk sources of exposure (Jacquez et al, 2005; 2006; Jacquez, 2008). Efforts are now underway to accommodate these additional dimensions in the analysis and to develop methods that can identify different morphological patterns of clusters beyond just the circular or elliptical shapes that are commonly produced in the current software packages.

4. Spatial prediction

So far, the analytical tests described above are not mutually exclusive tests. In many studies, researchers employ a combination of tests that consists of exploratory maps, ecological correlation analysis and cluster detection methods. Added to this mix are a number of spatial prediction methods. These methods extend beyond the traditional models of statistical prediction by incorporating the underlying spatial structure, notably spatial dependence, and heterogeneity into the analysis. Traditional regression models, for example, assume that the sample data are independent and uniformly distributed. Yet we know that this is not the case due to the likelihood of autocorrelation in the spatial data. Described below are some approaches used to incorporate the spatial structure of the data in statistical prediction.

a) Inverse distance weighting

One of the simplest methods that enable spatial prediction using the underlying spatial relationships is inverse distance weighting (IDW). This test produces a disease estimate at a given point (X) in space, by weighting and averaging out the known values obtained at neighbouring locations. The weights applied are inversely proportional to the distance between the two points, so neighbouring points that are closer will be more influential in the computation of the unknown estimate:

$$X = \frac{\sum_{i=1}^{n} Z_i/D_i}{\sum_{i=1}^{n} 1/D_i}$$

where X is the interpolated value at a unmeasured location; Z_i is the data value obtained from measured location adjacent to X, of which there are n in the neighbourhood; and D_i is the distance between point X and each data point in the neighbourhood. Figure 5.4b depicts a risk map of groundwater arsenic levels for Pennsylvania based on a total of 600 samples obtained from across the state between 1973 and 2001. The IDW technique was used to generate the continuous risk surface based on data acquired from the sampled points.

b) Kriging

Kriging is a more advanced predictive tool that is appropriate for situations in which there are inherent flaws in the data. Often we are faced with uncertainties in the data as a result of the small numbers problem, the presence of a large number of missing values in the data, evidence of spatial autocorrelation, or situations in which the variances obtained at each location are unstable resulting in a spatially heteroscedastic model. These data challenges can all be appropriately handled by the kriging technique. Like the traditional regression method, kriging has BLUE properties producing Best, Linear, Unbiased Estimators at unsampled sites along with their associated standard errors.

Analytically, kriging is a two step process that starts out with the computation of the semivariance model that is graphically summarized in a variogram (Cressie, 1993; Goovaerts, 2005; Goovaerts, 2009). The analysis is based on a regionalized variable Z, which is defined at each point within a region. So for N data locations $(x_i, i = 1 \ldots N)$, there is a value z_i at each location x_i. Assuming an intrinsic stationarity in the data, the expected mean between two places x, and $x + h$ (where h is the spatial lag) is zero, as denoted below:

$$E[z(x) - z(x + h)] = 0$$

The variance of the differences between these sites will also depend on the spatial lag, and will be calculated as follows:

$$
\begin{aligned}
E &= [\{z(x) - z(x + h\}^2] \\
&= E[\{\varepsilon'(x) - \varepsilon'(x + h\}^2] \\
&= 2\gamma(h)
\end{aligned}
$$

Where $\gamma(h)$ is the semivariance. Using sample data, the semivariance can therefore be calculated as follows:

$$\hat{\gamma}(h) = \frac{1}{2n} \sum_{i=1}^{n} \{z(x_i) - z(x_i + h)\}^2$$

where n represents the number of pairs of lag h. In ordinary kriging (OK), a graphical summary depicting the semivariance $\gamma(h)$ against the lag distance between pairs of data points is produced. This plot, often called a semivariogram (or variogram) captures the underlying spatial dependence (as well as the direction) between the data points. The graph has a definitive shape that is useful for diagnosing the extent of spatial autocorrelation in the data. If the variogram is the same at all distances and angles in the data, there is no autocorrelation at the spatial scales used in the analysis. Deviations from this pattern represent some degree of spatial autocorrelation with little or no random variation (white noise in the data). For example, Figure 5.4c shows the variogram obtained from a gaussian model of arsenic levels measured from 600 sampled points in Pennsylvania. The diagram shows evidence of spatial autocorrelation with a range of 1.19 and a nugget of 1.34, suggesting some random variability in the data.

Once these different parameters are captured from the variogram model, they are integrated into the kriging function to generate a continuous risk surface of the disease. The analysis produces several diagnostic measures that are useful in evaluating the overall performance of the kriged risk estimates,

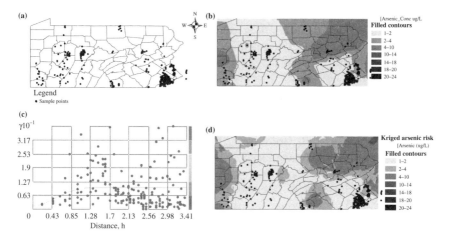

Source: USGS, groundwater quality samples obtained between 1973–2001

Figure 5.4 *Spatial interpolation of arsenic levels in groundwater*

including the ability to conduct cross-validation using a fresh batch of sampled points.

As with the other techniques reviewed earlier, there are several variants of this method, allowing users to select the most appropriate estimator for their study depending on the characteristics of the data at hand and the overall research objectives. Examples include: (i) *indicator kriging* which is global in scope, producing a distribution of values across an entire area, rather than the mean value of an area; (ii) *universal kriging* which is most applicable in cases where the data have a strong trend; (iii) *cokriging* which is used to produce risk estimates of a disease (or criterion variable) based on information obtained from covariates, or other variables that are believed to be strongly related to the criterion variable. More recently, following the input from Goovaerts (2006) and Goovaerts et al (2007), *Poisson kriging* has been applied extensively to the analysis of cancer morbidity and mortality outcomes in the United States.

Chapter summary

With increasing advances in computer technologies, geographic tools such as GIS and spatial statistical analysis now offer innovative approaches for data capture, analysis and mapping of environmental health disparities. This chapter has reviewed four of the approaches that are commonly used by spatial epidemiologists to study the health patterns and related disparities: disease mapping, ecological correlation analysis, cluster detection using space and time algorithms, and spatial prediction methods. As discussed in the chapter, the effective use of these approaches depends in part on the collection and integration of reliable data in a GIS environment. Using the hazard–exposure–outcome framework, a variety of databases and surveillance systems have been presented as potentially great data sources for evaluating the complex relationships between hazardous exposures and disease outcomes. Also highlighted in this chapter are the shortcomings of these databases as well as the strengths and inherent limitations of the analytical methods. Knowledge of these limitations is required to ensure their proper use in evaluating health disparities.

References

Anselin, L. (1995) 'Local indicators of spatial association – LISA', *Geographical Analysis*, vol 27, pp93–115

Beale, L., Abelian, J. J., Hodgson, S. and Jarup, L. (2008) 'Methodologic issues and approaches to spatial epidemiology', *Environmental Health Perspectives*, vol 116, no 8, pp1105–1110

Centers for Disease Control and Prevention (1998) 'Guidelines for evaluating surveillance systems', *Morbidity and Mortality Weekly Report*, vol 37, suppl S-5, pp1–18

Chakraborty, J. (2009) 'Automobiles, air toxics, and adverse health risks: Environmental inequities in Tampa Bay, Florida', *Annals of the Association of American Geographers*, vol 99, no 4, pp674–697

Cressie, N. (1993) *Statistics for Spatial Data*, Wiley, New York

Devesa, S. S., Grauman, D. G., Blot, W. J., Pennello, G., Hoover, R. N. and Fraumeni, J. F. Jr. (1999) *Atlas of Cancer Mortality in the United States, 1950–94*, US Govt Print Office, Washington, DC [NIH Publ No. (NIH) 99-4564]

Elliott, P. and Wartenberg, D. (2004) 'Spatial epidemiology: Current approaches and future challenges', *Environmental Health Perspectives*, vol 112, pp998–1006

Goovaerts, P. (2005) 'Analysis and detection of health disparities using geostatistics and a space–time information system: The case of prostate cancer mortality in the United States, 1970–1994', *Proceedings of GIS Planet 2005*, Estoril, 30 May–2 June, 2005d, available at http://home.comcast.net/~pgoovaerts/Paper148_PierreGoovaerts.pdf, accessed 15 July 2008

Goovaerts, P. (2006) 'Geostatistical analysis of disease data: Visualization and propagation of spatial uncertainty in cancer mortality risk using Poisson kriging and p-field simulation', *International Journal of Health Geographics*, vol 5, no 7, doi:10.1186/1476-072X-5-7

Goovaerts, P. (2009) 'Medical geography: A promising field of application for geostatistics', *Mathematical Geology*, vol 41, pp243–264

Goovaerts, P., Meliker, J. R. and Jacquez, G. M. (2007) 'A comparative analysis of aspatial statistics for detecting racial disparities in cancer mortality rates', *International Journal of Health Geographics*, vol 6, no 32, doi:10.1186/1476-072X-6-32

Greenberg, M. and Wartenberg, D. (1993) 'Solving the cluster puzzle: Clues to follow and pitfalls to avoid', *Statistics in Medicine*, vol 12, pp1763–1770

Jacquez, G. M. (2008) 'Spatial cluster analysis', Chapter 22 in Fotheringham, S. and Wilson, J. (eds) *The Handbook of Geographic Information Science*, Blackwell Publishing, Oxford, pp395–416

Jacquez, G. M., Kaufmann, A., Meliker, J., Goovaerts, P., AvRuskin, G. and Nriagu, J. (2005) 'Global, local and focused geographic clustering for case-control data with residential histories', *Environmental Health*, vol 4, no 4

Jacquez, G. M., Meliker, J. R., AvRuskin, G. A., Goovaerts, P., Kaufmann, A., Wilson, M. and Nriagu, J. (2006) 'Case-control geographic clustering for residential histories accounting for risk factors and covariates', *International Journal of Health Geographics*, vol 5, no 32

Kingsley, B. S., Schmeichel, K. L. and Rubin, C. H. (2007) 'An update of cancer cluster activities at the Centers for Disease Control', *Environmental Health Perspectives*, vol 115, no 1, pp165–171

Knox, E. G. (1964) 'The detection of space–time interactions', *Applied Statistics*, vol 13, pp25–29

Margai, F. M. (2003) 'Using Geodata techniques to analyze environmental health inequities in minority neighborhoods: The case of toxic exposures and low birth weights', in Frazier, J. W. and Margai, F. M. (eds) *Multicultural Geographies: The Changing Racial and Ethnic Patterns of the United States*, Global Academic Publishing, Binghamton, NY

Mather, F. J., Ellis White, L., Langlois, E. C., Shorter, C. F., Swalm, C. M., Shaffer, J. C. and Hartley, W. (2004) 'Statistical methods for linking health, exposure, and hazards', *Environmental Health Perspectives*, vol 12, no 14, pp1140–1145

Morello-Frosch, R., Pastor, M. and Sadd, J. (2001) 'Environmental justice and Southern California's "riskscape": The distribution of air toxics exposures and health risks among diverse communities', *Urban Affairs Review*, vol 36, pp551–578

Nsubuga, P., White, M. E., Thacker, S. B., Anderson, M. A., Blount, S. B., Broome, C. V., Chiller, T. M., Espitia, V., Imtiaz, R., Sosin, D., Stroup, D. F., Tauxe, R. V., Vijayaraghavan, M. and Trostle, M. (2006) 'Public health surveillance: A tool for targeting and monitoring intervention', in Jamison, D. T., Breman, J. G., Measham, A. R., Alleyne, G., Claeson, M., Evans, D. B., Jha, P., Mills, A. and Musgrove, P. (eds) *Disease Control Priorities in Developing Countries*, 2nd Edition, Oxford University Press, New York, pp997–1018, doi:10.1596/978-0-821-36179-5/Chpt-53

Olsen, S. F., Martuzzi, M. and Elliot, P. (1996) 'Cluster analysis and disease mapping: Why, when, and how? A step by step guide', *British Medical Journal*, vol 313, no 7061, pp863–870

Openshaw, S. (1984) 'Ecological fallacies and the analysis of areal census data', *Environmental Planning A*, vol 16, pp17–31

Oyana, T. and Margai, F. M. (2007) 'Geographic analysis of health risks of pediatric lead exposure: A golden opportunity to promote healthy neighborhoods', *Archives of Environmental and Occupational Health*, vol 62, no 2, pp93–104

Pew Commission Report (2000) *American's Environmental Health Gap: Why the Country Needs a National Health Tracking Network*, Pew Charitable Trusts, Baltimore, MD

TerraSeer, Inc, www.terraseer.com/products/clusterseer.html/, accessed 6 June 2008

Thacker, S. B., Stroup, D. F., Gibson, P. and Anderson, H. A. (1996) 'Surveillance in environmental public health: Issues, systems, and sources', *American Journal of Public Health*, vol 86, no 5, pp633–638

Thun, M. J. and Sinks, T. (2004) 'Understanding cancer clusters', *CA: A Cancer Journal for Clinicians*, vol 54, pp273–280

Wheeler, D. C. (2007) 'A comparison of spatial clustering and cluster detection techniques for childhood leukemia incidence in Ohio, 1996–2003', *International Journal of Health Geographics*, vol 6, no 13, doi:10.1186/1476-072X-6-13

PART II

ENVIRONMENTAL ASPECTS OF HEALTH DISPARITIES

6
Global Climate Change and Environmental Degradation: Place Vulnerability and Public Health Challenges

Introduction

Global climate change is now a widely accepted phenomenon among scientists, domestic and international policy makers despite ongoing debates over the proposed trajectories of change, and the validity and reliability of analytical models used to derive these probabilistic projections. Historical records dating as far back as the 1860s, together with more recent indisputable evidence of rising global average temperatures, changing sea levels, retreating glaciers and permafrost, and extreme weather events, all point towards a warming trend. Scientific studies along with evidence assembled by the United Nations Intergovernmental Panel on Climate Change (IPCC) have all arrived at similar conclusions. From 1900 to 2009, global average surface temperatures increased by approximately 0.7°C (1.3°F), and since the 1950s this climatological pattern has been induced primarily by anthropogenic greenhouse gas emissions. Figure 6.1 shows the anomalies in global mean temperatures when compared to mean temperatures observed in the 20th century. An upward trend is readily visible, with a faster and more sustainable rate of increase in temperatures observed during the last few decades. Human activities during this modern era of climate change have contributed more to the warming trend than naturally occurring processes such as solar or volcanic activities.

The purpose of this chapter is to examine the important sources of modern climate change, the real or anticipated impacts on health, and the geographical differentiation in population vulnerability to these impacts. We start with a discussion of the context and key drivers of global environmental change and then proceed to discuss the projected health impacts and differential levels of social vulnerability in various world regions.

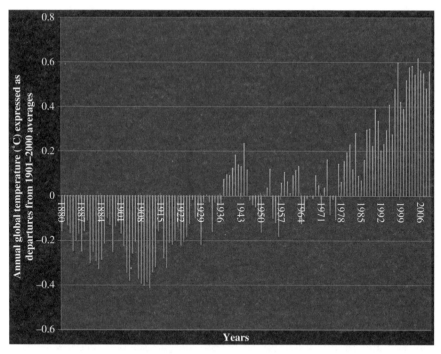

Data Source: National Climate Data Center www.climatewatch.noaa.gov/2009/articles/climate-change-global-temperature

Figure 6.1 *Global average temperature anomalies*

The human influence on global climate change

Climate change is formally described as 'the change in the state of the climate that can be identified by changes in the mean and/or variability of its properties, and that persists for an extended period, typically decades or longer' (Hegerl et al, 2007, p667). This definition reflects the extensive analytical work that goes into providing measurable evidence of climate change, first by compiling longitudinal data on various climatic properties such as temperature, precipitation and humidity, and then analysing these variables to uncover meaningful change in both the statistical mean and variability of the values.

For decades now, researchers have focused on estimating these trends primarily through the use of general circulation models (GCMs) and other climatological algorithms. Statistical analyses of the historical data have shown that over the last century or so, there has been a significant increase in global average temperatures by approximately 0.6°C to 0.8°C, with the 1990s being the hottest decade on record. Though the observed increase is partly the result of natural causes, scientific data now confirm that these recent changes in the Earth's climate are caused by the excess accumulation of greenhouse (heat-trapping) gases that are produced chiefly by the burning of fossil fuels during transportation, industrial and agricultural activities. Following below is a discussion of the effects of these human-induced factors on atmospheric greenhouse gases, along with the related effects from ozone depletion and land-use change.

1. The enhanced greenhouse effect

The greenhouse effect is a naturally occurring phenomenon that allows for global energy circulation and energy balance between the Earth and the atmosphere by transferring energy between these biospheric systems through the processes of insolation, absorption, reflection and reradiation. This process plays a critical role in human sustenance by moderating temperatures on the Earth's surface. Without it, temperatures would likely be 33°C (59°F) colder with significantly greater differences between daytime and night-time temperatures.

The greenhouse effect is largely driven by certain gases in the atmosphere. These gases allow incoming solar radiation during the day but retard the reradiation of some of this energy back into the upper atmosphere, thus causing the Earth's temperatures to rise. The primary greenhouse gases, when ranked in terms of their overall contribution to this process, are water vapour (which contributes 36–72 per cent), carbon dioxide (9–26 per cent), methane (4–9 per cent) and ozone (3–7 per cent).

During the last century, the greenhouse effect has been exacerbated by the atmospheric abundance of these gases, particularly carbon dioxide and methane, which have increased consistently over the years, reaching their highest observable levels in the 1990s. When compared to the pre-industrial era, the observable levels of atmospheric carbon dioxide concentration were nearly a third higher in the late 1990s. Figure 6.2 shows the annual mean levels of CO_2 measured at Mauna Loa since 1959. Globally, the current global atmospheric level is estimated to be approximately 387 ppm, and increasing at a rate of about 2 ppm per year. Nearly three-quarters of this increase has been attributed to the burning of fossil fuels.

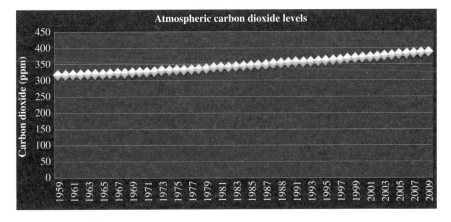

Data source: Tans, P. NOAA/ESRL (www.esrl.noaa.gov/gmd/ccgg/trends/)

Figure 6.2 *Annual atmospheric carbon dioxide levels*

Significant changes in the atmospheric concentration of methane have also occurred with more than a twofold increase in concentration levels when compared to the pre-industrial era. The globally averaged atmospheric surface abundance for this gas in the 1990s was 1745 parts per billion, originating from both natural sources (such as wetlands) and anthropogenic sources such as landfills, rice paddies and biomass burning. Other notable greenhouse gases include nitrous oxides (N_2O), and several classes of synthetic halogenated compounds such as chlorofluorocarbons (CFCs), hydrochloro-fluorocarbons (HCFCs) and bromofluorocarbons, that are the by-products of consumer and industrial activities. The increase in the atmospheric concentration of reactive gases such as carbon monoxide (CO), volatile organic compounds (VOC), and nitrogen oxides (NO and NO_2), have also been observed. The latter are often termed indirect greenhouse gases because they indirectly contribute to global warming by controlling the abundance of the direct greenhouse gases.

2. Ozone depletion

Researchers have found a strong synergistic interaction between the greenhouse effect and the stratospheric depletion of ozone, a problem that could potentially lead to more rapid climate change (Hartmann et al, 2000). Stratospheric ozone, lying between 15 and 40km (10–25 miles) above the Earth's surface, serves as a protective layer by absorbing most of the incoming ultraviolet radiation. As with the greenhouse effect, there has been a slow and steady modification of this natural layer over the last several decades due to human-induced changes in atmospheric composition. Specifically the addition of several synthetic substances such as CFCs, HCFCs, methyl bromide, carbon tetrachloride and methyl chloroform have contributed to the gradual depletion of the ozone layer at a rate of about 3 per cent per decade over the last 20 years.

The synergistic interaction between ozone depletion and the greenhouse effect is believed to be contributing to the pronounced changes in tropospheric and stratospheric climate during the last few decades. Both climatic processes are influenced by the increased concentration of halogenated substances in the atmosphere. However, based on data gathered from some atmospheric models, the trapping of heat in the troposphere by the greenhouse gases cools the stratosphere and allows the formation of ice crystals which enhance ozone-depleting chemical reactions (Patz et al, 2000). These trends in the stratosphere are, in turn, likely to influence the climatic conditions on the Earth's surface, producing a strong annular component in the middle and high latitudes of both the northern and southern hemispheres.

3. Deforestation and land conversion activities

A review of the primary sources of global climate change cannot be complete without addressing the problem of deforestation and land-use/land-cover change. Aside from the burning of fossil fuels, the single largest source of global warming is from deforestation and land-use conversion to make room for urbanization, agriculture and other anthropogenic activities. Current emissions of greenhouse gases from deforestation account for roughly 25 per cent of the enhanced greenhouse effect from anthropogenic sources (Houghton, 2005). As with other human activities, deforestation contributes directly and indirectly to the release of multiple greenhouse gases.

Among the greenhouse releases, carbon dioxide remains the most problematic gas for a number of reasons. First, carbon is stored primarily in forests, and forested regions account for about a third of the Earth's land surface, making such areas the most important global source of carbon. Though the precise amounts vary, carbon is about 20 to 50 times higher in forests than in cleared areas (Houghton, 2005). These carbon sinks vary further depending on the ecosystem, the type of region (tropical vs temperate), land-use and land-cover type. With increasing deforestation and land transformation activities in these areas, the carbon stored in the trees is released directly into the atmosphere through burning, or indirectly through the gradual decomposition of organic matter. Deforestation not only releases carbon dioxide, the absence of trees also reduces the amount of carbon dioxide uptake from the atmosphere.

Table 6.1 shows the percentage of initial stocks lost to the atmosphere by deforestation and land conversion activities. The largest losses are from agricultural and pastoral activities. Historical data show that during the 1750s, only about 7 per cent of the global land surface was devoted to these activities. However, there has been a fivefold increase and today agricultural and pastoral land uses account for more than 40 per cent of the global land surface. The earliest conversions took place in the temperate regions, primarily in Europe, China and the Indian subcontinent. Europe reportedly had cleared up to 80 per cent of its agricultural areas by the 1860s (Forster et al, 2007). Agricultural and land conversion activities in these regions continued up until the 1950s. In recent decades, however, the most significant changes have taken place in the tropical regions, with exponential rates of deforestation being recorded in Latin America, Africa, South and Southeast Asia. Experts warn that at these excessive rates of land conversion, forests are likely to be depleted in tropical Asia and West Africa within the next few decades. Unless major steps are taken soon to curb such activities, the changes in the forested landscapes would continue to amplify the greenhouse effect.

Table 6.1 *Carbon stocks lost to deforestation and land conversion activities*

Land use	Carbon lost to the atmosphere expressed as a % of initial carbon stocks
Cultivated land	90–100
Pasture	90–100
Degraded croplands/pasture	60–90
Shifting cultivation	60
Degraded forest	25–50
Logging	10–50
Plantations	30–50
Extractive reserves	0

Source: Houghton, 2005

Regional differentiation of the impacts of climate change

Scientists have predicted with a 90 per cent confidence that by the year 2100, the average global temperature will have risen anywhere from 1.7°C to 4.9°C (3.1°F to 8.8°F). This increase will be accompanied by sea-level rise, receding glaciers and melting of permafrost surfaces. Extreme weather events are also anticipated with more frequent heat waves, intense storm activities, prolonged droughts and related impacts such as wild fires and vegetation changes (Karl and Trenberth, 2003). There are indications that many of these environmental changes are already underway in many parts of the world.

As scientific evidence of these changes mounts, the accumulating information garnered from different world regions suggests an uneven distribution in the warming trend (Epstein, 2001; Hess et al, 2008). Specifically, there are diurnal, seasonal and regional differentiations in both the real and anticipated changes in climate. For example, the warming trend is currently occurring twice as fast during the winter months and at night-time. Further, the winter warming appears to be more pronounced in the high-latitudinal regions than the tropical regions (Houghton, 1995; Easterling et al, 2000). These observable trends are fairly consistent with the climatic scenarios postulated by some of the major climate models (The Met Office, 2009). A recent version of the Hadley Centre Coupled Model (HadCM3) projects a strong regional component in average winter temperatures by 2100 (see Figure 6.3a). Changes in precipitation levels are also likely to be spatially uneven with heavier levels expected around the tropical regions, while other areas are expected to see a decline in annual average precipitation (Figure 6.3b).

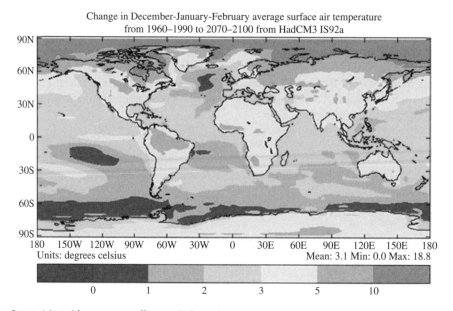

Source: Adapted from www.metoffice.gov.uk/climatechange/

Figure 6.3a *HadCM3 global winter temperatures*

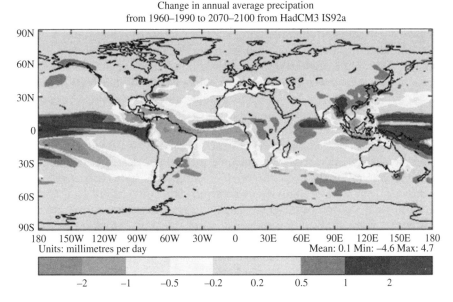

Change in annual average precipitation
from 1960–1990 to 2070–2100 from HadCM3 IS92a

Units: millimetres per day   Mean: 0.1 Min: −4.6 Max: 4.7

−2   −1   −0.5   −0.2   0.2   0.5   1   2

Source: Adapted from www.metoffice.gov.uk/climatechange/

Figure 6.3b *HadCM3 global precipitation levels*

As with natural biogeochemical cycles, the expected changes in climate will trigger a series of synergistic interactions and feedback loops among the basic components of the biosphere. Changes in temperature and precipitation will likely be accompanied by changes in annual average soil moisture content with an expected reduction in regions such as Amazonia, Southwestern Africa and in the lowland areas of northern Eurasia. Land and sea differences in the warming trend will result in an observable amount of heat retention within the oceans thus accelerating the melting of sea ice and ice shelves around the world. Evidence also shows that this accelerated heating of the land will lead to an unprecedented rate of thawing of permafrost surfaces in high-latitudinal regions, contributing further to the release of significant levels of methane into the atmosphere. Similarly, the intense heating of land/sea surfaces will alter the hydrological cycle by producing excess water vapour (another greenhouse gas) in the atmosphere, contributing further to a highly unstable climate system.

People, place and regional vulnerability to climate change

Vulnerability to climate change essentially implies the potential for loss of property or life as a result of exposure to the emerging environmental hazards that are associated with the changing climate. These hazards are expected to significantly disrupt the economic, political and social systems of many countries. The general consensus among researchers, however, is that some countries will likely bear the brunt of these impending hazards, and therefore the geographic context and place will serve as the key exposure determinants in assessing vulnerability (Adger, 1999; Patz and Kovats, 2002; Hess et al, 2008).

Like the anticipated climate change itself, the degree of vulnerability will vary from one place to another, and across time. Societal impacts would also be spatially differentiated with disparate risks among different population groups depending on their pre-existing levels of vulnerability. Within high-risk areas, some population groups will be more vulnerable than others. Specifically, children, the elderly population, pregnant or lactating women, refugees and migrant and displaced populations would be the most vulnerable. Their level of vulnerability would be compounded further by pre-existing disadvantages such as the racial/ethnic disparities and income inequalities described earlier in the preceding chapters. In the United States, for example, the 2005 Hurricane Katrina disaster uncovered the deep divide by race and class in the city of New Orleans. A geographical analysis of the environmental health hazards resulting from this catastrophic event showed that the most vulnerable populations residing in the maximum inundated areas were African American and low-income populations (Asomaning, 2008). An assessment of vulnerability to climate change hazards therefore requires a deeper understanding of the place-based risks, including the biophysical changes that are likely to occur in that location, the population characteristics, and the range of social, institutional, technological and behavioural measures taken, if any, to alleviate these challenges.

The model of place vulnerability to climate change hazards

The concept of place vulnerability has been researched extensively in the social sciences over the last few decades, with a number of conceptual frameworks developed to capture the physical and human dimensions of susceptibility. One of the most comprehensive geographic frameworks is the Hazards-of-Place model of vulnerability (Figure 6.4). This model was first proposed by Cutter (1996), and has since being applied in several studies of geoenvironmental hazards (Cutter et al, 2000; 2003).

In this model the potential for environmental hazards is largely dependent on the risks (the probability that the hazardous events will occur) and the measures taken to minimize those risks (mitigation). The hazard potential is then moderated or exacerbated by two major features of these places: (i) the geographic context (which reflects the site and situational characteristics of the places including their proximity to the source of the threat) and (ii) the social fabric of those places. Within the context of health inequities, the social fabric is probably the most important dimension to evaluate because it captures not only the demographic and socio-economic characteristics but also the pre-existing disparities by race, ethnicity and class, as well as chronic health conditions that may be exacerbated by climate change hazards. This social construct also includes the perception and previous experiences of residents in terms of dealing with such hazards, and their ability to cope, adapt or bounce back from such events.

Also relevant in the place vulnerability model are the critical infrastructural facilities such as transportation networks, dams, sewage treatment facilities,

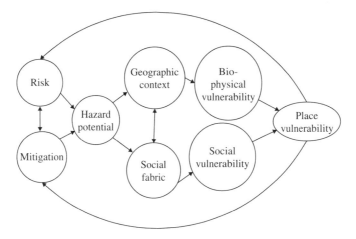

Source: Cutter (1996)

Figure 6.4 *Hazards-of-Place model*

industries, hospitals, utilities and other facilities that may serve to minimize or compound the level of social vulnerability to these hazards (Cutter et al, 2000). As shown in the model, all of these indicators collectively influence the vulnerability in a given place. The geographic context impacts the biophysical vulnerability whereas the social fabric accounts for social vulnerability. Both the biophysical and social indicators then interact to jointly influence the level of place vulnerability.

The use of biophysical and social indicators to assess place vulnerability to climate change hazards is suitable for finer geographic scales; however, there are examples of such applications at regional and global scales particularly since the initial assessments of climate change have been mostly completed at these aggregate levels. In exploring the potential for loss, biophysical assessments at the global and regional levels indicate that the most vulnerable places will be the high-latitudinal regions, the floodplains, river banks, coastal areas, small islands, deserts and arid areas, cities, and vector border regions where disease vectors are likely to expand their geographic range. In the United States, for example, Hess et al (2008) have identified the coastal counties consisting of 53 per cent of the US population as one of the most vulnerable areas for climate change. A rise in tropical cyclone intensity, attributed to elevated sea-surface temperatures during the last three decades, has already been observed around the areas. Along with the increased likelihood for waterborne, food-borne and vector-borne diseases, these areas are susceptible to shoreline erosion, wetland loss and land subsidence with significant impacts anticipated on housing, agricultural land and critical infrastructural facilities. The arid areas in the southwestern United States are also susceptible to these impeding hazards, with a warmer climate expected to result in permanent drought conditions.

When compared to the developed countries such as the United States, residents in the developing regions are clearly more vulnerable to climate change. These countries have less capacity to cope with the anticipated changes in biophysical characteristics of their environments. The societies are burdened further by significant rates of poverty, urbanization and rapid population growth in low-lying coastal areas that are susceptible to sea-level rise. Studies evaluating the regional impacts of climate change in these regions have identified specific sectors that are vulnerable.

In Asia, the sectors that are most likely to be adversely affected are linked to food security, coastal zones vulnerable to sea-level rise, the greater incidence of extreme weather events (monsoons, typhoons, floods and landslides), and the diffusion of vector-borne diseases. There are also concerns that climate change will exacerbate the threat to biodiversity in the region as a result of land conversion activities and growing pressure from burgeoning populations.

In Latin America, the impacts of climate change are projected to be wide ranging given the complex physiography of the region including its climatic heterogeneity and varying ecological systems. However, the key areas of concern are similar to the other developing regions, specifically in the areas of water resources, agriculture and plantation forestry, forest fragmentation and degradation resulting in biodiversity loss, sea-level rise and human health. An increase in El Niño-like mean conditions is expected, potentially resulting in prolonged droughts in regions such as Amazonia, Mexico and Central America with an increased likelihood of forest fires. El Niño and La Niña-like conditions are also likely to increase disease vector populations, with likely implications for human health.

Finally, Africa remains one of the most vulnerable regions to climate change and scientists are particularly worried about the likely impacts in the following sectors: (i) food security; (ii) water quality and scarcity; (iii) natural resource management and biodiversity loss; (iv) coastal vulnerability to sea-level rise; (v) amplification of desertification; (vi) emergence or re-emergence of water-borne diseases.

Current and anticipated health outcomes of global climate change

Scientists have identified a range of environmental health outcomes that are likely to emerge from the changing climate (Patz et al, 2000; Daszak et al, 2001; Greenough et al, 2001; Confalonieri et al, 2007). For the purposes of our discussion in this text, these outcomes are organized into six areas:

- Thermal stress
- Extreme events and meteorological hazards
- Air pollution
- Emergent and re-emergent infectious diseases
- Food insecurity
- Social and economic disruptions.

As summarized in Table 6.2, some of the anticipated health effects from these hazards will be direct, originating primarily from exposure to the changing

Table 6.2 *Current and anticipated health effects of climate change*

Hazards	Current/anticipated health effects
Direct effects on health	
Heatwaves	• Increased risk of death and serious illness principally in older age groups, those with pre-existing cardiorespiratory diseases, and the urban poor
	• Decrease in cold-related mortality (winter deaths) in many temperate countries
Extreme weather events: storms, floods, droughts, cyclones	• Loss of life, injury, psychological distress
	• Greater frequency of infectious disease
Air pollution	• Change in transportation of airborne pollutants (pollen, fossil fuel pollutants)
	• Increased concentration of ground-level ozone
	• Increase in pollutants from forest and rangeland fires, thereby increasing outpatient visits for respiratory disease and eye symptoms
Indirect effects on health	
Food production and supply	• Disruptions or local decreases in food supply lead to malnutrition, particularly in places with poor access to markets
Vector-borne infectious disease	• Altered range and seasonality of transmission of many vector-borne diseases (malaria, Lyme disease, encephalitis)
Waterborne infectious disease	• Heavy rainfall events can transport microbiological agents into drinking water sources (causing cryptosporidiosis, giardiasis, salmonellosis, amoebiasis, typhoid and other infections)
	• Surface temperature anomalies in coastal and inland lake waters have been associated with cholera epidemics
	• Changes in the marine environment may alter risks of bio-toxin poisoning from human consumption of fish and shellfish
Social and economic disruptions	• Displacement of island and coastal populations
	• Loss of shelter after extreme weather events
	• Damage to infrastructure for provision of health services
	• Increased demand for health services

Source: McMichael et al (2003) *Climate Change and Human Health: Risks and Responses*, WHO/WMO/UNEP

climatic elements such as excessive heat or cold temperature, atmospheric concentration of air pollutants or severe storms and flooding events. Other health outcomes will be indirect as a result of the multiple routes and pathways through which old or new disease pathogens are likely to impact people in their communities. For example, the changing climate may alter the ecological characteristics of certain areas, and in the process reduce the agricultural potential of residents in those areas. Changes in temperature and precipitation levels may contribute to the expansion of the geographic range of disease vectors, resulting in a greater incidence of transmissible diseases. These indirect changes may contribute to the displacement of people, economic instability and political unrest, all resulting in the social, psychological and cultural disruption of livelihoods as residents respond to these unexpected changes.

Currently, the availability of concrete data substantiating these health outcomes is relatively limited. The reasons for the delay in epidemiological evidence are due in part to the latency of human disease occurrence, but more importantly to the complex, multifactorial nature of environmental disease causation. The typology of environmental diseases that are likely to emerge from climate change also varies from acute and chronic illnesses, communicable and non-communicable diseases, to nutritional health outcomes and psychological disorders.

Despite the difficulties noted above, evidence regarding the health impacts of environmental and global climate change is gradually beginning to trickle into the public health literature. Accounts of record-breaking temperature extremes have been reported in several cities in the United States and across Europe. In Chicago for example, a five-day heatwave in 1995 resulted in 700 excess deaths, about 85 per cent higher than the number recorded during the same period of the preceding year (Patz et al, 2000). In another study of daily maximum temperature data for Western Europe, the researchers found that over the period 1880 to 2005, the length of summer heatwaves in the region doubled and the frequency of hot days almost tripled (Della-Marta et al, 2007). This was most evident in France where researchers observed that the 6452 excess deaths in 2003, and 2065 excess deaths in 2006 were both caused by heatwaves (Fouillet et al, 2008). These studies are now beginning to unravel the complex web of disease causation, and the specific linkages between climate change and health outcomes. By far the most progress so far has been in the study of emergent/re-emergent infectious diseases, an area that we shall turn to in the next chapter.

Chapter summary

Several environmental health challenges lie ahead as we face the long-term and possibly irreversible consequences of this modern era of climate change. As illustrated in this chapter, climate change along with its current and anticipated health impacts are geographically differentiated, with broad regional impacts but local contextual effects in specific places with disparate risks among various population groups. Tackling these challenges will require the knowledge and analytical expertise of geographers to work with public health professionals and policy makers to delineate the vulnerable areas and develop strategies that can be put in place to minimize, adapt or respond to these pressures. The sole use of computerized analytical tools will not be sufficient, however. Efforts to deal with this problem will require a deeper level of understanding of the local environments and population groups to devise meaningful and cost-effective strategies for global change. In the next chapter, we shall examine some of these efforts using cases studies drawn from the study of West Nile virus and malaria, two emergent and re-emergent diseases associated with global climate change.

References

Adger, W. N. (1999) 'Social vulnerability to climate change and extremes in coastal Vietnam', *World Development*, vol 27, no 2, pp249–269

Asomaning, S. (2008) 'Environmental health hazards: Spatial analysis of New Orleans after Katrina', MA Thesis, Department of Geography, Binghamton University, NY, p120

Confalonieri, U., Menne, B., Akhtar, R., Ebi, K. L., Hauengue, M., Kovats, R. S., Revich, B. and Woodward, A. (2007) 'Human health', in Parry, M. L., Canziani, O. F., Palutikof, J. P., van der Linden, P. J. and Hanson, C. E. (eds) *Climate Change 2007: Impacts, Adaptation and Vulnerability*, Contribution of Working Group II to the Fourth Assessment Report of the Intergovernmental Panel on Climate Change, Cambridge University Press, Cambridge, UK, pp391–431

Cutter, S. (1996) 'Vulnerability to environmental hazards', *Progress in Human Geography*, vol 20, no 4, pp529–539

Cutter, S. L., Mitchell, J. T. and Scott, M. S. (2000) 'Revealing the vulnerability of people and places: A case study of Georgetown county, South Carolina', *Annals of the Association of American Geographers*, vol 90, no 4, pp713–737

Cutter, S. L., Boruff, B. J. and Shirley, W. I. (2003) 'Social vulnerability to environmental hazards', *Social Science Quarterly*, vol 84, no 2, pp242–259

Daszak, P., Cunningham, A. A. and Hyatt, A. D. (2001) 'Anthropogenic environmental change and the emergence of infectious diseases in wildlife', *Acta Tropica*, vol 78, pp103–116

Della-Marta, P. M., Haylock, M. R., Luterbacher, J. and Wanner, H. (2007) 'Doubled length of western European summer heat waves since 1880', *J. Geophys. Res.*, vol 112, ppD15103 doi:10.1029/2007JD008510

Easterling, D. R., Meehl, G. A., Parmesan, C., Changnon, S. A., Karl, T. R. and Mearns, L. O. (2000) 'Climate extremes: Observations, modeling, and impacts', *Science*, vol 289, pp2068–2074

Epstein, P. R. (2001) 'Climate and emerging infectious diseases', *Microbes and Infection*, vol 3, pp747–754

Forster, P., Ramaswamy, V., Artaxo, P., Berntsen, T., Betts, R., Fahey, D. W., Haywood, J., Lean, J., Lowe, D. C., Myhre, G., Nganga, J., Prinn, R., Raga, G., Schulz, M. and Van Dorland, R. (2007) 'Changes in atmospheric constituents and in radiative forcing', in Solomon, S., Qin, D., Manning, M., Chen, Z., Marquis, M., Avery, K. B., Tignor, M. and Miller, H. L. (eds) *Climate Change 2007: The Physical Science Basis*, Contribution of Working Group I to the Fourth Assessment Report of the Intergovernmental Panel on Climate Change, Cambridge University Press, Cambridge, UK and New York, NY

Fouillet, A., Rey, G., Wagner, V., Laaidi, K., Empereur-Bissonnet, P., Le Tertre, A., Frayssinet, P., Bessemoulin, P., Laurent, F., De Crouy-Chanel, P., Jougla, E. and Hémon, D. (2008) 'Has the impact of heat waves on mortality changed in France since the European heat wave of summer 2003? A study of the 2006 heat wave', *International Journal of Epidemiology*, vol 37, pp309–317

Greenough, G., McGeehin, M., Bernard, S., Trtanj, J., Riad, J. and Engelberg, D. (2001) 'The potential impacts of climate variability and change on health impacts of extreme weather events in the United States', *Environmental Health Perspectives*, vol 109, no 2, pp191–198

Hartmann, D. L., Wallace, J. M., Limpasuvan, V., Thompson, D. W. J. and Holton, J. R. (2000) 'Can ozone depletion and global warming interact to produce rapid climate change?', *Proceedings of the National Academy of Sciences*, vol 97, no 4, pp1412–1417

Hegerl, G. C., Zwiers, F. W., Braconnot, P., Gillett, N. P., Luo, Y., Marengo Orsini, J. A., Nicholls, N., Penner, J. E. and Stott, P. A. (2007) 'Understanding and attributing climate change', in Solomon, S., Qin, D., Manning, M., Chen, Z., Marquis, M., Avery, K. B., Tignor, M. and Miller, H. L. (eds) *Climate Change 2007: The Physical Science Basis*, Contribution of Working Group I to the Fourth Assessment Report of the Intergovernmental Panel on Climate Change, Cambridge University Press, Cambridge, UK and New York, NY

Hess, J. J., Malilay, J. N. and Parkinson, A. J. (2008) 'Climate change: The importance of place', *American Journal of Preventive Medicine*, vol 35, no 5, pp468–478

Houghton, R. A. (2005) 'Tropical deforestation as a source of greenhouse gas emissions', in Moutinho, P. and Schwartzman, S. (eds) *Tropical Deforestation and Climate Change*, Amazon Institute for Environmental Research, Belém, Pará, Brazil, pp13–21

Karl, T. R. and Trenberth, K. E. (2003) 'Modern global climate change', *Science*, vol 302, pp1719–1723

McMichael, A. J., Campbell-Lendrum, D. H., Corvalan, C. F., Ebi, K. L., Githeko, A. K., Scheraga, J. D. and Woodward, A. (eds) (2003) *Climate Change and Human Health: Risks and Responses*, WHO document WHO/WMO/UNEP, World Health Organization, Geneva

Patz, J. A. and Kovats, R. S. (2002) 'Hotspots in climate change and human health', *British Medical Journal*, vol 325, no 7372, pp1094–1098

Patz, J. A., Engelberg, D. and Last, J. (2000) 'The effects of changing weather on public health', *Annual Review of Public Health*, vol 21, pp271–307

The Met Office (2009) 'Climate Projections', available at www.metoffice.gov.uk/climatechange/science/projections/, accessed 20 June 2009

7
A Spatial Analysis of Emergent and Re-emergent Public Health Risks

Introduction

Among the list of health challenges associated with global climate change and environmental degradation, the ones with potentially far-reaching health consequences are emerging and re-emerging infectious diseases (ERIDs). ERIDs are diseases of infectious origin that have either increased in incidence or geographic range, recently moved into new host populations, recently been discovered or are caused by newly evolved pathogens (Lederberg et al, 1992; Daszak et al, 2001). Central to the process of identifying such diseases also is the timeline, for which the focus is on those that have either increased since the 1970s or threaten to increase within the near future (Morse, 1995). Table 7.1 shows the timeline of new infections that emerged between the 1970s and 1990s. Added to this list are many re-emergent diseases such as malaria, dengue, tuberculosis, yellow fever and other infections that have surfaced since the initial compilation of these records.

This chapter examines the spatial epidemiological patterns of ERIDs, the ecological risk factors and processes that account for their incidence and the transmission channels through which they spread to new areas and host populations. Emphasis is placed on the geographic technologies that are used to develop the risk maps, evaluate the spatial and temporal dynamics of the diseases, identify the elements of the landscape that influence the disease risk, and how the derived information is used to address the impending health threats among different population groups. Geographic applications in disease control and intervention are illustrated using case studies of the West Nile virus in the United States, and malaria in Sierra Leone.

Spatial–temporal patterns and trends in the evolution of ERIDS

ERIDs have been in the limelight lately because of the recent and dramatic outbreaks of new and re-emerging infectious diseases such as SARs and the H1N1 virus, and the rapid pace with which they are diffusing globally. Severe Acute Respiratory syndrome (SARs) was the first pandemic disease to emerge in

Table 7.1 *Timeline in the identification of emergent diseases and their etiologic agents in the 20th century*

Year	Agent/disease
1973	Rotavirus. Major cause of infantile diarrhoea worldwide
1975	Parvovirus B19 Fifth disease; aplastic crisis in chronic haemolytic anaemia
1976	*Cryptosporidium parvum.* Acute enterocolitis
1977	Ebola virus. Ebola haemorrhagic fever
1977	*Legionella pneumophila.* Legionnaires' disease
1977	Hantaan virus. Haemorrhagic fever with renal syndrome (HFRS)
1977	*Campylobacter* sp. Enteric pathogens distributed globally
1980	Human T-cell lymphotropic virus-I (HTLV I) T-cell lymphoma – leukaemia
1981	*Staphylococcus* toxin. Toxic shock syndrome associated with tampon use
1982	*Escherichia coli* O157:H7. Haemorrhagic colitis; haemolytic uraemic syndrome
1982	HTLV II. Hairy cell leukaemia
1982	*Borrelia burgdorferi.* Lyme disease
1983	Human immunodeficiency virus (HIV). Acquired immunodeficiency syndrome (AIDS)
1983	*Helicobacter pylori.* Gastric ulcers
1988	Human herpesvirus-6 (HHV-6). Roseola subitum
1989	*Ehrlichia chaffeensis.* Human ehrlichiosis
1989	Hepatitis C. Parenterally transmitted non-A, non-B hepatitis
1991	Guanarito virus. Venezuelan haemorrhagic fever
1992	*Vibrio cholera.* O139 New strain associated with epidemic cholera
1992	*Bartonella* (= *Rochalimaea*) *henselae.* Cat-scratch disease; bacillary angiomatosis
1993	Hantavirus isolates. Hantavirus pulmonary syndrome
1994	Sabiá virus. Brazilian haemorrhagic fever

Source: Satcher, 1995

the 21st century. It was first reported in November 2002 in the southern Chinese province of Guangdong, and within six months, it spread globally to more than 30 countries. Approximately 8450 cases were diagnosed around the world with a 10 per cent case fatality rate. Within a couple of years, concerns about SARs were quickly overshadowed by the emergence of the H1N1 virus (swine flu), which was first detected in April 2009, and by August 2009 had infected 177,457 people, killing at least 1462. The disease diffused around the world at an unprecedented rate, originating in Mexico, then the southern United States, and later spread faster than SARs to more than 168 countries in less than six months. Commenting on this trend, Larry Brilliant, a prominent epidemiologist, declared the following:

> *The 2009 swine flu will not be the last and may not be the worst pandemic that we will face in the coming years. Indeed we might be entering the Age of Pandemics. In our lifetimes, or our children's lifetimes, we will face a broad array of dangerous emerging 21st-century diseases, manmade or natural, brand-new or old, newly resistant to our current vaccines and antiviral drugs. You can bet on it.* (Brilliant, 2009)

The Age of Pandemics is clearly on its way since more than 30 diseases have newly emerged or expanded their geographic territories within the last three decades. The incidents involving SARs and H1N1, along with other diseases preceding them such as mad cow disease (BSE) and the West Nile virus, have heightened public awareness of the significant risks for global health in this modern era of globalization, climate and environmental change.

Table 7.2 provides a sample listing of ERIDs, the pathogenic agents involved, the vectors and reservoirs associated with disease incidence and transmission. As noted earlier, one or more of the following parameters are essential in the classification of these diseases:

- raised incidence rates within the last three decades;
- new geographic territories;
- new host populations;
- new scientific discoveries; and
- genetic adaptation of the pathogenic agents.

Diseases such as malaria or yellow fever were once thought to have been contained or eradicated in most regions, but have reappeared, and are now afflicting even greater numbers of people around the world. Others such as the West Nile virus were previously confined to certain world regions, but are now spreading into other areas. SARs, Ebola, BSE, and H1N1 are all relatively new to the human species.

The microbial or pathogenic agents responsible for these diseases are also wide ranging, as illustrated in Table 7.2. The term *microbial traffic* describes the process through which these microbes diffuse from animals to humans, or move from isolated areas to new geographic territories (Morse, 1995). The traffic may be channelled through different processes as depicted in Figure 7.1. The most frequent transmission process for ERIDs is by *zoonosis* as microbial agents move either directly from animal hosts to humans (*direct zoonosis*) or through vectors, primarily arthropods (such as mosquitoes, ticks, flies and fleas) and rodents. Some diseases such as yellow fever are channelled through *anthropo-zoonosis*, a process that is characterized by parallel transmission chains within human and animal hosts, with a likelihood of cross-interaction between the two populations.

Table 7.2 *Examples of ERIDs and the agents and organisms involved in their transmission*

	Disease	Pathogen	Major vector	Reservoir
VIRUSES	West Nile Encephalitis	Flavivirus	Mosquitoes	Birds
	Yellow fever	Togavirus B	Mosquitoes	Monkeys
BACTERIA	Bubonic Plague	*Yersinia pestis*	Fleas	Rodents
	Lyme Disease	*B. burgdorferi*	Ticks	Deer
PROTOZOA	Malaria	Plasmodium	Mosquitoes	Humans
	Trypanosomiasis	*T.gambiense*	Tsetse Fly	Humans/cattle
NEMATODES	Onchoerciasis	*O.volvulus*	Black Fly	Humans
	Elephantiasis	*Brugia malayi*	Snails (*Intermediate Host*)	None

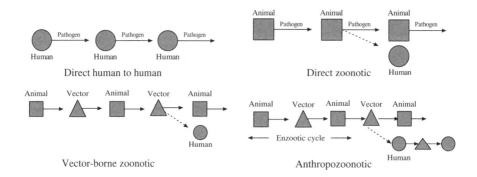

Figure 7.1 *Transmission modes for ERIDs*

Factors contributing to the emergence/re-emergence of infectious diseases

Scientists are continuing to piece together the causal factors that are responsible for the emergence of these diseases (Lederberg et al, 1992; Morse, 1995; Gubler, 1998; Daszak et al, 2001; McMichael et al, 2006; Gayer et al, 2007; Jones et al, 2008). As shown in Table 7.3, one of the leading causes is global environmental degradation and climate change. Climate influences all of the key players in the incidence and transmission of these diseases including the pathogens, vectors, the reservoirs, hosts, and the habitats in which they reside. As Epstein (2001) argues:

> *Climate constrains the range of infectious diseases, while weather affects the timing and intensity of outbreaks. A long term warming trend is encouraging the geographic expansion of several important infections, while extreme weather events are spawning 'clusters' of disease outbreaks and sparking a series of surprises. Ecological changes and economic inequities strongly influence disease patterns. But a warming and unstable climate is playing an ever-increasing role in driving the global emergence, resurgence and redistribution of infectious diseases.* (p747)

Alongside climate change, environmental disturbances, human demographics and risky behaviours are key drivers in the global transmission of ERIDS. Traditional agricultural practices coupled with the poor hygienic conditions in many low-income communities contribute to the ongoing prevalence and, in some areas, the resurgence of endemic diseases such as ascariasis and other geohelminths that together affect billions of people around the world. Deforestation, land conversions, suburban sprawl and encroachment into natural habitats have led to diseases such as Ebola, Marburg, rabies and Lyme disease. There are many more factors and underlying processes at work, however. Global commerce and travel enable the transfer of infectious agents around the world at a pace that exceeds even the incubation periods of the diseases, allowing individuals in the infective stages to transmit the disease.

Table 7.3 *Driving forces and probable factors in the emergence and re-emergence of diseases*

Driving forces	Contributing factors and processes	Emerging or re-emerging diseases
Climate change / environmental disturbances, and ecological changes	Global and regional climate change Weather anomalies: El Niño/ENSO	Malaria and West Nile virus Hantavirus pulmonary syndrome (HPS)
	Drought amplification; natural disasters such as floods	Asthma
	Agriculture/unsanitary household environments lacking access to improved water and sanitation	Geohelminths such as ascariasis
	Pig–duck agriculture: genetic variants and re-assortment of avian and mammalian influenza strains	Pandemic influenza: SARs, H1N1 and other strains
	Irrigation and dam building	Schistosomiasis, onchocersiasis, elephantiasis (filariasis)
	Urban sprawl, land encroachment into natural habitats	Rabies, Lyme disease, Ebola, Marburg
Human demographics and behaviour	Population growth Urbanization, poverty	Malaria Tuberculosis,
	Urban decay, overcrowding	Yellow fever, Lassa fever
	Risky behaviours and lifestyles	HIV/AIDS
	Unprotected sex, intravenous drug use	Hepatitis B and C
	Transfusions, transplantations, contaminated hypodermic apparatus	
Global travel and commerce	Population mobility and migration	Airport malaria, tuberculosis, cholera
	Worldwide movement of goods	Dengue fever, SARs, H1N1,
	Globalization of food supplies	Trypanosomiasis (Chagas)
Technology and industry	Changes in food processing and packaging	Bovine spongiform encephalopathy (BSE)
Microbial adaptation	Drugs causing immune-suppression	Re-emergence of resistant strains of pathogens such as malaria plasmodium parasite
	Widespread use of antibiotics	XDR tuberculosis
	Evolution of new microbes due to adaptation and response to the environment	
Breakdown in public health measures	Curtailment or reduction in prevention programmes. Inadequate sanitation and vector control measures	Resurgence of tuberculosis, cholera, etc.

Source: Morse, 1995

Technology and industry including changes in food production, processing and distribution place more people at risk of contamination. Within the health sector, one also finds several medical practices that have contributed to these challenges such as organ transplantations and blood transfusions, the overuse of antibiotics, along with the breakdown of public health measures in many countries.

Table 7.3 offers examples of ERIDs that have surfaced or resurfaced as a result of all of the aforementioned factors. More recently, additional causes fuelling the expansion of these diseases have been famine, intentional harm or bioterrorism (as in the case of anthrax), conflict situations in many world regions, persistent poverty and social inequalities among population groups, and the lack of political will on the part of governments to take on these challenges (Gayer et al, 2007). Human susceptibility to these emergent diseases has also increased due to the aging population (longer life expectancies) in many developed countries, and the adverse effects of the HIV pandemic which places the infected populations at greater risk of contracting other infectious diseases.

Using geographic perspectives to target vulnerable groups and places

The diffusion of ERIDs at unprecedented levels during this modern era of globalization and environmental change demands the use of innovative approaches to ensure the timely identification of transmissible zones. Along these lines, geographers can assist with the development of public health strategies to cope with these environmental health threats, globally, regionally or locally. In a call for public health preparedness for global change, Hess et al (2008) recently advocated the need to formally incorporate a place-based approach in all frameworks and public health planning strategies that are geared toward addressing these environmental threats. A focus on place, they argued, would emphasize the local nature of both the human exposures and responses to the hazards. A geographical perspective would bring attention to the local areas where the potential effects of climate change would be most acutely felt, and where the motivation to address these issues would be strongest. Such a perspective would also showcase the strengths of local people, enabling these communities to participate in the decision making process by adopting measures that promote sustainability (Hess et al, 2008, p476).

A place-based perspective also enables the use of geographic tools and technologies (geographic information systems (GIS), global positioning systems (GPS), remote sensing, spatial statistics and cartography) to identify the high-risk areas for disease surveillance and intervention. A specific example of how this can be accomplished is through the *landscape epidemiology* approach which relies on geospatial methodologies to delineate the geographic territories of transmissible diseases for disease control and intervention. This approach was first presented by a Russian parasitologist, Eugene Pavlovsky, in the 1960s, during which he made the case that every disease has its own territorial extent (or geographic regionalization). Referring to this as the *doctrine of nidality*, Pavlovsky proposed that the natural habitat (*nidus*) of each transmissible disease can be delineated by overlaying the spatial distribution of the pathogenic agent (virus, bacteria, parasite) with the distribution of the disease vectors, and host populations. Within this distribution range, one can then determine the favourable biophysical and social conditions that favour the survival and transmission of the disease (Pavlovsky, 1966). Pavlovsky's approach is supported by many scholars who argue for a *spatially explicit* approach in the study of emerging diseases (Kitron, 1998; 2000; Plantegenest et al, 2007). As Ostfeld et al (2005) contend, maps that capture both the abiotic and biotic conditions can be used to predict both the contemporaneous risk of the disease and the future change in risks.

With advances in computerized technologies, landscape epidemiological analysis is now commonly performed within a GIS environment. The biophysical characteristics of the landscape that are necessary for maintaining the disease, such as elevation, slope, hydrology, soils, vegetation, temperature and precipitation, are integrated into the GIS database. Also relevant are the demographic indicators and social characteristics such as population density, income, home ownership patterns, racial/ethnic characteristics, land-use patterns and other cultural attributes that favour the transmission of the disease. Using these data layers, the geo-analytical tools are applied to identify, predict or model the spatial patterns of disease risk. The visual associations between the landscape properties and the disease distributions are then validated using statistical methodologies.

Within the literature one comes across many recent examples of the use of this approach in monitoring the spatio-temporal characteristics of ERIDs (Kitron, 1998; 2000; Ostfeld et al, 2005). The landscape epidemiological approach is most valuable when studying diseases that are channelled through haematophagous arthropods with ecological habitats that conform to broad regional patterns. For example, applications could be based on mosquito-borne diseases in warm and humid regions, tick-borne disease in the high latitudes and altitudes, and diseases transmitted by fleas in dry arid environments. Knowledge of the geographic distribution of these vectors, their abundance, vectorial capacity and the ecological niche of the pathogens that they transmit can be incorporated into the spatial analytical applications. Such efforts assist in delineating the territorial extent of disease risks as well as designing the appropriate disease prevention and intervention strategies. Below are examples of such applications in the study of West Nile virus and malaria.

Targeting the high-risk areas for West Nile virus

The West Nile virus (WNv) is a mosquito-borne flavivirus and a human neuropathogen that was first identified in the West Nile district of Uganda in 1937. Though indigenous to several world regions (Africa, the Middle East, Europe, central and west Asia, and Australia), significant outbreaks of the disease have occurred only within the last two decades. Outbreaks of WNv were recorded in Algeria in 1994, Romania 1996, Czech Republic 1997, the Democratic Republic of Congo 1998, Russia 1999 and Israel 2000. In terms of its geographic scope, the most recent public health threat came from the introduction and spatial diffusion of the disease in the United States. The disease first appeared on the east coast of the United States in 1999, and over the course of the next decade, it spread to all states except Hawaii, Alaska and Oregon.

In its new geographic environment, the WNv is maintained primarily by corvid birds (primarily crows and jays), and transmitted to humans and other mammals through the bite of infected adult mosquitoes (mostly the culex species in the United States). Humans and horses are incidental hosts of the disease. However, person to person transmission has been reported in a few instances, occurring through organ transplantation and via mother to child transplacentally or through breastfeeding (Huhn et al, 2003). The most serious clinical manifestation of the disease has been encephalitis (inflammation of the brain) with greater risks of mortality among individuals aged 50 years and older.

The rapid expansion of WNv across the United States in recent years has spurred the development of several GIS-based models to monitor its spatial and temporal spread and predict future outbreaks. One of earliest applications was by Theophilides et al (2003) in which they used a dynamic monitoring system consisting of human and avian fatality records to monitor the changing geography of WNv in New York City. The Dynamic Continuous-Area Space–Time (DYCAST) system was developed as an early warning system for targeted public response to the emerging public health threat in the city. In 2004, Ruiz and others examined the disease risk in the Greater Chicago area, using biophysical attributes such as vegetation cover, elevation range and physiographic regions (Ruiz et al, 2004). Another study used environmental data such as hydrology, slope, soil permeability, vegetation and climate, and road density, as well as avian fatality rates (Cooke et al, 2006). They developed a GIS landscape-based model along with seasonal climatic models to delineate the vulnerable areas in Mississippi. These high-risk areas were characterized by low stream density, gentle slopes and high road density. In Georgia, the study by Gibbs et al (2006) revealed that the spatial patterning of WNv was primarily influenced by physiography, temperature, housing density and urbanization.

In a recent application, Ozdenerol et al (2008) applied GIS and spatial statistical methods, specifically Mahalanobis distance statistics, to identify the areas that are ecologically suitable for sustaining WNv. The study was completed in Shelby county, Tennessee using data layers such as elevation, slope, land use, vegetation density, temperature and precipitation. Avian and mosquito surveillance data along with socio-economic data (race, income and housing occupation) were integrated into the analysis. The study revealed that along with the environmental characteristics, human attributes such as the high percentage of blacks, low income, high rental occupation, old structures and vacant housing were associated with the focal areas of WNv infection cases.

Finally, under the supervision of Margai, Elwell (2006) examined the spatial patterns of the WNv diffusion in Colorado, one of the hardest hit states in the United States in 2003. A total of 2947 cases of the disease were reported that year, constituting almost 30 per cent of the nationwide caseload. In this study, zoonotic and human case count data were integrated into a GIS along with social characteristics (population distribution, urbanization) and physical environmental data (elevation, precipitation, temperature, geological bedrock, soil texture, hydrology and drainage patterns). The spatial pattern of the disease was assessed using two geostatistical methods, Oden's I pop and Kulldorf's Spatial Scan Statistics, to determine whether the cases were randomly distributed or clustered in space. A disease cluster was detected in the eastern half of the state, following which a battery of statistical tests was then performed to determine the ecological and cultural factors behind the observed pattern. The prevalence of the disease was strongly associated with moderate temperatures, and areas with lower elevations. The lack of precipitation, amplified by drought conditions, was also linked to the disease transmission.

The studies reported above represent a small fraction of the geographic applications in recent years to uncover the emerging risk zones of WNv and population vulnerability within the United States. By applying these analytical techniques, geographers have been able to assist public health officials in targeting areas that are ecologically capable of sustaining the disease pathogens and vectors. These efforts have also led to the development of disease control measures based on the location of high infection rates and human case counts. Health education and outreach materials aimed at changing the behaviour of residents to minimize exposure to the disease vectors have been implemented.

Geographical targeting of high-risk areas for malaria transmission

Malaria is a vector-borne parasitic disease that is much more problematic than the West Nile virus. Each year, the disease causes more than 300 million clinical cases, killing nearly 1 million people in addition to other negative health conditions such as low birth weights, maternal anaemia, neurological impairments and other developmental delays in young children. The disease is caused by a single-celled plasmodium parasite. Of the four different plasmodium species, *P. falciparum* is the most widespread and dangerous pathogen. It is transmitted primarily by infective female *Anopheles* mosquitoes. The clinical symptoms of *P. falciparum* malaria include fever, chills, headache, nausea, flu-like symptoms. More adverse effects include anaemia, renal failure, coma and possibly death.

As of 2008, the World Health Organization (WHO) reports that malaria is now endemic in 109 countries, with nearly half of the world's population (3.3 billion) at risk, mostly in sub-Saharan Africa where roughly 90 per cent of all malaria deaths occur. The changing global climate, rising levels of poverty, armed regional conflicts and the scourge of the HIV/AIDs pandemic have all contributed to the persistence of this disease in this region.

Malaria was successfully eradicated in the temperate regions in the 1960s. However, there is a strong possibility of disease resurgence because of the changing physical environment, the remaining presence of the disease vectors, along with increasing international travel. In the United States, for example, malaria is now the most frequently imported disease, with more than 1200 cases reported annually (Skarbinski et al, 2006). Surveillance data summaries obtained for the last two decades indicate a 200 per cent increase in incidence, from 481 imported cases in 1997 to slightly more than 1500 cases in 2007 (see Figure 7.2). The highest incidence of malaria importation often occurs among US civilians (73 per cent) travelling to malarious regions and failing to follow the proper guidelines for prophylactic treatment and disease prevention (Mali et al, 2009). Those visiting Africa (64 per cent), especially West Africa, are at greatest risk of contracting the disease, when compared to travellers to Asia (21 per cent), the Americas (11.3 per cent) and Oceania (2.3 per cent).

Malaria risk assessment using geospatial models

Biological and geospatial models have been used to predict the global transmission of malaria, providing informative data regarding the emergent patterns of the disease (Martens et al, 1995; 1999; Martin and Lebfevre, 1995). Overall, these models have predicted net increases in the global transmission zone of malaria, with a projected rise in the population at risk to about 8 billion by 2080. It is important to note, however, that many of the models have been generated at aggregate (macro) scales, limiting their usefulness at more localized levels. They have also been faulted for overly emphasizing the anticipated changes in temperature without incorporating the contributory role of other factors that influence transmission dynamics such as rainfall, humidity, host exposures and other demographic and socio-economic characteristics (McMichael and Githeko, 2001). Notwithstanding these limitations, the models, overall, provide a valuable starting point for countries to begin

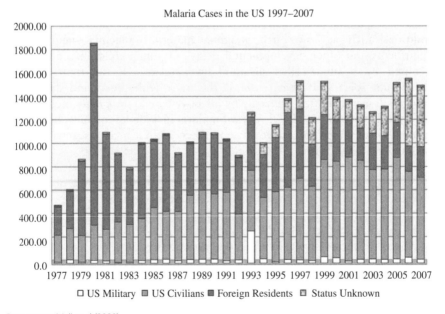

Data source: Mali et al (2009)

Figure 7.2 *Number of cases based on asymptomatic and symptomatic illness in persons with laboratory-confirmed malaria parasitaemia*

developing public health strategies for tackling future malaria risks. Below are more details regarding the spatial transmission patterns predicted in the world's most vulnerable regions.

Models of malaria transmission in developing regions

a. Africa

In a regionally based model developed for Africa, Tanser et al (2003) estimated a 5–7 per cent potential increase (mainly altitudinal) in malaria distribution with only a slight increase anticipated in the latitudinal extents of the disease by 2100. Transmission is projected to decrease in some countries, however; an overall potential increase of 16–28 per cent in person-months of exposure is anticipated, of which a large proportion will be seen in areas of existing transmission.

With the anticipated changes in climate, specifically changes in temperature, rainfall and humidity, the transmission of malaria is likely to expand beyond the low latitudinal areas of the continent to the southern and highland regions. Within the tropical areas, a potential warming trend with higher temperatures exceeding the tolerable limits of the disease agents (pathogens and vectors) is likely to lower transmission rates. However, in cooler parts of these countries, a slight to moderate increase in temperature will potentially increase the risk of transmission. Thus, the predicted warming trend is more likely to heighten the disease risk in the mid-latitudinal and high altitudinal regions, than the low latitudes of Africa.

The results obtained at the more localized geographic scales are much more nuanced both in terms of the projected increase in malaria risk and the drivers of the disease risk. For example, in the highland regions of Africa, several studies conducted during the last decade have linked malaria outbreaks to transient increases in either temperatures and/or rainfall. In the highland regions of Rwanda, Loevinsohn (1994) attributed the localized outbreaks to the observed warming associated with El Niño conditions. In Uganda, highland epidemics were attributed to increases in rainfall, whereas excessive rainfall (associated with El Niño) in Tanzania was credited for flushing out the breeding sites of the anopheles mosquitoes, resulting in lower infection rates. In yet another study conducted in southern Africa, the seasonal changes in malaria cases were significantly linked to climatic variables; however, the long-term trends in the disease were not significantly associated with climate (Craig et al, 2004).

More recently, Li et al (2009) examined the impact of climatic variability on the distribution of mosquito larval habitats in the highlands of Western Kenya. Using geostatistical methods, this study showed significant inter-seasonal and annual variability in the location and distributional patterns of the larval habitats. Similar efforts involving the development of GIS-based malaria information systems have provided more localized trends in malaria risk within African countries (Martin et al, 2002). These research findings underscore the effective use of geographical tools at micro-spatial scales for disease control.

b. Latin America

The linkages between malaria risk and climate change are yet to provide definitive results in Latin America. The results are mixed with limited evidence due to the paucity of historical data on climate and malaria, the complexity of malaria transmission dynamics and the growing importance of non-climatic factors such as socio-economic development, immunity and drug resistance (Confalonieri et al, 2007). In one study of the relationship between El Niño Southern Oscillation (ENSO) events in South America and malaria epidemics, a statistically significant relationship was found in Colombia, Guyana, Peru and Venezuela (Gagnon et al, 2002). The authors concluded that flooding engenders malaria epidemics in the dry coastal region of northern Peru, while droughts favour the development of epidemics in Colombia and Guyana, and epidemics lagged behind a drought by one year in Venezuela. On the other hand in Brazil, French Guiana and Ecuador, they did not detect an ENSO/malaria signal, and non-climatic factors such as insecticide sprayings, variation in availability of anti-malaria drugs, and population migration played a stronger role in malaria epidemics than ENSO-generated climatic anomalies. More detailed investigations are needed in these countries to confirm the influential role of climate change on malaria.

c. Asia

Studies in Asia have been geared more towards malaria risk mapping and vector control. In India, Srivastava et al (2001) used GIS to develop a predictive habitat model for forest malaria vector species. Thematic maps based on forest cover, temperature, rainfall and altitude were used to delineate the areas of disease occurrence at the micro level to enable the implantation of species-specific disease control measures. Klinkenberg et al (2003) also utilized a GIS-based malaria risk mapping approach in Sri Lanka for epidemic forecasting and planning of malaria control activities. Focusing on an irrigated agricultural area, they mapped the malaria cases at the smallest spatial level based on monthly observations over a ten-year period. The analysis revealed that the areas of high risk were best characterized by higher than average rainfall, greater forest coverage; slash and burn cultivation as a predominant agricultural activity; presence of many abandoned irrigation reservoirs; and poor socio-economic status.

Overall, the spatial patterning and the predictive risks of malaria in the world's tropical regions in Africa, Latin America and Asia remain strongly associated with climatic variability and socio-economic factors though there is some disagreement in the scientific evidence garnered so far.

Malaria in Sierra Leone: A case study of prevention and intervention efforts

Geographers have played a major role in the fight against malaria in developing countries. As evident in the preceding section, the bulk of the work completed so far has been through the use of GIS and other spatial analytical tools to produce malaria risk maps and identify the underlying risk factors of the disease (MARA, 1998). Along with the development of these predictive malaria risk models, many scholars are increasingly involved in fieldwork activities to uncover the contextual attributes of the disease including the social, economic and behavioural factors that influence the transmission dynamics of the disease, and the treatment-seeking practices and therapies used by residents in these high-risk communities. One such study was recently undertaken in Sierra Leone, and the results used to develop an intervention programme (Minah and Margai, 2008).

a. Political and socio-economic context

Combating malaria in Sierra Leone has historically been, and continues to be a major challenge. Having emerged recently from a brutal civil war (1991–2002), the country currently is burdened by high poverty levels with very low rankings in global economic classifications such as the Human Development Index (HDI). The war resulted in more than a million immigrants to neighbouring countries of Guinea and Liberia, and roughly 250,000 internally displaced persons (IDPs). With assistance from international organizations, efforts are underway to rebuild the country. However, the progress is very slow and it is widely believed that by 2015, the country will not reach any of the Millennium Development Goals (MDGs) and associated targets. One of those goals (Goal 6) is to combat malaria, with a set target for halting its spread and reversing the currently high prevalence levels.

Malaria is endemic in Sierra Leone with an annual average of one malaria episode per person. The transmission risk of the disease is highest during the months of May through September. In Freetown, the capital city, the outpatient morbidity rate is 40 per cent, with significantly higher rates for pregnant women and under-five children. Although the disease vector density has been shown to be significantly lower in urban areas, residents in these environments are consistently at high risk of contracting the disease.

Sierra Leone participates in an international roll-back malaria programme with the support of various development partners including the WHO, World Bank, United Nations Children's Fund (UNICEF) and United Nations Development Programme (UNDP). But there are many constraints and barriers that hinder the country's progress towards achieving these goals. Rapid urbanization, poverty, low educational attainment, transportation barriers, limited number of health facilities, and outmigration and brain drain of the few reliable health practitioners are only a few of the driving forces.

Recent efforts to combat malaria have been centred largely on the use of insecticide treated nets and conventional drugs. However, given the high rates of poverty, most residents cannot afford the recommended drug therapies (Table 7.4). Instead, many rely on drugs such as chloroquine or fansidar, which are no longer efficacious for *P. falciparum* parasites in this region. The recommended drugs, such as artesunate and lariam, are relatively expensive for residents in poor, endemic regions, with some treatments costing up to $60 per malaria episode.

b. Implementing a community-based intervention programme

In the quest for safe, affordable and effective therapies for malaria, a community-based intervention programme was implemented in 2006

Table 7.4 *Health care costs / efficacy / potential side effects of conventional malaria therapies*

Resochin (chloroquine)	$2.00 – Poor – Hearing impairment
Pyrimenthamin + sulphadoxine (fansidar)	$6.00 – Poor – Allergic reactions
Mefloquine/lariam	$60.00 – High – Cardiac failure, psychosis
Atovaquon + proguanil (malarone)	$60.00 – Limited data – Abdominal problems

(Minah and Margai, 2008). With funding from the Blackie Foundation Trust, the one-year pilot programme was implemented in Kroo Bay, a large urban slum settlement located in the heart of Freetown, the capital city. Kroo Bay, a community with nearly 12,000 people, was selected because of its status as the poorest and most distressed area in the city with significant health risks and high rates of poverty. The community is characterized by unhealthy living conditions with poorly constructed, overcrowded housing, open sewers and unsanitary environmental conditions that heighten the overall risks of infectious diseases (see Figures 7.3a–c).

In an effort to reduce the malaria burden among residents in Kroo Bay, the specific goals of this study were to (i) examine the prevalence of malaria, the severity and duration of the episodes before and after health intervention; (ii) assess the levels of awareness of risk factors, health effects, and knowledge of treatment therapies; and (iii) evaluate the efficacy, costs and benefits of using alternative treatment therapies.

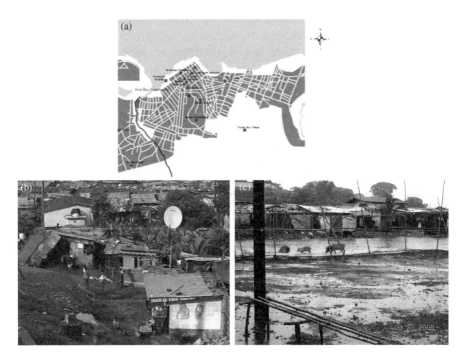

Figure 7.3a to c *The locational and community context of Kroo Bay*

A total of 731 participants registered for the project during the baseline phase. About 73 per cent were females, and the average age was 38.6 years. The participants were first required to complete a questionnaire detailing their personal case histories. They were also asked questions about the symptoms of fever and malaria, the frequency of malaria episodes, and their treatment-seeking patterns during the previous 12 months. Upon completion of the survey, they underwent a comprehensive physical exam including the collection of blood samples to test for malaria.

The baseline results confirmed the prevalence of malaria in the community. Self-reports from patients suggested an average of 3.24 episodes per year, which was high but credible given the environment risk factors of the community. Based on the blood samples, 29 per cent tested positive for malaria with a mean parasitic density of 401/*ul*. About eight of these were clinical cases based on the diagnostic threshold established in the study.

An analysis of the treatment-seeking sources showed that the three most common places they visited were the government hospital (23.8 per cent), local pharmacies (29.6 per cent) and itinerant drug vendors (19.2 per cent). Evidence from the baseline survey also showed ongoing reliance on ineffective malaria therapies. More than half (56.9 per cent) of the participants indicated they used chloroquine and 17.5 per cent used fansidar, both of which were known to have increased parasitic resistance. Only 10 per cent of the patients reported using quinine, the state-recommended therapy at the time (Figure 7.4).

Subjects were also asked about the use of bednets and other devices that assist in malaria prevention. Only 16 per cent had bednets, and other devices used to ward off mosquitoes such as mosquito coils and insecticides were less commonly used in the community.

The information generated in the first phase of the study was used to develop an interventive programme. This was implemented four months later during the second phase of this study. This involved the use of complementary and alternative treatment therapies including homeopathic prophylaxis

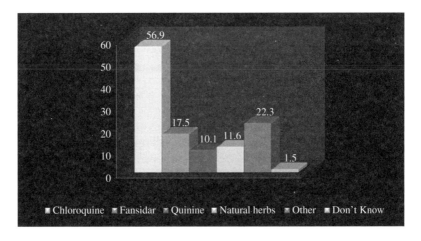

Figure 7.4 *Malaria treatment therapies in Kroo Bay at baseline phase*

Table 7.5 *Comprehensive analysis of blood samples tests across all phases*

Measure: PARASITE				
		PHASES		
			95% Confidence Interval	
PHASES	Mean	Std Error	Lower Bound	Upper Bound
1	76.355	19.790	37.309	115.402
2	23.099	6.786	9.710	36.488
3	18.508	3.432	11.737	25.279
4	7.740	2.143	3.511	11.969

Note: Valid N = 195; results show significant difference in parasitic density between phase I and IV t = 4.125 $p < 0.001$***

(Tropica nosode pellets). Subjects testing negative for malaria were randomized into a treatment and control group and monitored during the next two phases of the study. The treatment effort was also accompanied by intense educational campaigns and community outreach to promote greater public awareness of the dangers and symptoms of malaria, more testing, diagnosis and treatment for malaria, and greater access and utilization of the health care system.

Analysis of the clinical data compiled in the third phase following the intervention revealed promising results with a decline in the mean density of malaria parasites. Over a one-year period, the mean density of malaria parasites decreased from 76.35/*ul* to 7.74/*ul* among all patients (see Table 7.5). A test of the differences observed between the pre- and post-intervention phase confirmed that the observed reduction in malaria parasitic density was statistically significant.

Overall, the results of this pilot intervention programme were promising and provided some indication of the likely benefits of integrating community outreach efforts with affordable treatments and prophylaxes to reduce the burden of malaria in endemic communities. The observed reduction in malaria burden was attributable partly to the aggressive educational campaigns and outreach in the community. Greater public awareness of the dangers and symptoms of malaria, more testing, diagnosis and treatment for malaria, and greater utilization of the health care facilities were all critical to the positive health outcomes observed during the study.

Chapter summary

The emergence/re-emergence of infectious diseases and the rapid pace at which they are diffusing around the world provide a glimpse of the kinds of public health challenges that lie ahead as we begin to face the long-term and possibly irreversible consequences of climate change. Tackling these challenges will require the knowledge and analytical expertise of geographers to work in tandem with public health professionals and policy makers to map out the vulnerable areas and design strategies that can be put in place to minimize, adapt or respond to these pressures. The sole use of computerized analytical tools will not be sufficient, however. Efforts to deal with these challenges will require a deeper level of understanding of the local communities and environmental contexts through fieldwork and site visits. This chapter illustrates the combined use of both strategies for disease control and prevention.

References

Brilliant, L. (2009) 'The Age of Pandemics', *The Wall Street Journal*, 2 May, http://online.wsj.com/article/SB124121965740478983.html, accessed 10 May 2009

Confalonieri, U., Menne, B., Akhtar, R., Ebi, K. L., Hauengue, M., Kovats, R. S., Revich, B. and Woodward, A. (2007) 'Human health', in Parry, M. L., Canziani, O. F., Palutikof, J. P., van der Linden, P. J. and Hanson, C. E. (eds) *Climate Change 2007: Impacts, Adaptation and Vulnerability*, Contribution of Working Group II to the Fourth Assessment Report of the Intergovernmental Panel on Climate Change, Cambridge University Press, Cambridge, UK, pp391–431

Cooke, W., Katarzyna, G. and Wallis, R. C. (2006) 'Avian GIS models signal human risk for West Nile virus in Mississippi', *International Journal of Health Geographics*, vol 5, no 36, doi:10.1186/1476-072X-5-36

Craig, M. H., Kleinschmidt, I., Le Sueur, D. and Sharp, B. L. (2004) 'Exploring 30 years of malaria case data in KwaZulu-Natal, South Africa: Part II. The impact of non-climatic factors', *Tropical Medicine and International Health*, vol 9, no 12, pp1258–1266

Daszak, P., Cunningham, A. A. and Hyatt, A. D. (2001) 'Anthropogenic environmental change and the emergence of infectious diseases in wildlife', *Acta Tropica*, vol 78, no 2, pp103–116

Elwell, G. (2006) 'Spatial analysis of West Nile virus in Colorado, using geographical information systems', MA Thesis, Department of Geography, Binghamton University, NY

Epstein, P. R. (2001) 'Climate and emerging infectious diseases', *Microbes and Infection*, vol 3, pp747–754

Gagnon, A. S., Smoyer-Tomic, K. E. and Bush, A. B. G. (2002) 'The El Niño Southern Oscillation and malaria epidemics in South America', *International Journal of Biometeorology*, vol 46, pp81–89

Gayer, M., Legros, D., Formenty, P. and Connolly, M. A. (2007) 'Conflict and emerging infectious diseases', *Emerging Infectious Diseases*, vol 13, pp1625–1631, available at www.cdc.gov/EID/content/13/11/1625.htm

Gibbs, S. E. J., Wimberly, M. C., Madden, M., Masour, J., Yabsley, M. J. and Stalknecht, D. E. (2006) 'Factors affecting the geographic distribution of West Nile virus in Georgia, USA: 2002–2004', *Vector-Borne and Zoonotic Diseases*, vol 6, no 1, pp73–82

Gubler, D. J. (1998) 'Resurgent vector-borne diseases as a global health problem', *Emerging Infectious Diseases*, vol 4, no 3, pp442–450

Hess, J. J., Malilay, J. N. and Parkinson, A. J. (2008) 'Climate change: The importance of place', *American Journal of Preventive Medicine*, vol 35, no 5, pp468–478

Huhn, G. D., Sejvar, J. J., Montgomery, S. P. and Dworkin, M. S. (2003) 'West Nile Virus in the United States: An update on an emerging infectious disease', *American Family Physician*, vol 68, no 4, pp653–660

Jones, K. E., Patel, N. G., Levy, M. A., Sterygrad, A., Balk, D., Gittleman, J. L. and Daszak, P. (2008) 'Global trends in emerging infectious diseases', *Nature*, vol 451, no 21, pp990–994

Kitron, U. (1998) 'Landscape ecology and epidemiology of vector-borne diseases: Tools for spatial analysis', *J. Med. Entomol.*, vol 35, pp435–445

Kitron, U. (2000) 'Risk maps: Transmission and burden of vector-borne diseases', *Parasitol. Today*, vol 16, pp324–325

Klinkenberg, E., van der Hoek, W. and Amerasinghe, F. P. (2003) 'A malaria risk analysis in an irrigated area in Sri Lanka', *Acta Tropica*, vol 89 (2004), pp215–225

Lederberg, J., Shope, R. E., Oaks, S. E. (eds) (1992) *Emerging Infections: Microbial Threats to Health in the United States*, Committee on Emerging Microbial Threats to Health, Institute of Medicine, National Academy Press, Washington, DC

Li, L., Bian, L., Yakob, L., Zhou, G. and Yan, G. (2009) 'Temporal and spatial stability of *Anopheles gambiae* larval habitat distribution in western Kenya highlands', *International Journal of Health Geographics*, vol 8, no 70

Loevinsohn, M. E. (1994) 'Climate warming and increased malaria in Rwanda', *Lancet*, vol 343, pp714–748

Mali, S., Steele, S., Slutsker, L. and Arguin, P. M. (2009) 'Malaria surveillance: United States', *MMWR Surveillance Summaries*, vol 58 (SS02), pp1–16

MARA (1998) *Towards an Atlas of Malaria Risk. First Technical Report of the MARA/ARMA Collaboration*, Mapping Malaria Risk in Africa / Atlas du Risque de la Malaria en Afrique (MARA/ARMA), Durban, South Africa, p31

Martens, W. J. M., Jetten, T. H., Rotmans, J. and Niessen, L. W. (1995) 'Climate change and vector-borne diseases: A global modelling perspective', *Global Environmental Change*, vol 5, pp195–209

Martens, W. J. M., Kovats, R. S., Nijhof, S., de Vries, P., Livermore, M. T. J., Bradley, D., Cox, J. and McMichael, A. J. (1999) 'Climate change and future populations at risk of malaria', *Global Environmental Change*, vol 9 (supp), S89–107

Martin, C., Curtis, B., Fraser, C. and Sharp, B. (2002) 'The use of a GIS-based malaria information system for malaria research and control in South Africa', *Health and Place*, vol 8, no 4, pp227–236

Martin, P. H. and Lefebvre, M. G. (1995) 'Malaria and climate: Sensitivity of malaria potential transmission to climate', *Ambio*, vol 24, pp200–207

McMichael, A. J. and Githeko, A. (2001) 'Human health', in McCarthy, J., Canziani, O., Leary, N., Dokken, D. and White, K. (eds) *Climate Change 2001: Impacts, Adaptation, and Vulnerability*, Contribution of Working Group II to the Third Assessment Report of the Intergovernmental Panel on Climate Change, Cambridge University Press, New York

McMichael, A. J., Woodruff, R. E. and Hales, S. (2006) 'Climate change and human health: Present and future risks', *Lancet*, vol 367, pp859–869

Minah, J. and Margai, F. M. (2008) 'The use of malaria nosodes to reduce the prevalence of malaria in depressed communities', *International Coethener Exchange ICE 7.InHom 2008*, pp25–29

Morse, S. S. (1995) 'Factors in the emergence of infectious diseases', *Emerging Infectious Diseases*, vol 1, no 1, pp7–15

Ostfeld, R. S., Glass, G. E. and Kessing, F. (2005) 'Spatial epidemiology: An emerging (or re-emerging) discipline', *Trends in Ecology and Evolution*, vol 20, no 6, pp328–336

Ozdenerol, E., Bialkowska-Jelinska, E. and Taff, G. N. (2008) 'Locating suitable habitats for West Nile virus-infected mosquitoes through association of environmental characteristics with infected mosquito locations: A case study in Shelby County, Tennessee', *International Journal of Health Geographics*, vol 7, no 12, doi:10.1186/1476-072X-7-12

Pavlovsky, E. N. (1966) *The Natural Nidality of Transmissible Diseases*, Leveine, N. D. (ed) University of Illinois Press, Urbana, IL

Plantegenest, M., Le May, C. and Fabre, F. (2007) 'Landscape epidemiology of plant diseases', *Journal of the Royal Society Interface*, vol 4, pp963–972

Ruiz, M. O., Tadesco, C., McTighe, T. J., Austin, C. and Kitron, U. (2004) 'Environmental and social determinants of human risk during a West Nile virus outbreak in the greater Chicago area', *International Journal of Health Geographics*, vol 3, no 8

Satcher, D. S. (1995) 'Emerging infections: Getting ahead of the curve', *Emerging Infectious Diseases*, vol 1, no 1, pp1–6

Skarbinski, J., Eliades, M. J., Causer, L. M., Barber, A. M., Mali, S., Nguyen-Dinh, P., Roberts, J. M., Parise, M. E., Slutsker, L. and Newman, R. D. (2006) 'Malaria surveillance: United States, 2004', *MMWR Surveillance Summaries*, 26 May, vol 55 (SS04), pp23–37

Srivastava, A., Nagpal, B., Saxena, R. and Subbarao, S. (2001) 'Predictive habitat modeling for forest malaria vector species *An. dirus* in India: A GIS-based approach', *Current Science*, vol 80, no 9, pp1129–1134

Tanser, F. C., Sharp, B. and le Sueur, D. (2003) 'Potential effect of climate change on malaria transmission in Africa', *Lancet*, vol 362, pp1792–1798

Theophilides, C. N., Ahearn, S. C., Grady, S. and Merlino, M. (2003) 'Identifying West Nile virus risk areas: The Dynamic Continuous-Area Space-Time System', *American Journal of Epidemiology*, vol 157, no 9

8
Toxic Chemicals: Disparate Patterns of Exposure and Health Outcomes

Introduction

One of the mainstays of the modern global economy is the chemicals industry with sales grossing over $1500 billion a year, and accounting for roughly 10 per cent of the trade between countries (OECD, 2001). Using raw materials such as metals, minerals and fossil fuels, this industry produces nearly all synthetic consumer products, including materials that serve as input into a wide array of industrial, agricultural, transportation and construction activities. Estimates show that since the 1930s, global production has increased exponentially, from 1 million to more than 400 million tons a year. At this rate, chemical production is expected to far outpace the world population growth rate in the 21st century, resulting in a higher global chemical output per capita (OECD, 2001).

Alongside the projected rise in the production of chemicals, there are questions regarding their pervasive use and the potentially adverse impacts on human and environmental health. This chapter examines these issues including the properties for characterizing the chemicals and the basis for identifying those chemicals that pose the most serious risks to human health. Using dichlorodiphenyltrichloroethane (DDT) and lead (Pb) as examples, the global production and use of these toxic substances are discussed in relation to their adverse health effects. A case study is presented to illustrate the use of geospatial approaches in evaluating the distributional patterns of the chemicals and population health disparities.

Global chemical production and use: Key concerns about public safety

The increasing production and use of synthetic materials from the chemicals industry is a global economic activity with widespread appeal in all countries regardless of the level of development. An Organisation for Economic Co-operation and Development (OECD) report released earlier this decade showed a large inventory of products consisting of: (i) basic chemicals and commodity chemicals; (ii) consumer care products (such as soaps, detergents, cosmetics, household cleaning agents); (iii) speciality chemicals (such as sealants, adhesives, catalysts, plastic additives, etc.); and (iv) more advanced materials derived from the life science industries (such as pharmaceuticals, pesticides and biotechnology). Some of these materials are reformulated to generate additional products or sold to other industries (OECD, 2001, p10).

Nearly every country now has a chemical industry with some producing only the basic necessities for their populace, while others offer more advanced and varied products for global export. The bulk of the production (80 per cent) and trade occurs among the developed countries with the United States, Germany and Japan serving as the leading producers. However, as more countries become technologically advanced, the demand, production and use of these chemicals will grow even faster, increasing the risks of human exposure and the likelihood of chemically induced diseases. The major concerns regarding their use are noted below:

1. Increasing volume and complexity of the chemicals

For nearly two decades now, scientists have raised questions about the unbridled growth and environmental safety of these chemicals (NRC, 1984; Greenberg, 1986; Moore, 1999). Each year, about 1500 to 2000 new formulations are produced globally in addition to the current inventory of between 80,000 to 100,000 chemicals in regular use (Holt, 2000). The problem is compounded further by the increasing complexity of the chemicals as the industry responds to growing demand and pressure for innovative and life-saving products.

2. Inadequate screening of chemicals

A second and related area of concern has to do with the inadequate screening of the new chemicals prior to consumer use. Though many of the chemicals are believed to be hazardous and are increasingly being detected in humans based on biomonitoring studies, minimal research is done prior to market release to evaluate their toxicological effects, or the synergistic effects that might arise following their combined use with other consumer products. Among the few chemicals that are tested, knowledge regarding their toxicity is sometimes incomplete, requiring the collection of more data over a longer time period. In other situations, the research findings are unreliable due to the use of animal experiments. It is difficult to fully extrapolate the experimental results to humans because the physiological characteristics, metabolic and immunologic systems of lab animals differ significantly from human beings (Greenberg, 1986). Similarly, while useful for screening the chemicals, in-vitro science may not be entirely helpful in extrapolating the direct effects of these chemicals on humans.

These scientific concerns were first brought to light in 1984 when the National Research Council (NRC) examined a select inventory of 65,725 chemicals used in the United States. The listing consisted of several categories of chemicals regulated by the federal government including pesticides and related by-products, drugs and other formulations in the health care industry, food additives, cosmetics and several other chemicals used in commerce. A stratified random sample of 675 of these chemicals was then selected for more detailed investigation. Overall, the study revealed that a significant proportion of the substances in the various categories had no toxicity information. The category that was most affected, for which 82 per cent of information was lacking, was associated with chemicals used in commerce. Virtually no testing had been done to evaluate their toxicological profiles, particularly for chronic and reproductive/developmental health effects. The study also showed that toxicity information was missing for 25 per cent of consumer drugs or related formulations, as with 38 per cent of the pesticides and related products, 46 per cent of food additives and 56 per cent of the cosmetics (NRC, 1984).

Since the completion of the NRC study nearly two decades ago, remarkable improvements have occurred in the field of toxicity testing. An updated report released by the NRC (2007) points to advances in bioinformatics, development of toxico-kinetic models and computational toxicology, all of which have now expanded the knowledge base regarding the hazardousness of chemicals and their potential health impacts. The scientists acknowledged that more work still lies ahead, however, to keep up with the rapid pace of production and annual release of new products in the global marketplace.

3. Global ubiquity of chemicals

Natural geochemical processes such as weathering, volcanism and hydrothermal activities contribute to environmental releases; however, the majority of the chemicals in use today are produced anthropogenically (Holt, 2000). These releases occur at several stages of the life cycle of the chemicals, literally from cradle to grave. Emissions occur from the extraction/mining stage, to manufacturing and formulation of the products. The chemicals are also released through different end-uses, industrial, agricultural, transportation and construction activities, leading to the eventual disposal in illegal dumps or landfills. During each of these stages, environmental discharges are likely to occur through volatilization, site leaching, hazardous spills and accidents. Individuals are exposed to these chemicals through the different environmental media or pathways: indoor and outdoor air pollution, contaminated surface or groundwater, soil, food, medications, consumer products or any combination of these. The routes or modes of entry of these chemicals into the human body include inhalation, ingestion, dermal absorption and radiation. Some chemicals are of greater concern than others because of the multiple exposure pathways and routes of entry into the human body. Following below is a discussion of the key properties used to characterize their likely impacts on human health.

Chemicals of concern: Evaluating toxicity, persistence and bioaccumulation

Among the thousands of substances that are produced yearly by the chemical industry, there are definitely some that are more harmful than others. The most important properties used to differentiate among the chemicals in terms of their overall impacts on human health and ecosystems are (i) persistence; (ii) bioaccumulation; and (iii) toxicity (PBT). This PBT model is used extensively in the international, regional and national policy arena to screen chemical hazards and designate priority contaminants for environmental monitoring and regulation. In the United States, about 650 chemicals are included on a list that is monitored by the Environmental Protection Agency (EPA), the first national governmental agency to institute a toxic chemical regulatory programme. A chemical is added to this list if it poses unreasonable risk to human and environmental health because of its toxicity, persistence or tendency to bioaccumulate in the environment. This list is continually upgraded to incorporate new substances as knowledge of their inherent risks becomes known. For example, in 2009, the EPA added four new synthetic chemicals deemed to be of serious risk to human health: phthalates, long-chain perfluorinated chemicals (PFCs), polybrominated diphenyl ethers (PBDEs) in products, and short-chain chlorinated paraffins (SCCPs). These chemicals are used in many consumer products: as plasticizers to improve the durability and flexibility of plastics, as flame retardants, coolants, lubricants and sealants, and as non-stick coatings and stain/water resistant surfacing in cooking utensils, textiles and food packaging (USEPA, 2009). Along with other substances on the regulatory list compiled by the government, biomonitoring studies show that these chemicals are environmentally persistent and bioaccumulative, with toxic effects on human health, laboratory animals and wildlife. Following is a brief discussion of these properties.

Toxicity

A chemical is classified as a toxic substance if it is known to cause significantly adverse health consequences when it interacts with humans, animals or the environment. The health effects that are typically under consideration are cancer and other teratogenic effects, serious or irreversible health problems (such as reproductive dysfunctions, developmental disabilities, genetic mutations, neurological disorders) and other chronic conditions. The toxicological effects depend on the properties of the chemical, the dose and concentration level, the duration and route of exposure, the personal characteristics of the individual exposed, and the additive, interactive or synergistic interactions with other chemicals in the human body (Moore, 1999).

Scientific evidence suggests that children are the most susceptible to chemical toxicity and the most likely to suffer irreparable harm from exposure (Margai et al, 1997; Moore, 1999; Landrigan et al, 2004). Among the features that make children uniquely vulnerable to these toxicants are their physiological and metabolic systems. Children breathe faster and consume more food and water per pound of their body weight than adults. Their kinetic processes, along with their increased hand to mouth activity, and their ability to play close to the ground enhance their risk of greater rate of uptake and ingestion of toxins in their surroundings than adults (Landrigan et al, 2004). The physiological characteristics of children also place them at greater risks of toxic exposure. Specifically, when compared to adults, the neurological systems, endocrine systems, detoxifying systems (liver, kidneys) and metabolic pathways of children are not fully developed (Moore, 1999). Consequently, they are more likely to retain larger proportions of toxins than their adult counterparts.

The physiological disadvantages of children are most evident during the fetal and perinatal stages of development and disappear gradually with age. Children also have many more future years of life than adults and thus their exposure to environmental agents in early life is more likely to translate into poor health outcomes in the latter stages of life. These paediatric health risks are even greater among low-income, underrepresented populations residing in urbanized environments where toxic chemicals are widely used in different sectors. Scientists concerned about these paediatric health geographies have recently called for new approaches that incorporate the unique vulnerabilities of children in toxicity testing (Landrigan et al, 2004).

Persistence

Many of the toxic substances included on governmental watch lists are also very stable chemically and biochemically. The term *persistence* is used to describe the degradation half-life of such chemicals, or their average residence time within the environment or the human body. Persistence reflects how long a given chemical is likely to remain within the human body, or its ability to remain unchanged in its original form in any environmental medium. The most commonly used metric for evaluating this chemical property is the half-life, $t_{1/2}$, which is the time required for the concentration of the chemical to diminish to half of its original value within a single medium (such as human tissue, blood, hair, contaminated soil, air or water), or multiple media. Scientific studies using multimedia models show that depending on the fate processes, the half-life of a chemical is most likely to be independent of the quantity introduced in the environment and whether the introduction is in a steady (continuous) or unsteady state (Mackay and Webster, 2006). Generally, the longer the half-life of a chemical, the more resistant and more stable it is in the body or the environment (Ray and Trieff, 1980). Such chemicals are therefore more likely to pose serious risks to human health and ecosystems than those that are easily biodegradable.

Bioaccumulation

The third metric used by government agencies to evaluate the hazardousness of chemicals is bioaccumulation. This is the process through which a chemical increases in concentration within a person (or other living organisms) as it makes its way through multiple routes and environmental pathways. The result is a higher concentration of the contaminant within the person (or organism) over time, when compared to the observed concentration level in his/her surrounding environment. Kinetic processes such as absorption, distribution, metabolism and elimination (ADME) determine the extent to which chemicals accumulate in various organisms (Nichols et al, 2009). Certain compounds are more likely to bioaccumulate when they are absorbed and stored faster than the rate at which they are metabolized or eliminated from the body.

Chemical solubility and lipophilicity are also important properties that influence the extent to which a given chemical is bioaccumulative. A chemical that is highly soluble in water is more likely to be quickly removed in the urine, rather than be incorporated into the bodily tissues of an organism. On the other hand, a chemical that exhibits the property of lipophilicity is soluble in fat. Examples include DDT and other hydrocarbons, which are more easily transported and distributed across various membranes in the human body, including the placental barrier and the blood–brain barrier. They also tend to accumulate easily in the fatty tissues of the body, resulting in greater concentrations over time (Ray and Trieff, 1980).

A concept related to bioaccumulation is biomagnification, which occurs when the concentration of a chemical increases as it goes through successive levels of the food web. Among the many factors that impact this process are: the number of links in the food web; the kinds of organisms in the web; the type of compound that is being bioaccumulated; the dose of each substance at each level of the food web and the amount of time that the organism was in contact with the contaminant (Ray and Trieff, 1980). Many chemicals exhibit the dual properties of bioaccumulation and biomagnifications: PCB (polychlorinated biphenyls) and DDT are two great examples.

In the remaining sections of this chapter, we shall discuss the health risks associated with two substances: DDT, a synthetic compound, and lead (Pb), a naturally occurring heavy metal. These have been selected as examples of chemicals exhibiting the properties of persistence, bioaccumulation and toxicity. We shall discuss the trends in global production and use, and the related health impacts documented in both developed and developing countries.

DDT: Global trends in production and use, and the environmental health implications

Like some of the biological emerging and re-emerging infectious diseases (ERIDS) discussed previously in Chapter 7, DDT is a chemical pathogen that is re-emerging globally as a public health threat (see Figure 8.1). Concerns about this chemical hazard have resurfaced as a result of its growing use to fight malaria and other arthropod-borne diseases (Van den Berg, 2008). Recent statistics suggest a gradual rise in global production of DDT from 5000 tons in 2005 to nearly 6500 tons in 2007. The increase is occurring mostly in anticipation of the growing demand for insecticide applications in developing countries (Van den Berg, 2008).

India, China and North Korea are the main producers of DDT; however, the chemical is being used for disease control in at least 14 countries, and plans are underway to reintroduce it in others. The revival of DDT is largely due to a position statement issued by the World Health Organization (WHO) in 2006 promulgating the use of indoor residual spraying (IRS) as a major interventive approach for malaria control. DDT was among the list of 12 insecticides recommended for IRS (WHO, 2007). The chemical is deemed the least expensive in combating malaria in holoendemic regions with long/continuous transmission periods. It has a long residual efficacy of about 6–12 months when sprayed indoors.

In a cost comparison study, the average cost of DDT use was estimated at only $1.6 per house per six months, more than ten times lower than other

Global status of DDT: Production and usage

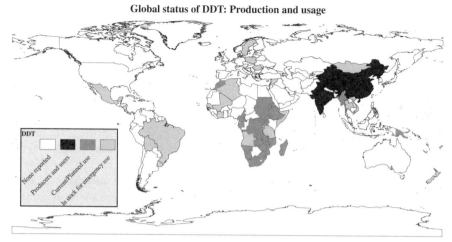

Data source: Van den Berg (2008) 'Global status of DDT and its alternatives for use in vector control to prevent disease', prepared for the Secretariat of United Nations Environment Programme, UNEP/POPS/DDTBP.1/2. Stockholm Convention

Produced by Margai (2009)

Figure 8.1 *DDT global production and usage*

chemicals recommended by WHO (Sadasivaiah et al, 2007). Proponents of DDT cite additional benefits such as its ability to repel mosquitoes. By deterring the entry of mosquitoes into treated dwellings, the end result will be lower feeding rates, shorter resting periods and subsequently lower disease transmission rates. Further support for the use of this chemical in disease prevention efforts has come from other international agencies and programmes like the Presidential Malaria Initiative (PMI) established in 2005 by the former US President, George W. Bush. DDT use has subsequently increased as reflected in 2007, the year for which the most recent data are available; nearly 4000 tons of the chemical were sprayed on the ceiling and walls of residential structures in malarious regions, mostly in Africa and India.

Prior to the 2006 WHO endorsement, the global production and use of DDT was prohibited under the 2001 Stockholm Convention, an international agreement designed to eliminate the use of persistent organic pollutants (POPs). DDT was one of 12 chemicals or compounds included on the priority list of POPs. However, amid concerns regarding the intractable burden of malaria and its likely re-emergence with changing global climate, a decision was made to rescind the ban on DDT and allow its limited production and use within the public health sector.

Knowledge of the ensuing controversy over the reintroduction of DDT in the global market requires some understanding of its history, chemical properties and potential health risks. This chemical dates as far back as the 1870s when it was first formulated (Turusov et al, 2002). However, it was not until the late 1930s, nearly six decades later, that its beneficial properties as a powerful insecticide were first realized. Subsequent testing confirming its efficacy led to its widespread use in the 1940s, during and after WWII. In the

United States, DDT use increased to as high as 80 billion pounds in 1959, with applications in different economic sectors. Additional formulations of the chemical led to at least 334 registered products in agriculture alone (Ray and Treiff, 1980; Sadasivaiah et al, 2007).

Concerns about the safety of DDT gained national and global attention after the 1962 publication of the *Silent Spring* by Rachel Carson. Mounting evidence from many studies thereafter confirmed that DDT, along with its primary metabolite DDE (*dichlorodiphenyldichloroethylene*), embodies all of the dangerous properties of hazardous chemicals discussed earlier. It is highly persistent in all environmental media with a half-life of three to ten years within soils. The risk of exposure to humans was first thought to be highest within residues in agricultural produce. However, more recent findings suggest that the exposure levels from indoor spraying in malarious areas are significantly greater through inhalation and dermal contact with sprayed walls, in addition to the traditional routes of entry through the ingestion of contaminated food and water (Sadasivaiah et al, 2007). DDT, and its metabolites, also exhibit the property of lipophilicity, implying a greater tendency to bioaccumulate and biomagnify within organisms and the food web. Studies documenting these impacts in the developed world have shown how the concentration levels would start off as low as 0.00005 ppm (parts per million) in water, and subsequently rise to measurable quantities at successive levels of the food chain, from plankton to fish, reaching as high as 27 ppm in predatory birds (Ray and Treiff, 1980). Impacts on wildlife, including the thinning of bird egg shells, the shrinking of their brains and other poor outcomes have been attributed to these higher concentration levels. In humans, the health effects attributed to DDT and related metabolites include adverse reproductive outcomes (early pregnancy loss, birth defects, pre-term births, low birth weights, impaired semen quality in men), leukaemia, pancreatic cancer and breast cancer, diabetes and neuro-developmental deficits. Evidence about the toxicological effects of these chemicals, though conflicting at times, led to a US federal ban on most applications in 1972. Many countries followed suit thereafter, resulting in the aforementioned Stockholm agreement.

Today, the resurgence of DDT as a valuable chemical for malaria control is contentious. While it is considered to be cost-effective in developing regions, many believe that priority should be given to safer alternatives and DDT should only be used a last resort. Sadly, the individuals who are at risk of suffering irreparable harm are the poor who are largely unaware of the inherent dangers of the chemicals. The few studies completed so far in these marginalized communities corroborate the health effects documented earlier in the developed world. These risks are unlikely to be confined to the poor rural communities, however. Increasing news accounts from reporters around the world, including a recent United Nations Environment Programme (UNEP) report (Van den Berg, 2008) suggest the illegal trafficking and use of DDT in other sectors. There are reports of DDT being traded on local markets for use in agriculture, being used for pest control in other settings such as libraries, and in fishing. The presence of DDT residues in fruits and vegetables have also been reported in countries such as India (Jayashree, 2009), a clear indication of an emerging cycle of poison.

Data from UNEP also show that many other countries, beyond those who currently produce or use the chemical, have purchased and retained measurable quantities of the chemical for use in the event of a malaria outbreak (Van den Berg, 2008). Syria reportedly has about 1575 tons, Poland 404 tons, Japan 943 tons and Cote d'Ivoire 1125 tons of the chemicals. Over time, these stockpiles will become obsolete, limiting their effectiveness for disease control. But even more disconcerting is the fact that there is no systematic means of tracking these stockpiles. Further, many of these countries do not have legislation in place nor the technological know-how to properly dispose of these materials. So overall, while the original intent of the WHO to reintroduce DDT for malaria control is well meaning and good, it has reopened the door to a global environmental health problem that is likely to remain with us for decades. A silver lining is that the WHO hopes to reduce its reliance on the chemical for IRS over time, with a proposed 30 per cent cut in the application worldwide by 2014 and a total phase-out by the early 2020s. Along with this, biomonitoring studies are needed to track the long-term health of residents in the countries where the DDT-based IRS approaches are being used. A concerted effort to prevent the use of this chemical in non-medical sectors is also necessary to minimize its re-entry into the food chain.

Global trends in environmental lead contamination and related health impacts

Like DDT, lead (Pb) embodies all of the distinctive properties of the world's most significant chemical hazards. It is the second most important chemical health hazard (after indoor pollution), causing about 1 per cent of the global burden of disease (Levy and Sidel, 2006). It is ubiquitous, persistent and bioaccumulative, and has long been recognized as a protoplasmic poison with the ability to interfere with several functions of the human body. The health impacts of lead exposure have been known for centuries, yet it remains one of the most commonly used substances around the world.

Unlike DDT, which is a synthetic chemical, lead is a naturally occurring heavy metal found within the Earth's crust. It is dispersed in small amounts by natural biogeochemical processes; however, human activities dating as far back as the Roman times account for the bulk of the environmental releases. Specifically, lead's versatility as a primary and secondary material accounts for its widespread use and application in nearly every human activity: industrial and commercial operations, mining, transportation, agriculture, domestic, cosmetic and medical applications. Until recently, industrial emissions from foundries, smelters and battery recycling plants, and gasoline additives contributed the most to these releases. Other significant sources worldwide included lead-based paints, lead pipes in homes, cooking utensils and food storage containers, cosmetics and folk remedies. Global consumption of lead increased steadily for decades reaching about 5.6 million tons by 1990, with the largest increases occurring more recently among the developing countries (Tong et al, 2000).

A comparison of the human lead burden shows a dramatic increase in lead risk over the last several centuries with a 500–1000 times difference between the lead levels observed in human bodies now, and those observed in the skeletal remains of humans during the pre-industrial age (0.0016μg/dl). The major route of lead absorption for both children and adults is the gastrointestinal tract with 90 per cent of the uptake occurring via food and water, and 10 per cent from the air. Within the human body, lead has no known biological function other than to mimic the biochemical effects of calcium and iron. It is persistent, with a long half-life of ten or more years, and bioaccumulative, with a tendency to be deposited primarily in the bones and teeth of individuals (Pier and Bang, 1980; Meyer et al, 2008).

The toxic impacts of lead are widespread in the human body with significant effects on the nervous, haematopoietic, endocrine, renal and reproductive systems (Centers for Disease Control and Prevention (CDC), 1991). As with most chemicals, the severity of these effects depends on the amount of exposure, the rate of absorption and the extent to which it is circulated within the human body. With low concentration levels, the preliminary effects may be asymptomatic but get progressively worse with cumulative levels of exposure. Evidence of the health effects of lead exposure have been garnered primarily from developed countries. These impacts include blood disorders and long-term irreversible health problems such as cognitive, neurological, learning and developmental impairments, behavioural disorders, juvenile delinquency and criminal behaviour (Needleman et al, 1990; Schwartz, 1994; Lanphear et al, 2000; Canfield et al, 2003; Margai and Henry, 2003; Needleman, 2004; Lidsky and Schneider, 2006).

Lead toxicity in the United States and other developed countries

A wealth of data collected by scholars in many disciplines has shown that children, especially in marginalized communities, are more vulnerable to lead toxicants than adults. Disparities in lead exposure exist by location, race, ethnicity, housing and economic status (Sargent et al, 1995; Margai and Henry, 2003; Oyana and Margai, 2007). The risks are greatest in the global cities with old housing stock in historic neighbourhoods and those with a legacy of heavy manufacturing and transportation activities (Bailey et al, 1994; Griffith et al, 1998; Jacobs et al, 2002). Children from low-income, migrant or minority families who reside in these older and often poorly maintained rental properties face the greatest risks of lead poisoning.

In the United States, the characterization of lead as a public health hazard and the designation of the federal threshold level above which medical action is required went through several iterations. The first official acknowledgement of lead as an environmental health hazard was in 1967, when the Surgeon General recommended an early screening programme for children. As new information regarding the hazardous effects of the chemical became available, the federal threshold for 'elevated' blood lead level (BLL) was lowered from 60 micrograms per decilitre (μg/dl) in the 1960s, to 40μg/dl in 1971, to 30μg/dl in 1978, to 25μg/dl in 1985, and finally to 10μg/dl in 1991 (the limit also recommended by the WHO in 1995). The passage of the Lead-Based Paint Poisoning Prevention Act in 1972 also resulted in a mandatory mass blood lead screening of children, followed by a 1978 amendment banning the use of lead-based paint in homes.

Additional measures taken over the years have included lead awareness and prevention programmes in local communities, and regulatory and voluntary bans on the use of consumer products containing lead.

Surveillance data garnered from different health agencies across the United States show a steep decline (84 per cent) in childhood elevated BLLs (Jones et al, 2009). Only 1.4 per cent of these children are now estimated to have blood lead levels $\geq 10\mu g/dl$. There are still widespread health disparities by race and ethnicity, however. Black children continue to have higher levels relative to white children. In Chicago Oyana and Margai (2010) documented some overall success in reducing childhood elevated BLLs but the racial/ethnic disparities remain. The study examined the temporal and spatial dynamics of the disease among children aged five years and less. Using large-scale screening data covering 1 January 1997 through 31 December 2003, the results showed a significant reduction in elevated BLL ($\geq 10\mu g/dl$) during the study period. However, children residing in neighbourhoods on the city's west and south sides with a high concentration of minorities consistently had the highest prevalence rates of elevated BLLs.

In other developed countries, though many of the studies conducted so far have failed to address BLL prevalence levels by race, ethnicity or class, reports of geographical disparities in the distribution of lead contaminants have been documented (Zeitz et al, 2001; Chandramouli, 2009). Zeitz et al (2009) examined the regional differences in the frequency of tap water contamination found in the lower Saxony region of Germany. At least 7.5 per cent of the homes had lead concentrations above the recommended threshold limit of $10\mu g/dl$. Families residing in multi-family houses were more frequently affected than those residing in single and double family dwellings.

Lead toxicity in developing countries

Researchers have also explored the distributional patterns of lead poisoning hazards in developing countries. Elevated BLLs in these countries are even more disturbing with more varied sources of exposure than those observed in the developed countries. Lead mining, smelting, lead-acid battery processing factories, metal recyclers, flour mills, cottage industries, and until recently, leaded gasoline, have been the most commonly reported sources of exposure. Poor zoning laws with industrial facilities located next to residential areas, high population density near transportation corridors, near-obsolete, old and poor quality vehicles, hot climates and dusty conditions amplify the risks (Falk, 2003). The risks of exposure are high in both the poor communities and the more traditional urbanized centres.

In rapidly industrializing countries such as China and India, high lead levels have been observed in the urbanized environments, as well as the small communities that host the cottage industries, small factories and recycling workshops. Risks of lead exposure in China, in particular, are being closely followed by the international media due to the increasing number of lead tainted consumer products, especially children's toys and jewellery. Part of the problem in China is linked to the large volume of lead in the country. China leads the world in both the mining and production of lead (Lee and Chen,

2008). In 1999, leaded gasoline was banned, but there are still reports of its availability in the western provinces (Washam, 2002). Significant amounts of lead also originate from the processing of electronic wastes (e-wastes), a primary source of income in some of the communities in southern China. For example, in Giuyu, a popular destination of global e-wastes, about 60–80 per cent of the families work in e-waste cottage industries. Hou et al's (2007) study of BLL prevalence levels in this community found 81 per cent of the children (aged six years and above) had unsafe BLLs. Regional variations in lead levels have also being reported, with exposure levels higher among those residing in the urban and industrial areas than those in the rural areas (Wang and Zhang, 2006).

In Latin America and the Caribbean Islands, vehicular lead emissions were previously a major health risk but a 1997 study revealed that at least 46 per cent of the countries, mostly in Latin America, had introduced unleaded gasoline (Romieu et al, 1997). At the time, other countries in Central America and the Caribbean were working toward the implementation of a gasoline lead control programme. The other primary risk sources of lead were from fixed sources (lead battery processing, lead wire and pipe factories, metal foundries, petrochemical plants, scrap and metal solid wastes, and mines), lead-based paint, ceramic-glazed food containers and water pollution (Romieu et al, 1997; Mañay et al, 2008). The analysis of lead content in environmental samples collected from 14 countries in this region showed that some of the levels far exceeded international standards. Prevalence data showed that the proportion of children with elevated BLLs ($10\mu g/dl$) ranged from 45 per cent to 100 per cent, with the highest levels observed among those residing in close proximity to fixed sources of lead emissions (Romieu et al, 1997).

In Africa, the study by Nriagu et al (1996) was among the first to provide a glimpse of the inherent risks of childhood lead poisoning across the continent. The primary risk sources of lead pollution identified in this study were from mining and smelting operations (54 per cent) and from the use of leaded gasoline (41 per cent). At the time of the study, Nriagu et al (1996) reported that the use of leaded gasoline in Africa was the highest globally, due in part to the large volume of used and near-obsolete vehicles imported from the developed world. Further, the predominance of home-lead cottage industries and the use of unregulated paint formulations contribute to the high levels of environmental lead. Lead is also used in certain folk medicines and cosmetics with related formulations known as 'tiro', 'kohl uhie', or 'moju' among different ethnic groups. Some of these products reportedly have lead concentration levels as high as 81 per cent (Healy et al, 1984; Nnorom et al, 2005).

Though limited in scope, studies of lead prevalence among the residents in African communities reveal alarming rates. Nriagu et al (1996) summarized the results of several studies including one report of a 100 per cent elevated BLL prevalence among children up to two years old, and 82 per cent among three to five year olds residing in an urbanized area. In another study, 93 per cent and 100 per cent of the children in Cape Province, South Africa had elevated lead levels. Among school children in Kumasi, Ghana, the lead levels observed ranged from 28 to $32\mu g/dl$, far greater than the allowable levels.

A decade has gone by since these preliminary studies were conducted in Africa. Since then, significant strides have been made by these countries to phase out leaded gasoline. Starting out initially in 2003, and continuing on till 2007, many countries have shifted to fully unleaded gasoline. However, given the persistence of lead in the environment, it will likely take decades before the beneficial effects of these measures are realized. Olewe et al's (2009) study of the Kibera slums in Nairobi provides encouraging results with only 7 per cent of the children tested having elevated BLLs. But ongoing exposure to low but cumulative doses of this neurotoxicant will undoubtedly produce long-term irreparable health problems in the population. Experts warn that given the prevalence of sickle cell anaemia in this region, increasing levels of childhood lead toxicity will likely exacerbate the anaemic conditions suffered by those afflicted with the disease, resulting in even worse clinical symptoms than those manifested in the developed countries.

Eliminating the use of lead gasoline is only a first step toward the reduction of the exposure risks. Health agencies in these African countries must follow the lead taken by the developed countries to implement lead hazard abatement programmes that target all of the primary risk sources. Following below in this final section of this chapter is a case study documenting the use of geographic and statistical approaches to monitor the multiple pathways of lead exposure and paediatric health impacts.

Assessing the risk sources and health effects of paediatric lead exposure: A case study

While there has been progress in reducing the elevated BLLs among children, there are still significant sources of lead in the environment in both the developed and developing countries. These sources (including lead in paint, soil and dust) are closely linked to the historical processes of urbanization and industrialization and account for the variations in lead poisoning across geographic landscapes. Figure 8.2 illustrates the relationships between the various sources of paediatric exposure as documented in the studies reviewed earlier. There are also a number of spatial indicators or associative factors that may indirectly show where the risk areas are. These include the socio-economic attributes, dwelling type, age and quality, proximity to major transportation corridors, and proximity to sites emitting lead into the atmosphere. In this final section of the chapter, we shall examine the approaches used in a previous study to explore the associations between these multiple sources of childhood lead contamination in a built-up urban environment.

The project had both short-term and long-term goals. First, we sought to show the distributional pattern of elevated BLLs among children and test for possible associations with demographic and environmental factors. Second, we intended to use this framework to narrow down the contaminated environments spatially, through the identification of geographic clusters of the disease, and associatively, through the identification of important environmental factors linked to the high BLLs. We conducted more micro analysis of the locations and associations revealed through our efforts above.

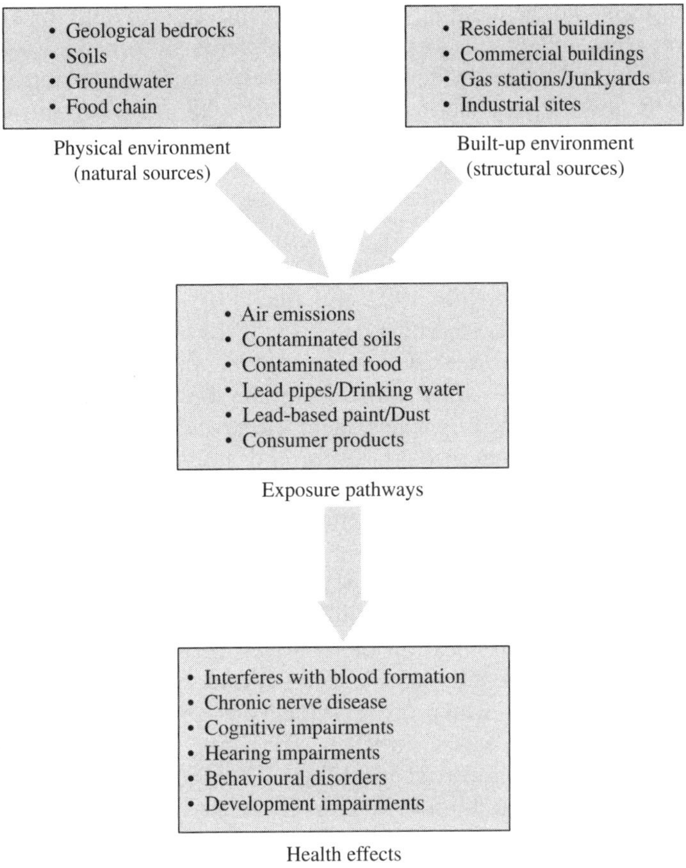

• Geological bedrocks • Soils • Groundwater • Food chain

Physical environment
(natural sources)

• Residential buildings • Commercial buildings • Gas stations/Junkyards • Industrial sites

Built-up environment
(structural sources)

• Air emissions • Contaminated soils • Contaminated food • Lead pipes/Drinking water • Lead-based paint/Dust • Consumer products

Exposure pathways

• Interferes with blood formation • Chronic nerve disease • Cognitive impairments • Hearing impairments • Behavioural disorders • Development impairments

Health effects

Source: Adapted from Oyana and Margai, 2010

Figure 8.2 *Sources of environmental lead and health outcomes*

Our longer term goal was to link these results to a larger database of childhood learning disabilities in the school district. A full description of the research methodology, data collection efforts and findings were subsequently published in journal articles (Margai et al, 1997; Lansana-Margai, 1998), including the collection of additional data sets and follow-up studies of long-term childhood disabilities (Margai and Henry, 2003; Margai and Tuck, 2004).

1. The study area

This study was conducted in Binghamton, the most urbanized area in the southern tier of New York State. Once a thriving urban and industrialized centre, the population size of the city has dwindled to only about 49,965 people of which 8.1 per cent are minorities (US Census, 2000). Like other northern US cities, the city has experienced economic declines. Several industries have closed or downsized their workforce to cope with economic difficulties. There has also been a drop in downtown activities and service functions due to suburbanization and the building of shopping centres in the outlying areas. The downtown areas reflect the characteristic patterns of urban decay despite attempts to rebuild and attract new businesses. Several neighbourhoods are inhabited by low- to middle-income families, with many of the large old properties in the inner city subdivided to serve as low-income rentals and as university student units.

2. Data sources

The primary data consisted of longitudinal health statistics data on all children screened for lead between July 1991 and June 1995. The data, consisting of 1840 records, included the screening dates, the BLLs observed and the location of the children. Another set of data, consisting of all socio-demographic variables relevant to the study came from the US Census. The variables, collected at census block group levels, included median income, poverty levels, minority populations, educational levels and housing quality. Additional information on the age of individual housing units was obtained from the real property records provided by Binghamton City Department of Planning, Housing and Community Development (BCHD). Data from the New York State Department of Transportation (NYDOT) consisted of the location and types of roads (interstate or highway) and rail lines (main, siding). We also had access to data sets on the location of industrial facilities in the city such as hazardous waste sites, service stations, lead-emitting industries and junkyards.

Some information on water and soil quality was provided by BCHD. The data set on soil quality was insufficient, consisting only of soil lead levels obtained from selected industrial locations. We augmented this information with primary data from additional samples taken from residential areas across in the city. Finally, base maps consisting of boundary and street data were obtained from the US Census. These files were useful for geocoding and portrayal of the information contained in the other data files.

Using the multiple data sets listed above, the key steps undertaken in the study were: (i) identifying the geographic patterns and variations in elevated blood lead incidences using health screening records; (ii) exploring possible associations between elevated BLLs and the socio-economic and demographic characteristics of the population; (iii) evaluating the relationships between childhood lead contamination and various indicators of environmental lead including housing stock, soil and water quality, transportation corridors and commercial facilities dealing with leaded gasoline on a daily basis (such as service stations, automobile repair shops and dealerships); and (iv) using the results from the preceding tasks to identify high-risk areas that require further analysis and possibly environmental remediation.

3. Data preprocessing and sample profile

The health screening records were queried to identify all children with BLLs at or above 10μg/dl, the CDC recommended threshold level of concern. A total of 316 children were identified – approximately 17 per cent of all children tested in the city. Figure 8.3 illustrates the location of the childhood lead incidences at the block group level. Based on the geographic location of these cases and the

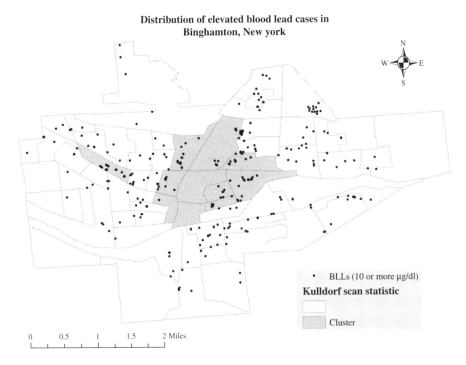

**Distribution of elevated blood lead cases in
Binghamton, New york**

Figure 8.3 *Distribution of BLLs in Binghamton 1991–1995*

at-risk population in each census block group, the prevalence rate of BLL was computed per 1000 children in each spatial unit.

The geographic patterning of the elevated BLLs was assessed using one of the geostatistical algorithms described earlier in Chapter 5. Using the Kulldorf's Spatial Scan Statistic in the ClusterSeer software, a spatial cluster was identified in the centre-north end of the city consisting of 11 census block groups ($p < 0.001$). The average disease frequency in this cluster was 7.85 per cent, when compared to an average of 2.6 per cent for the city at large. Further analysis involved an examination of the relationships between the elevated cases of BLL, the geographic clusters and the socio-demographic and environmental risk factors.

a. Socio-demographic variables

Additional characteristics of relevance in the study included the age and sex of each subject, the period of initial testing and the ethnic composition. The majority of the children with elevated BLLs were white, but there was an over-representation of minority children relative to the composition of the general population in the study area (see Table 8.1).

Twelve variables were selected to explore the relationships between BLL prevalence levels and poverty, ethnicity and housing quality. Correlation analysis showed that 9 of the 12 variables were significantly related to paediatric lead poisoning rates (Table 8.2). Housing quality and poverty

Table 8.1 *Sample profile*

Variable	Frequencies	%	
Blood lead concentration levels			
Class IIa (10–14.9µg/dl)	190	60.1	
Class IIb (15–19.9µg/dl)	75	23.7	
Class III (20–44.9µg/dl)	49	15.6	
Class IV (45–69.9µg/dl)	2	0.6	
Class V (Over 70µg/dl)	0	0.0	
Age of child at initial test			
Under 12 months	21	6.6	
12 to 24	119	37.7	
25 to 36	70	22.2	
37 to 48	46	14.6	
49 to 60	35	11.1	
61 to 72	20	6.3	
Over 72	3	0.9	
Unknown	2	0.6	
Period of initial test			
7/91 to 6/92	70	22.2	
7/92 to 6/93	105	33.2	
7/93 to 6/94	86	27.2	
7/94 to 6/95	55	17.4	
Sex of child			
Female	150	47.5	
Male	166	52.5	
Ethnic composition	*Frequency*	%	*Population %**
White	201	63.6	87.8
Black	56	17.1	5.6
Asian	23	7.3	3.4
Hispanic	17	5.4	2.5
Unknown	19	9.0	n/a
			$N = 316$

* Reflects the composition of the city.

variables had the strongest coefficients. Block groups with low-income groups, low rental values and low housing values were more likely to have high lead cases. Lead poisoning cases were also strongly associated with block groups with a large proportion of pre-1940s housing, rented property and subdivided structures. No associations were found between the variables measuring race/ethnicity, single family composition and lead poisoning.

b. Transportation corridors

Within the GIS, buffers were drawn around the roads and railway corridors in the city (Figure 8.4). The first was a 500 feet buffer around all of the major roads (ROADBUF). A second buffer using a distance of 1000 feet was drawn around the railroads (RAILBUF). Each buffer was then divided into smaller polygons whose boundaries corresponded to the block group boundaries of Binghamton. The area of each buffered portion was then divided by the area of the

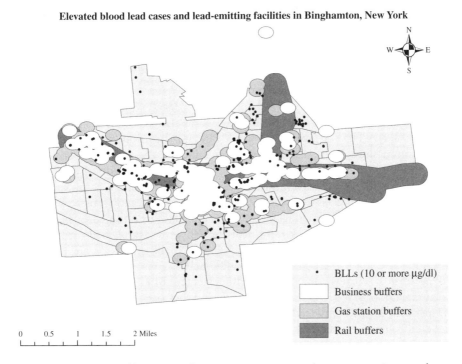

Elevated blood lead cases and lead-emitting facilities in Binghamton, New York

•	BLLs (10 or more µg/dl)
▫	Business buffers
▨	Gas station buffers
▦	Rail buffers

0   0.5   1   1.5   2 Miles

Figure 8.4 *Buffers around transportation corridors, gas stations and lead-emitting facilities*

Table 8.2 *Correlation between socio-demographic variables and lead cases/cluster occurrences*

Criterion variable: Lead cases per 1000 Children (n = 316) Predictor variables	Pearson's r coefficient	p
PCTBLK (% of African Americans)	0.24	ns
PCTHISP (% of Hispanics)	−0.08	ns
PCT1PARF (% of households with single parent – female)	0.07	ns
P25EDDR (% of persons aged 25 + with at most HS educ.)	0.57*	.001
PPUBAST (% of households receiving pub. assistance)	0.53*	.001
PVACRT (% of housing units rented or vacant)	0.59*	.001
PLE4RM (% of housing units with more than four rooms)	0.61*	.001
PMUHH (% of subdivided housing: 'multiunits' or apts)	0.62*	.001
PCT40HH (% of housing built before 1940)	0.40	.01
MEDHINC (Median household income)	−0.54*	.001
MEDRENT (Median household rent)	−0.39	.01
MEDHVAL (Median household value)	−0.42	.001

* Retained for canonical correlation analysis

corresponding block group to arrive at a percentage of each block group covered by either rail (RAILBUF) or major roadways (ROADBUF). These variables were used in the statistical analysis to determine the degree of correlation with lead poisoning cases in the city. The correlation coefficient for lead cases and major road buffers was 0.30, and 0.46 for railroads. Both coefficients were statistically significant ($p < 0.05$); however, given the strength of the relationship between RAILBUF and childhood lead poisoning, the latter was retained for further statistical analysis.

c. Industrial and commercial sites

The relationships between lead prevalence levels and the location of lead-emitting industries and businesses were also examined in this study (Figure 8.4). The database consisted of all business locations within Binghamton since 1890. The businesses included in the database consisted of only those whose operations were likely to incorporate the use of lead or lead by-products. These included industries such as machine-shops, foundries, paint manufacturers and glass manufacturers. The buffer zone and statistical analysis of these sites was performed using the same approach as outlined earlier for the transportation variables. A 500 feet buffer was established around the industries as the reasonable distance over which the effects of airborne lead would be felt on the landscape. The variable BUSBUF was formed and later used to perform a correlation analysis with elevated BLLs. A highly significant relationship ($r = 0.61$; $p < 0.05$) was found between the variables. About 41 per cent of the confirmed lead cases fell within the industrial buffers which covered roughly 20 per cent of the city's areal extent.

d. Automobile-related sites

A similar approach was followed by creating a 500 feet buffer around gas stations, repairs shops, dealerships, junkyards and other areas with permanent vehicle storage. Following the same steps as outlined above, the newly created variable GASBUF was strongly linked to lead poisoning cases ($r = 0.59$; $p < 0.05$). In all, about 53 per cent of all confirmed cases fell within the buffered areas.

e. Incorporating soil lead samples into the analysis

As part of a comprehensive approach to explain the observed lead cluster in Binghamton, this next phase of the research focused on the potential effects of soil quality. The soil lead levels for the targeted residential areas in Binghamton were determined by a detailed soil sampling procedure. The data collection process was based on the lead clusters identified earlier in the study. Two sets of soil samples were taken: (1) a study group consisting of 40 samples within the high-risk areas (clusters); and (2) a control group consisting of ten samples outside the lead clusters. Overall, 50 soil samples were obtained mostly from the front, rear and side yards of the selected properties. The soil samples were then sent to a professional laboratory to test for lead levels using the EPA 6010 method.

The soil test results were added to the GIS database. Later, the inverse distance weighting (IDW) method was used to develop a continuous risk surface for soil lead contamination (Figure 8.5). A query was performed to identify all sites that exceeded the EPA standards of 500 parts per million (ppm). A correlation analysis to determine whether the soil lead levels were significantly linked to childhood blood lead levels showed that there was no relationship.

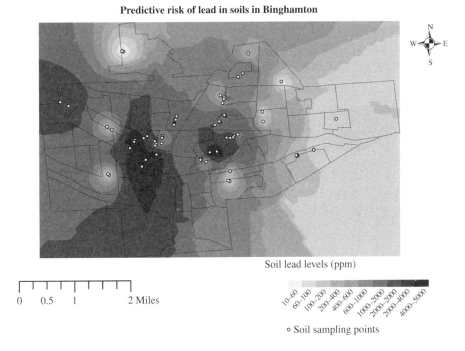

Figure 8.5 *Predictive risk of soil lead levels*

Geospatial characterization of high-risk areas

In the preceding section the primary risk sources and contextual factors of lead exposure were examined: demographic factors, transportation corridors, industrial sites, automobile-related sites, and soil contamination levels. Strong relationships were observed between most of the variables and the rate of lead poisoning among the children. In an effort to spatially characterize and map the areas of high risk, the variables with the strongest linkages were retained for subsequent analysis using canonical correlation. This additional evaluation was designed to develop scores that would provide the most explanation for the location of the observed lead clusters. Two sets of variables were utilized in the analysis. The first set consisted of the three variables that measured the effects of railroads, businesses and automobile-related sites. The second set included the six demographic variables that were best associated with the location of lead poisoning cases. The canonical correlation coefficients derived from the analysis were very high with $r = 0.83$ (at 18 and 153 degrees of freedom); implying that at least 80 per cent of the observed cases of elevated BLLs could be explained by these variables.

Canonical correlation scores, representing the aggregate values of the two sets of variables, were also obtained for each block group. Scores with values greater than zero were classified as HIGH and those with values less than zero were classified as LOW. The results were then mapped to show the relationships between both sets of variables within the city (Figure 8.6).

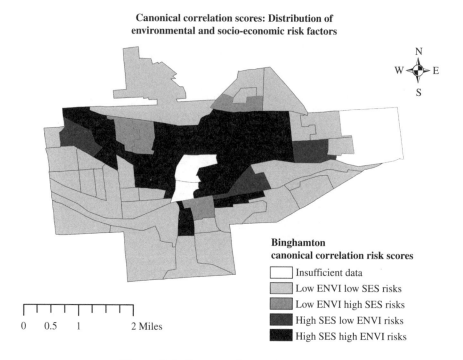

Canonical correlation scores: Distribution of environmental and socio-economic risk factors

Binghamton
canonical correlation risk scores
☐ Insufficient data
☐ Low ENVI low SES risks
☐ Low ENVI high SES risks
☐ High SES low ENVI risks
■ High SES high ENVI risks

0   0.5   1   2 Miles

Figure 8.6 *Canonical correlation scores*

As expected, block groups with high scores were found mainly in the centre of the city and along the rail corridor going westward. Those with low scores on both groups of variables were along the outskirts of the city, almost forming a continuous ring. A few block groups showed dissonant canonical correlation scores (high/low or low/high). These are areas characterized by industrial and commercial activities as well as low- and middle-income families. They reflect neighbourhoods where the middle class and senior residents have not migrated to the suburban areas perhaps due to proximity to employment and various functions provided by the city.

In an attempt to associate the block groups with the confirmed lead cases, some interesting results were found. Among the 26 block groups with high scores on both variables, 191 cases of lead poisoning were reported, a rate of 7.3 occurrences per block group. Among the 29 with low scores on both sets of variables about 85 cases were found with a rate of 2.9 cases per block group. These results demonstrate the strength of the two sets of variables in identifying high-risk areas for childhood lead poisoning.

Overall, through the use of GIS and statistical approaches the study confirmed the presence of a geographic cluster of lead poisoning cases in the city of Binghamton. Statistical analysis of the neighbourhoods (census block groups) identified nine demographic variables that were linked to the distributional patterns of the disease. Both housing quality and poverty levels were strong indicators of the areas with high BLL prevalence. GIS buffering methods around lead-emitting sources illustrated that railroads, certain industries and gasoline-related locations were also significantly linked to blood lead clusters. Canonical correlation analysis revealed that block groups that were in close proximity to the railroad, industries and gasoline-related operations were areas of high risk. These block groups had proportionately higher numbers of cases of child lead poisoning than their counterparts. These findings demonstrate the effectiveness of geographic tools in assessment of the paediatric lead prevalence and the potential risk factors.

Chapter summary

The increasing global dependence on the chemical industry for consumer products implies greater risks of chemical-induced diseases among residents in both the developed and developing world. The most hazardous chemicals are often those that are persistent, toxic and bioaccumulative. This chapter has examined two such chemicals, DDT and lead, in terms of the global production patterns, usage and health impacts. As various countries grapple with ways to minimize the risks of exposure to these chemicals, more environmental health research, including biomonitoring studies, is required to track the long-term impacts on residents – particularly children, who are known to be the most vulnerable. The use of GIS and other geographical and statistical approaches in linking multiple databases in a computerized environment, and monitoring the disease patterns and trends through maps and related visuals will go a long way in mounting effective campaigns against these chemical hazards.

References

Bailey, A. J., Sargent, J. D., Goodman, D. C., Freeman, J. and Brown, M. J. (1994) 'Poisoned landscapes: The epidemiology of environmental lead exposure in Massachusetts children 1990–1991', *Social Science Medicine*, vol 39, no 6, pp757–766

Canfield, R. L., Henderson, C. R., Cory-Slechta, D. A., Cox, C., Jusko, T. A. and Lanphear, B. P. (2003) 'Intellectual impairment in children with blood lead concentrations below 10 µg per deciliter', *New England Journal of Medicine*, vol 348, pp1517–1526

Centers for Disease Control and Prevention (CDC) (1991) 'Preventing lead poisoning in young children: A statement by the Centers for Disease Control', US Department of Health and Human Services, Public Health Service, Atlanta, GA

Chandramouli, K., Steer, C. D., Ellis, M. and Emond, A. M. (2009) 'Effects of early childhood lead exposure on academic performance and behavior of school age children', *Archives of Disease in Childhood*, vol 94, no 11, pp844–848

Falk, H. (2003) 'International environmental health for the pediatrician: Case study of lead poisoning', *Pediatrics*, vol 112, no 1, pt 2, pp259–264

Greenberg, M. R. (1986) 'Health effects of environmental chemicals', *Journal of Planning Literature*, vol 1, no 1, pp1–13

Griffith, D. A., Doyle, P. G., Wheeler, D. C. and Johnson, D. L. (1998) 'A tale of two swaths: Urban childhood blood-lead levels across Syracuse, New York', *Annual Association of American Geographers*, vol 88, pp640–665

Healy, M. A., Aslam, M. and Bamgboye, O. A. (1984) 'Traditional medicines and lead-containing preparations in Nigeria', *Public Health London*, vol 98, pp26–32

Holt, M. S. (2000) 'Sources of chemical contaminants and routes into the freshwater environment', *Food and Chemical Toxicology*, vol 38, S21–S27

Hou, X., Peng, L., Xu, X., Zheng, L., Qiu, B., Qi, Z., Zhang, B., Han, D. and Piao, Z. (2007) 'Elevated blood lead levels of children in Guiyu, an electronic waste recycling town in China', *Environmental Health Perspectives*, vol 115, no 7, pp1113–1117

Jacobs, D. E., Clickner, R. P. and Zhou, J. Y. (2002) 'The prevalence of lead-based paint hazards in US housing', *Environmental Health Perspectives*, vol 110, no 10, pp599–606

Jayashree, B. (2009) 'Pesticide level in veggies, fruits rises', *Economic Times*, 10 June, http://economictimes.indiatimes.com/Markets/Commodities/Pesticide-level-in-veggies-fruits-rises/articleshow/4637527.cms, accessed 12 January 2010

Jones, R. L., Homa, D. M., Meyer, P. A., Brody, D. J., Caldwell, K. L., Pirkle, J. L. and Brown, M. J. (2009) 'Trends in blood lead levels and blood lead testing among US children aged 1 to 5 years, 1988–2004', *Pediatrics*, vol 123, no 3, e376–e385

Landrigan, P. J., Kimmel, C. A., Adolfo, C. and Eskenazi, B. (2004) 'Children's health and the environment: Public health issues and challenges for risk assessment', *Environmental Health Perspectives*, vol 112, no 2, pp257–265

Lanphear, B. P., Dietrich, K., Auinger, P. and Cox, C. (2000) 'Cognitive deficits associated with blood lead concentrations <10μg/dl in US children and adolescents', *Public Health Reports*, vol 115, pp521–529

Lansana-Margai, F. M. (1998) 'Geographic information analysis of pediatric lead poisoning', *Proceedings of GIS in Public Health*, August

Lee, D. and Chen, J. (2008) 'Growing up in a leaded environment: Lead pollution and children in China', A research brief produced as part of the China Environment Forum's partnership with Western Kentucky University on the USAID-supported China Environmental Health Project, www.wilsoncenter.org/topics/docs/lead_may08.pdf, accessed 12 January 2010

Levy, B. S. and Sidel, V. W. (2006) *Social Injustice and Public Health*, Oxford University Press, Oxford

Lidsky, T. I. and Schneider, J. S. (2006) 'Adverse effects of childhood lead poisoning: The clinical neuropsychological perspective', *Environmental Research*, vol 100, no 2, pp284–293

Mackay, D. and Webster, E. (2006) 'Environmental persistence of chemicals', *Environmental Science and Pollution Research*, vol 13, no 1, pp43–49

Mañay, N., Cousillas, A. Z., Alvarez, C. and Heller, T. (2008) 'Lead contamination in Uruguay: The "La Teja" neighborhood case', *Reviews of Environmental Contamination and Toxicology*, vol 195, pp93–115

Margai, F. M. and Henry, N. (2003) 'Community-based assessment of learning disabilities using environmental and contextual risk factors', *Social Science and Medicine*, vol 56, no 5, pp1073–1085

Margai, F. M. and Tuck, L. (2004) 'Exploratory analysis of learning disabilities and environmental risk factors', *Research in Contemporary and Applied Geography: A discussion series*, vol XXXVIII, no 3

Margai, F. M., Walter, S. G., Frazier, J. W. and Brink, R. (1997) 'Exploring the potential environmental sources and associations of childhood lead poisoning', *Applied Geographic Studies*, vol 1, no 4, pp253–269

Meyer, P. A., Brown, M. J. and Falk, H. (2008) 'Global approach to reducing lead exposure and poisoning', *Mutation Research*, vol 659, no 1–2, pp166–175

Moore, G. S. (1999) *Living with the Earth: Concepts in Environmental Health Science*, Lewis Publishers, New York

Needleman, H. (2004) 'Lead poisoning', *Annual Review of Medicine*, vol 55, pp209–222

Needleman, H. L., Schell, A., Bellinger, D., Leviton, A. and Allred, E. N. (1990) 'The long-term effects of exposure to low doses of lead in childhood. An 11-year follow-up report', *New England Journal of Medicine*, vol 322, no 2, pp83–88

Nichols, J. W., Bonnell, M., Dimitrov, S. D., Escher, B. I., Han, X. and Kramer, N. I. (2009) 'Bioaccumulation assessment using predictive approaches', *Integrated Environmental Assessment and Management*, vol 5, no 4, pp577–597

Nnorom, I. C., Igwe, J. C. and Oji-Nnorom, C. G. (2005) 'Trace metal contents of facial (make-up) cosmetics commonly used in Nigeria', *African Journal of Biotechnology*, vol 4, no 10, pp1133–1138

NRC (National Research Council) (1984) *Toxicity Testing: Strategies to Determine Needs and Priorities*, The National Academies Press, Washington, DC, http://books.nap.edu/openbook

NRC (2007) *Toxicity Testing in the 21st Century: A Vision and a Strategy*, The National Academies Press, Washington, DC, http://books.nap.edu/openbook

Nriagu, J. O., Blankson, M. L. and Ocran, K. (1996) 'Childhood lead poisoning in Africa: A growing public health problem', *The Science of the Total Environment*, vol 181, pp93–100

OECD (Organisation for Economic Co-operation and Development) (2001) *Environmental Outlook for the Chemicals Industry*, OECD Environment Directorate, Environment, Health and Safety Division, Paris

Olewe, T. M., Mwanthi, M. A., Wang'ombe, J. K. and Griffiths, J. K. (2009) 'Blood lead levels and potential environmental exposures among children under five years in Kibera slums, Nairobi', *East African Journal of Public Health*, vol 6, no 1, pp6–10

Oyana, T. J. and Margai, F. M. (2007) 'Geographic analysis of health risks of pediatric lead exposure: A golden opportunity to promote healthy neighborhoods', *Archives of Environmental and Occupational Health*, vol 62, no 2, pp93–104

Oyana, T. J. and Margai, F. M. (2010) 'Spatial patterns and health disparities in pediatric lead exposure in Chicago: Characteristics and profiles of high-risk neighborhoods', *The Professional Geographer*, vol 62, no 1, pp46–65

Pier, S. M. and Bang, K. M. (1980) 'The role of heavy metals in human health', in Trieff, R. (ed) *Environment and Health*, Ann Arbor Science Publishers, Ann Arbor, MI, pp367–409

Ray, S. M. and Trieff, N. M. (1980) 'Bioaccumulation of anthropogenic toxins in the ecosystem', in Trieff, R. (ed) *Environment and Health*, Ann Arbor Science Publishers, Ann Arbor, MI, pp93–120

Romieu, I., Lacasana, M. and McConnell, R. (1997) 'Lead exposure in Latin America and the Caribbean, Lead Research Group of the Pan-American Health Organization', *Environmental Health Perspectives*, vol 105, no 4, pp398–405

Sadasivaiah, S., Tozan, Y. and Breman, J. G. (2007) 'Dichlorodiphenyltrichloroethane (DDT) for indoor residual spraying in Africa: How can it be used for malaria control?', *The American Journal of Tropical Medicine and Hygiene*, vol 77, no 6 (suppl), pp249–263

Sargent, J. D., Brown, M. J., Freeman, J. L., Bailey, A., Goodman, D. and Freeman, D. H. (1995) 'Childhood lead poisoning in Massachusetts communities: Its association with sociodemographic and housing characteristics', *American Journal of Public Health*, vol 85, pp528–534

Schwartz, J. (1994) 'Low-level lead exposure and children's IQ: A meta-analysis and search for a threshold', *Environmental Research*, vol 65, no 1, pp42–55

Tong, S., Von Schirnding, Y. E. and Prapamontol, T. (2000) 'Environmental lead exposure: A public health problem with global dimensions', *Bulletin of the World Health Organization*, vol 78, no 9, pp1068–1077

Turusov, V., Rakitsky, V. and Tomatis, L. (2002) 'Dichlorodiphenyltrichloroethane (DDT): Ubiquity, persistence, and risks', *Environmental Health Perspectives*, vol 110, pp125–128

USEPA (US Environmental Protection Agency) (2009) 'Existing Chemical Action Plans', www.epa.gov/oppt/existingchemicals/pubs/ecactionpln.html, accessed 12 January 2010

Van den Berg, H. (2008) 'Global status of DDT and its alternatives for use in vector control to prevent disease', prepared for the Secretariat of United Nations Environment Programme, Stockholm Convention, UNEP/POPS/DDTBP.1/2

Wang, S. and Zhang, J. (2006) 'Blood lead levels in children, China', *Environmental Research*, vol 101, pp412–418

Washam, C. (2002) 'Lead challenges China's children', *Environmental Health Perspectives*, vol 110, no 10, A567

WHO (2006) *Indoor Residual Spraying: Use of indoor residual spraying for scaling up global malaria control and elimination*, Global Malaria Programme, World Health Organization, Geneva, Switzerland

WHO (2007) *The Use of DDT in Malaria Vector Control*, Position Statement, Global Malaria Programme, World Health Organization, Geneva, Switzerland

Zietz, B., de Vergara, J. D., Kevekordes, S. and Dunkelberg, H. (2001) 'Lead contamination in tap water of households with children in Lower Saxony, Germany', *The Science of the Total Environment*, vol 275, no 1–3, pp19–26

Zietz, B. P., Lass, J., Dunkelberg, H. and Suchenwirth, R. (2009) 'Lead pollution of drinking water in lower Saxony from corrosion of pipe materials', *Gesundheitswesen*, vol 71, no 5, pp265–274

9
Geographic Principles of Environmental Justice and Equity

Introduction

The previous chapter examined the increasing global production of chemicals along with their toxicological properties, persistence and tendency to bioaccumulate in the human body and ecological systems. Also discussed was the ubiquity of these chemical hazards and the potential for environmental releases from the extraction phase, product generation, storage, use and final disposal. As a follow up in the present chapter, we shall examine the geographical distribution of the facilities that handle such operations and the variability in exposure risks. Even though the risks are pervasive, too often they are not distributed equitably across communities. Rather, social and economically disadvantaged communities tend to bear the brunt of the exposures while reaping limited or none of the larger societal benefits. Studies addressing these concerns have collectively contributed to the environmental justice (EJ) literature, a fast growing area in the study of environmental hazards (USGAO (Government Accountability Office), 1983; UCC (United Church of Christ), 1987; Bullard, 1990; Mohai and Bryant, 1992; Burke, 1993; Adeola, 1994; Been, 1994; Bowen et al, 1995; Cutter, 1995; Yandle and Burton, 1996; Pulido, 2000; Harner et al, 2002; Maantay, 2002; Mennis, 2002; Margai, 2003; Chaix et al, 2006; Chakraborty, 2009).

The chapter examines the underlying principles and goals of EJ, the root causes and processes that account for the observed disparities in exposure risks and the efforts by governmental and non-governmental entities to correct the imbalances. This discussion is accompanied by the presentation of a conceptual framework of environmental equity that weaves together the driving forces, the environmental and health outcomes and societal responses to these problems. Given the origin and long history of EJ activism in the United States, nearly all of the examples of host communities that are currently grappling with these environmental concerns are drawn from this country. Studies reporting similar situations in other wealthy industrialized countries are presented in the final section.

Principles of environmental justice, classism, racism and equity

Environmental justice, environmental classism, environmental racism, and environmental equity are all part of a growing body of literature documenting the existence of racial, ethnic and socio-economic disparities in the distribution of environmental hazards. We begin the discussion in this chapter by pinpointing the important differences between these different perspectives.

Environmental justice

Environmental justice is the most popular term in the literature and is widely used by human and civil rights activists, environmental organizations and governmental institutions. EJ is both a societal aspiration, and a movement that seeks the fair treatment, inclusion and representation of all people (regardless of race, ethnicity, class or culture) in the development, implementation and enforcement of environmental laws, regulations and policies (Higgs and Langford, 2009; USEPA, 2009).

Historically, the EJ movement can be traced to a low-income black community called Afton, in Warren County, North Carolina. In 1982, the state selected the community to host a hazardous landfill to dispose of polychlorinated biphenyl (PCB) contaminated soils. This decision triggered dissent among community members resulting in a series of demonstrations, arrests and, later, several court proceedings. The community's campaign did not halt the completion of the landfill; however, this experience laid the foundation for a national grassroots movement, which later became known as the Environmental Justice movement.

After the Warren County incident, ongoing concerns about the unfair distribution of environmental hazards were validated by two landmark studies produced by the USGAO (1983), and the United Church of Christ Commission for Racial Justice (1987). In the UCC (1987) study, researchers examined the location of hazardous waste treatment, storage and disposal facilities (TSDF) relative to the demographic attributes of the residential zip codes. The study concluded that, while there was a possibility for income to be a significant factor, '*race was consistently a more prominent factor in the location of commercial hazardous waste facilities than any other factor examined*' (UCC, 1987, p13). These findings, along with many studies published a few years later, provided conclusive evidence of significant relationships between the location of toxic waste facilities and the disadvantaged status of the residents in the host communities (Bullard, 1983; 1990; Mohai and Bryant, 1992; Burke, 1993; Adeola, 1994; Been, 1994).

Subsequent studies affirming the national scope and extent of these environmental disparities led to the formal establishment of the Office of Environmental Justice in 1992. Two years later, in 1994, this was followed by the enactment of Presidential Executive Order 12898 outlining the following principles of EJ:

1   To raise awareness of EJ issues among federal agencies, bringing their attention to human health and environmental conditions in minority and

low-income communities with the overarching goals of achieving environmental justice;
2 To ensure that there is no discrimination is involved in federal programmes that substantially impact human health and the environment; and
3 To provide greater opportunities for residents in racial/ethnic and socio-economically disadvantaged communities to participate in, and have access to public information on, all matters relating to their health and environment.

These guidelines established the framework for EJ in the United States, requiring all public institutions to incorporate an EJ mindset into their operations.

Environmental racism (ER) and environmental classism (EC)

Closely related to the EJ movement are concerns about *environmental racism* (ER) and *environmental classism* (EC) as the root causes of environmental disparities. Claims of ER include all instances in which racial and ethnic minority groups are disproportionately targeted in site selection decisions and environmental deliberations. Corporations have been known to purposely site noxious facilities and locally unwanted land uses (LULUs) in areas where they are least likely to face political resistance from the minority communities. ER concerns have also surfaced in situations where public entities, local, state and federal institutions, differentially formulate or enforce environmental regulations, zoning laws and policies based on the racial/ethnic composition of the host communities (Brown, 1995; Maantay, 2001). Similar concerns exist in instances of EC where low-income and working-class communities bear the brunt of these negative externalities and receive limited response for remedial action from the polluters or the governmental agencies.

Of the two concepts, ER is a more politically charged term, and is more widely used by civil rights activists to draw attention to institutional forms of racism in which corporate environmental practices adversely impact communities of colour. For example, in the recently revised UCC report which first raised this issue, Bullard et al (2007) appropriately defined ER as '*any policy, practice or directive that differentially affects or disadvantages individuals, groups or communities based on race or color*' (p134). Along these lines, the situation in Warren County, discussed earlier, may be described as a clear case of environmental racism because it involved the deliberate targeting of an impoverished black community by the State of North Carolina for the location of a hazardous landfill. Bullard et al (2007) also cite the example of Dickson County, Tennessee, as another poster child for ER. Blacks make up less than 5 per cent of the county's population and occupy less than 1 per cent of the county's land mass, yet all of the state permitted landfills are located in their community. Many health problems have been reported among these residents as a result of four decades of waste disposal. Overall, many studies show that race remains the strong demographic attribute of communities that are unfairly targeted. However, given the strong overlap between race and class, particularly within the US context, it is commonplace to find situations in which both factors are at play, with the vulnerable communities consisting predominantly of both low-income and minority populations. This certainly appears to be the case for Kettleman City in California.

Kettleman City: A case of environmental racism, classism or both?

Kettleman City has been in the national spotlight lately as another example of a vulnerable host community that is dealing with environmental health challenges as a result of excessive exposures to toxic contaminants. The community is located in the San Joaquin Valley, in Kings County between the metropolitan areas of Los Angeles and San Francisco, California. The community's history, settlement geography, racial/ethnic composition of the residents, and their lack of political representation in decision making partly account for the current environmental health challenges. Kettleman City was first established as a ranching community in the 1850s. It went through a period of significant growth during the oil boom in the 1920s, and later transitioned (in the 1950s) into a predominantly agricultural community. The agricultural sector attracted Latino migrant workers, many of whom later settled permanently in the community. By 2000, 93 per cent of the town's population was of Hispanic descent, with high unemployment rates, and nearly half of the population below the poverty line.

Though known for its aesthetic landscape, in 1979 Kettleman City became a host to a 1600-acre TSDF which is now operated by one of the nation's largest waste corporations, Waste Management, Inc. The site, located just four miles southwest of the city, had previously been used to dispose of oil drilling waste. It is the fifth largest TSDF in the country and the largest waste facility west of the Mississippi. Over the last decade, the total volume of wastes disposed on-site has quadrupled ranging from about 4 million pounds in the 1990s to nearly 16 million pounds in 2008 (Figure 9.1). The facility accepts many types of waste

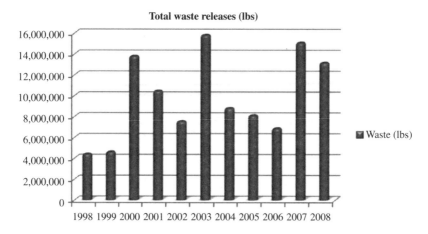

Data source: US EPA's Toxic Release Inventory database (TRI)

Figure 9.1 *Total waste releases by Waste Management Inc in Kettleman City*

with reportedly more than 200 20-ton truck deliveries per day consisting of hazardous materials originating from all over the country (Invisible.Org, 2009). A statistical query of the Toxic Release Inventory (TRI) database shows a wide array of hazardous chemicals including many carcinogenic and teratogenic compounds (Table 9.1).

Table 9.1 *Hazardous substances disposed of by Chemical Waste Management Inc (Kettleman City, California), 2008*

Chemicals disposed of in 2008	Pounds
Asbestos (friable)	4,330,678
Zinc compounds	2,632,699
Lead compounds	2,426,347
Aluminium (fume or dust)	1,262,304
Nickel compounds	1,018,338
Barium	693,764
Anthracene	615,178
Chromium compounds	530,550
Cobalt compounds	455,534
Naphthalene	423,487
Copper compounds	376,200
Vanadium compounds	297,087
Cyanide compounds	166,678
Arsenic	121,439
Molybdenum trioxide	113,132
Antimony compounds	91,592
Ethylene glycol	48,413
Polycyclic aromatic compounds	38,391
Manganese compounds	37,934
Toluene	34,956
Nitrilotriacetic acid	28,218
Cadmium	23,107
Aluminium oxide (fibrous forms)	22,810
Tetrachloroethylene	19,558
Xylene (mixed isomers)	19,201
Benzene	18,415
Hydrogen fluoride	16,520
Methanol	15,265
Mercury	14,062
Phenanthrene	13,113
1,3-Phenylenediamine	12,455
Silver	12,370
Decabromodiphenyl oxide	11,287
Selenium	10,565
Polychlorinated biphenyls (PCBs)	9,884
Benzo(g,h,i)perylene	4,288
Chlordane	318
Methoxychlor	112
Heptachlor	28
Total Volume	15,966,277

Data source: US EPA's Toxic Release Inventory database (TRI)

In the 1990s, a proposal to build a hazardous waste incinerator adjacent to the existing landfill was fiercely contested by the residents, forcing the company to scale back its plans. More recently, in 2009, the facility sought permission to expand its operations and Kings County Board of Supervisors granted the request.

Suspicions about the facility's operations and likely health impacts on the local residents had lingered for years, attracting attention from environmental activists, the media and, more recently, the federal government. Among the health concerns facing residents, birth defects, particularly facial deformities, have been the most worrisome. Between September 2007 and November 2008, five of the 20 children born in the community had cleft palates, three of whom later died, suggesting the possibility of a disease cluster (Schwartz, 2010). Additional health concerns consist of disproportionately high rates of asthma and environmentally induced cancers. In January 2010, US Environmental Protection Agency finally agreed to conduct an EJ investigation. It remains unclear whether the observed health outcomes are linked to pesticide exposures in the agricultural fields or to the exposure to hazardous contaminants from the TDSF. However, residents are hopeful that the federal investigation will help uncover the root causes of their problems, following which the necessary remedies can be put in place to undo the environmental damage in their community. Efforts to identify the underlying causes of toxic contamination, to assess the negative impacts on the environment and human health, and to implement the appropriate remedies constitute the realm of environmental equity.

Environmental equity (EE)

While the EJ movement deals with the political and grassroots activities, and EC and ER are linked to the more pernicious practices of private and public institutions, environmental equity (EE) is used to describe a broader and more encompassing objective that lends itself to geographical applications. EE acknowledges the injustices in the spatial distribution of environmental risks, the claims of ER, and the impacts on marginalized groups. The emphasis, however, is on using the knowledge gained from the root causes and impacts of these activities to develop interventive and remedial measures that redress these challenges and achieve a more equitable distribution of the hazards. EE efforts revolve around the core principles of EJ as a fundamental human rights issue that ensures fairness and equal protection from environmental hazards. As with our discussion of health inequities in Chapter 3, advocates of EE argue that the observed differences in the geographic distribution of environmental hazards are unjust, and steps must be taken to correct the inequities if and when they do occur. The case of Kettleman City reviewed in the previous section clearly falls within this context.

A conceptual framework of environmental equity

In a previous study Margai (2003) proposed a conceptual model of EE that offers a geographical context for examining the inequities in environmental health hazards in terms of the driving forces, the impacts and responses to these challenges. This model has since been refined to include four dimensions of EE: process equity, state equity, impact (or outcome) equity and response equity (Figure 9.2). Each dimension is characterized by a set of measurable indicators that describe i) the root causes of the environmental hazards observed in disadvantaged communities; ii) the poor state and quality of the environment in these communities; iii) the negative impacts on human health; and iv) societal response to mitigate these problems.

The EE conceptualization is rooted in the pressure–state–response (PSR) framework (OECD, 1993), a perspective that contends that in any given place, community, region or country, poor environmental decision making, institutional choices, and anthropogenic activities (PROCESS) exert pressure on the environment. These activities alter the state and quality of the environment, producing a series of environmental hazards (STATE). The poor state of the environment contributes directly to the negative health impacts observed among those residing close to these activities with greater exposure risks than their counterparts in other communities (IMPACT). People may respond to these negative outcomes through protests, demonstrations, grassroots activism or legal action. Governmental institutions may respond by holding the companies accountable for their actions, implementing and

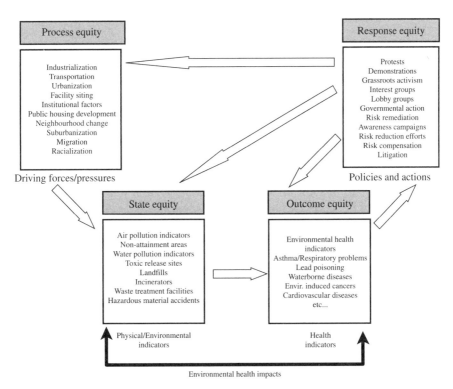

Figure 9.2 *The four dimensions of environmental equity*

enforcing regulations, or cleaning up the contaminated sites. Companies may decide to scale back their activities, compensate the victims or relocate elsewhere (RESPONSE). All of these efforts form a feedback loop to the original driving forces and processes, and may produce a cleaner environment and more positive health outcomes that collectively meet the core goals of EE. Following below is a description of each dimension and the empirical measures used to document the problems in host communities.

Process equity

Figure 9.2 provides a comprehensive listing of the empirical indicators that are used to evaluate each of the four dimensions of EE. At the root of it all, is the first dimension, PROCESS equity, which captures all of the driving forces of environmental injustice, the causal processes and mechanisms that contribute to the current landscapes of environmental inequality. To measure this dimension, one would have to rely on the historical sequence of events, including the political, economic and social forces that account for the present distributions of the hazards. Along these lines, a question that is typically raised by many scholars is: Which came first? The people or the hazard? In other words, were the hazardous facilities deliberately located in pre-existing disadvantaged communities, or did low-income and minority populations move into the hazardous areas after the facilities had been sited, thus placing these populations at risk?

Without the relevant historical data on the facility, and demographic records of the host community that date as far back as the establishment of the facility, it is often difficult to validate claims of ER, EC or siting discrimination. However, some studies have addressed these questions with measurable success. In the United States, these studies have been done mostly in urbanized settings such as Houston, Boston, Los Angeles, Cleveland, Chicago, St Louis and Detroit, many of them identifying a broad range of processes, factors and ineffective governmental policies that account for the inequities (Bullard, 1983; Mohai and Bryant, 1992; Bowen et al, 1995; Krieg, 1995; Pulido et al, 1996). It is important to note, however, that though most of the historical investigations documented patterns of injustice, a few studies of process equity concluded otherwise. That is, in some communities, the proportion of minorities or low-income families in an area with a waste site increased only *after* a facility was sited. For example, in a national study, Oakes et al (1996) conducted a longitudinal analysis of minorities before and after the siting of TSDFs. They found that the percentage of minorities increased significantly after a TSDF was sited, a change they attributed to white flight. Bullard (1983) and Yandle and Burton (1996) also found that white flight dramatically heightened the composition of minorities in neighbourhoods with TSDFs. Krieg (1995) found that as TSDF sites increased, the number of minorities in the vicinity increased. These findings led to the conclusion by some scholars that increases in the proportion of minorities or low-income families after a facility was sited did not necessarily constitute environmental injustice, rather it was caused by the migration of these groups into the high-risk areas to take advantage of the newly created jobs and low real estate costs (Kriesel et al, 1996).

Recently, a more comprehensive analysis by Fisher et al (2006) confirmed that historical laws and practices such as the one-drop rule, Jim Crow laws, racial discrimination and zoning laws are the primary forces that have impacted land ownership and settlement patterns to produce the present landscapes of environmental hazards. Beyond the historical forces, the political factors that continue to drive these processes include the lack of representation or participation of these groups in environmental decision making, their lack of lobbying power, the NIMBY (not in my backyard) syndrome, corporate greed and illicit deals with political organizations, and inadequate laws that protect communities (Fisher et al, 2006).

The economic and social processes also include historical and ongoing drivers of environmental degradation in low-income and minority communities. Urbanization and industrialization, and the agglomeration of the manufacturing activities in prime areas to take advantage of land use, access to transportation corridors and favourable market and regulatory conditions contribute mostly to these problems. Neighbourhood transitions and housing market dynamics also impact property values, along with suburbanization, white flight, immigration and other demographic shifts (Been, 1994; Liu, 1997). All of these activities collectively produce differential patterns of environmental quality.

State equity

Beyond process equity are the dimensions of state and impact equity (Figure 9.2). Here too, one finds measurable attributes that are useful in geographic applications to confirm or deny claims of inequity. Specific parameters that reflect the state and quality of the environment in terms of the location of landfills, incinerators, toxic release facilities and hazardous materials accidents can be calibrated. Indicators of air quality, water quality, resource depletion and degradation, soil contamination and related hazards are included in this second dimension (STATE). All of the these variables are accessible through the hazardous surveillance databases described earlier in Chapter 5 such as the Aerometric Information Retrieval System (AIRS), the National Drinking Water Contaminant Occurrence Database and the Safe Drinking Water Information System (SDWIS), the Emergency Release and Notification System (ERNS) and the Toxic Release Inventory (TRI). Each of these will provide relevant data for mapping the spatial distribution of environmental toxicants in communities, and evaluating claims of environmental inequity.

Impact equity

The third component, IMPACT (or OUTCOME) equity, focuses on the health outcomes and disparate patterns of morbidity and mortality observed among residents as a result of their proximity to these contaminated sites. The indicators for this dimension are also available within the health outcome databases (HODs) described earlier in Chapter 5. Incidence or prevalence rates of paediatric asthma levels, lead poisoning and other environmental health outcomes are available through the nationwide surveys described earlier such as the National Health and Nutrition Examination Survey (NHANES), the National Health Interview Survey (NHIS), the national hospital discharge data, National Vital Statistics System (NVSS), and the Behavioral Risk Factor Surveillance System (BRFSS).

Response equity

Finally, the fourth dimension, RESPONSE, forms an integral part of environmental equity efforts. It incorporates all of the societal activities including policy responses by governments to reduce, ameliorate and prevent further damage to the environment and the health of residents in the host communities. This would include empirical indicators that evaluate the presence or absence of governmental laws to protect residents from pollution, the enforcement of those laws, and the existence of proper mechanisms that penalize polluters, holding them accountable for the clean-up of the contaminated communities.

Response equity may also take the form of grassroots activism, protests and demonstrations with support from well known national and international environmental organizations and interest groups such as Greenpeace, Sierra Club, Public Research and Interest Group (PIRG), and the National Toxics Campaign (NTC). These efforts bring attention to the problem, enabling the local residents to mount an effective campaign against the polluting companies in their neighbourhoods. Studies examining the general characteristics of these groups, including their struggles, tactics and accomplishments, report that such campaigns are often faced with formidable challenges (Bullard, 1992; Capek, 1993; Greenberg, 2000). Too often, they are going against establishments that are firmly entrenched in these communities, and have deep pockets as well as political connections. The success of grassroots campaigns therefore depends on factors such as the timing of the protests, and an early framing of the protest ideology that appeals to the wider public (Walsh et al, 1993). Also relevant is whether there is a *protest infrastructure* in place that is rooted in a strong community network with residents' prior participation and affiliation with civic clubs, neighbourhood associations, community improvement and empowerment groups, anti-poverty and anti-discrimination organizations (Bullard, 1992). Communities with a stronger social capital are therefore more likely to mount an effective campaign against corporate polluters. Finally, as shown in Figure 9.2, relief from environmental injustices may also be attained through litigation and risk compensation packages to offset some of the disproportionate environmental costs incurred by the host populations.

Overall, the proposed EE conceptualization offers a geographic framework for understanding the root causes and processes, the differential impacts and responses to environmental injustices and inequities. The desired goal is not only to describe the primary dimensions of these inequities, but to offer empirical measures through which these claims can be validated, and steps taken to redress the challenges facing vulnerable communities. Given the scope of the framework, no study has simultaneously examined all four dimensions and the relationships between them. To date, most investigations have focused on only one or two dimensions at a time. Further, the initial studies have been met with a number of data limitations and methodological challenges hampering the ability to develop a full blown multidimensional analysis of EE. Summarized below are these limitations and recent efforts to resolve them.

Methodological challenges and accomplishments in EJ research

For nearly three decades now, scholars in many social science disciplines have examined the various EE dimensions identified above. In the process, they have produced a vast literature that ranges from descriptive accounts of inequities to more comprehensive studies that are based on fairly robust methodologies. Many of the initial EE studies were plagued with a few methodological challenges. As with most geographic applications, one of the initial challenges was choosing the appropriate spatial scale of the analysis (the modifiable areal unit problem (MAUP)) and statistical validation measures. Most of the original EJ studies were based on large spatial units such as counties or zip codes (Bullard, 1983; Mohai and Bryant, 1992). Anderton (1996) was among the first to caution against the use of these coarse units, noting that the aggregation may not accurately demonstrate the existence or non-existence of environmental inequities. Subsequent studies have since utilized smaller and less aggregated units such as census tracts or block groups, but these scales are also problematic for analysing process (historical) equity due to the variations in size and temporal changes in boundaries (Bowen et al, 1995; Cutter et al, 1996; Bowen, 2002). Fortunately, the use of software packages such as GeoLytics now enable the clipping of newer census boundaries to conform to the older spatial boundaries. The package offers a neighbourhood change database (NCDB) with access to socio-demographic data that are consistent across the census tract levels used for all four decades 1970, 1980, 1990 and 2000, and possibly also 2010 following the release of the most recent census data. Additional efforts to meet these challenges have included the use of multiple scales to explore the inequities at different geographies (Fisher et al, 2006), and the modification of the various population estimation techniques such as polygon, centroid and buffer containment methods (Higgs and Langford, 2009).

Another research flaw identified in the original EJ studies was the tendency to disregard the general proportion of minorities to whites, in the region under study. For instance, given the documented patterns of hypersegregation of black communities, there are generally more blacks in some regions than others. Far more blacks reside in South Atlantic states than in the Midwestern states, or in major metropolitan areas such as Detroit than in more rural areas. Yet in some of the previous EJ studies (such as USGAO, 1983; Mohai and Bryant, 1992) these demographics patterns were not taken into consideration when evaluating the proximal relationships with the pollution sources (Anderton, 1996).

Some of the earlier EJ studies also lacked statistical credibility and others relied on simplistic measures to supply evidence of environmental equity or inequity. More rigorous statistical measures have since been developed and are now being used to establish significant connections between poverty, race and hazardous wastes sites. For example, following a comprehensive review of the existing measures, Harner et al (2002) proposed a series of benchmark indicators for evaluating environmental injustices. These included measures such as the Comprehensive Environmental Risk Index (CERI), the Toxic Demographic Quotient Index (TDQI), the Toxic Concentration Equity Index (TCEI) and the Toxic Equity Index (TEI). These measures were compared using data for three metropolitan areas in the United States. These authors concluded that the CERI and the TDQI were the most consistent measures. Both also produced EJ statistics that were meaningful and easily interpretable.

Table 9.2 summarizes the formula used to compute these measures for poor and minority populations. Both the CERI and TDQI are quotients (a ratio of ratios that could also be expressed as percentages). The higher the derived index, the greater the disparity in environmental risk observed between the groups. Also included is the Toxic Demographic Difference Index (TDDI) which has been used before in other studies (see Margai, 2001; 2003). The TDDI is based on the independent samples t-test which compares the average values of the population groups observed in risk groups to determine if the distributions are comparable or statistically different. It is easily quantifiable and is a statistical significance test allowing the analyst to validate the patterns of inequity with a certain degree of confidence in the findings.

Over the years, EJ studies have also grappled with the types of approaches use to delineate the risk zones (buffers) around the hazardous facilities. In

Table 9.2 *Basic measures of environmental justice*

Index	Computation of risk for minority and poor populations in a study area
Comparative Environmental Risk Index (CERI)	$\text{CERI Poor} = \dfrac{\text{at-risk poor population/total poor population}}{\text{at-risk non-poor population/total non-poor population}}$
	$\text{CERI Minority} = \dfrac{\text{at-risk minority population/total minority population}}{\text{at-risk non-minority population/total non-minority population}}$
Toxic Demographic Quotient Index TDQI	$\text{TDQI Minority} = \dfrac{\text{at-risk minority population/total population at risk}}{\text{not at-risk minority population/total population not at risk}}$
	$\text{TDQI Poor} = \dfrac{\text{at-risk poor population/total population at risk}}{\text{not at-risk poor population/total population not at risk}}$
Toxic Demographic Difference Index	$t \equiv \dfrac{\bar{x}_1 - \bar{x}_2}{\sqrt{\frac{(n_1-1)s_1^2+(n_2-1)s_2^2}{n_1+n_2-2}\left(\frac{1}{n_1}+\frac{1}{n_2}\right)}}$

For any two population groups under investigation (for example when comparing poor vs non-poor, or minority vs non-minority groups), the means for the two population groups are represented by $\bar{x}_1$ and $\bar{x}_2$; the population variances are represented by s_1^2 and s_2^2; and the sample sizes are denoted as n_1 and n_2.

The analysis is based on a significance test (t) with $n_1 + n_2 - 2$ degrees of freedom.

The Toxic Demographic Difference Index is $(1 - p)$ where p is the significance level obtained for the variable.

general, two major approaches have been used, often depending on whether the risk sources are fixed (routine releases or point sources such as TSDFs, landfills, industrial sites) or mobile sources (such as transportation hazards, hazardous accidents and other non-routine releases). For fixed sources, proximity-based measurements have been used with a specified radius ranging anywhere from 0.5 kilometres to 5 kilometres around the facilities. Some researchers have followed the guidelines proposed by the USEPA for delineating these buffers (Harner et al, 2002). For non-routine releases, some have utilized dispersion-based models (Chakraborty and Armstrong, 1996; Margai, 2001; Fisher et al, 2006) that delineate the plume or footprint over which the contaminants are likely to disperse based on the toxicological properties of the chemical, the volume released and the atmospheric conditions at the time of release. This derived information is then integrated into a GIS and superimposed on a demographic layer to determine the profile of the residents that are at risk of environmental contamination. More recently also, spatial regression and geographically weighted regression (GWR) analyses have been used to account for spatial dependence and non-stationarity in the relationships between mobile and fixed pollution sources and the demographic attributes of the host communities (Mennis and Jordan, 2005; Chakraborty, 2009). All of these studies have, for the most part, generated consistent results that point to race and class inequities in the distribution of the environmental health hazards.

Finally, studies of EJ and EE have evolved beyond concerns regarding TSDFs and the contamination of minority communities in the United States to include other population groups and broader areas of injustice in other world regions. In Europe, EJ studies have focused primarily on the socio-economic characteristics of residents (Chaix et al, 2006; Fairburn et al, 2009; Higgs and Langford, 2009). The study by Fairburn et al (2009) used GIS to examine the cumulative impacts of environmental pollution on the socio-economically deprived population in South Yorkshire, UK. A modified Index of Multiple Deprivation was first used to classify the population into different groups. Two environmental indices were then derived: a CERI, and an Impact Intensity Index based on multiple environmental risk sources. The association between the environmental and the demographic data layers showed that the risks were highest in the urban areas, though some inequities also emerged in the rural areas. Overall the most socially deprived areas had the highest number of environmental emissions. The highest intensity scores were also skewed towards the most socially vulnerable areas.

Another interesting EJ study in Europe was conducted in Sweden by Chaix et al (2006). These researchers used a large database of 29,133 school-aged children to examine the relationships between socio-economic status (SES) and exposure to outdoor pollution in their school and residential environments. Using the spatial scan statistics, the authors identified eight clusters of children with low SES. All of these clusters were located in the most polluted areas. Four clusters of affluent children were identified, and none of those were located in the polluted areas. Based on these findings, the authors concluded that there is evidence of environmental injustice even in countries such as Sweden that are known for their egalitarian goals and interventive efforts to promote social equity.

Chapter summary

Concerns about the differential spatial distribution of environmental hazards are expressed in many ways as witnessed by the different terminologies in the literature such as environmental injustice, environmental racism, environmental classism and environmental inequity. In this chapter, we examined these issues including many studies in the United States seeking to validate these claims. The health challenges facing residents in host communities were also documented with some communities, such as Afton, North Carolina, achieving relative success in environmental justice while the struggles continue for others, such as Kettleman City. Using the EE framework, the comprehensive goal of identifying the driving forces of these inequities, their impacts on the environment and human health, and the response to these challenges to promote distributional parity was also presented. The empirical evaluation of these issues has not been easy, as documented by the methodological pitfalls associated with several of the initial studies. However, as illustrated in this chapter, geographers have been at the forefront of efforts to develop more rigorous approaches to study and validate these issues.

References

Anderton, D. L. (1996) 'Methodological issues in the spatiotemporal analysis of environmental equity', *Social Science Quarterly*, vol 77, no 3, pp508–515

Been, V. (1994) 'Locally undesirable land uses in minority neighborhoods: Disproportionate siting or market dynamics?', *Yale Law Journal*, vol 103, no 6, pp1383–1422

Bowen, W. (2002) 'An analytical review of environmental justice research: What do we really know?', *Environmental Management*, vol 29, no 1, pp3–15

Bowen, W. M., Salling, M. J., Haynes, K. E. and Cyran, E. J. (1995) 'Toward environmental justice, spatial equity in Ohio and Cleveland', *Annals of the Association of American Geographers*, vol 84, no 4, pp641–663

Brown, P. (1995) 'Race, class, and environmental health: A review and systemization of the literature', *Environmental Research*, vol 69, pp15–30

Bullard, R. D. (1983) 'Solid waste sites and the black Houston community', *Sociological Inquiry*, vol 53, no 2/3, pp273–288

Bullard, R. D. (1990) *Dumping in Dixie: Race, Class and Environmental Quality*, Westview Press, Boulder, CO

Bullard, R. D. (1992) 'Environmental blackmail in minority communities', in Bryant, B. and Mohai, P. (eds) *Race and the Incidence of Environmental Hazards*, Westview Press, Boulder, CO, pp82–95

Bullard, R. D., Mohai, P., Saha, R. and Wright, B. (2007) 'Toxic Waste and Race at twenty: 1987–2007: Grassroots struggles to dismantle environmental racism in the United States', Report prepared by the United Church of Christ, www.ejnet.org/ej/twart.pdf

Burke, L. (1993) 'Race and environmental equity: A geographic analysis in Los Angeles', *Geo Info Systems*, vol 3, no 9, pp44–47

Capek, S. M. (1993) 'The environmental justice frame: A conceptual discussion and an application', *Social Problems*, vol 40, pp5–24

Chaix, B., Gustafsson, S., Jerrett, M., Kristersson, H., Lithman, T. and Boalt, A. (2006) 'Children's exposure to nitrogen dioxide in Sweden: Investigating environmental injustice in an egalitarian country', *Journal of Epidemiology and Community Health*, vol 60, pp234–241

Chakraborty, J. (2009) 'Automobiles, air toxics, and adverse health risks: Environmental inequities in Tampa Bay, Florida', *Annals of the Association of American Geographers*, vol 99, no 4, pp674–697

Chakraborty, J. and Armstrong, M. P. (1996) 'Using geographic plume analysis to assess community vulnerability to hazardous accidents', *Computers, Environment, and Urban Systems*, vol 19, nos 5/6, pp341–356

Cutter, S. L. (1995) 'Race, class and environmental justice', *Progress in Human Geography*, vol 19, no 111, pp111–122

Cutter, S. L., Holm, D. and Clark, L. (1996) 'The role of geographic scale in monitoring environmental justice', *Risk Analysis*, vol 16, no 4, pp517–526

Fairburn, J., Butler, B. and Smith, G. (2009) 'Environmental justice in South Yorkshire: Locating social deprivation and poor environments using multiple indicators', *Local Environment*, vol 14, no 2, pp139–154

Fisher, J. B., Kelly, M. and Romm, J. (2006) 'Scales of environmental justice: Combining GIS and spatial analysis for air toxics in West Oakland, California', *Health & Place*, vol 12, no 4, pp701–714

Greenberg, D. (2000) 'Reconstructing race and protest: Environmental justice in New York City', *Environmental History*, vol 5, no 2, pp223–250

Harner, J., Warner, K., Pierce, J. and Huber, T. (2002) 'Urban environmental justice indices', *Professional Geographer*, vol 54, no 3, pp318–331

Higgs, G. and Langford, M. (2009) 'GIscience, environmental justice, and estimating populations at risk: The case of landfills in Wales', *Applied Geography*, vol 29, pp63–79

Invisible.Org (2009) 'Invisible-5 audio project: Kettleman City', www.invisible5.org/?page=kettlemancity, accessed 29 December 2009

Krieg, E. J. (1995) 'A socio-historical interpretation of toxic waste sites: The case of Greater Boston', *The American Journal of Economics and Sociology*, vol 54, no 1, pp1–14

Kriesel, W., Centner, T. J. and Keeler, A. J. (1996) 'Neighborhood exposure to toxic releases: Are there racial inequalities?', *Growth and Change*, vol 27, pp479–499

Liu, F. (1997) 'Dynamics and causation of environmental equity, locally unwanted land uses, and neighborhood changes', *Environmental Management*, vol 21, no 5, pp643–656

Maantay, J. (2001) 'Zoning, equity, and public health', *American Journal of Public Health*, vol 91, pp1033–1041

Maantay, J. (2002) 'Mapping environmental injustices: Pitfalls and potential of geographic information systems in assessing environmental health and equity', *Environmental Health Perspectives*, vol 110, pp161–171

Margai, F. Lansana (2001) 'Health risks and environmental inequity: A geographical analysis of accidental releases of hazardous materials', *The Professional Geographer*, vol 53, no 3, pp422–434

Margai, F. M. (2003) 'Indicators of environmental inequities and threats to minority health in urban America', in Frazier, J., Margai, F. and Tettey-Fio, E. (eds) *Race and Place: Equity Issues in Urban America*, Westview Press, Boulder, CO, pp189–212

Mennis, J. (2002) 'Using geographic information systems to create and analyze statistical surfaces of population and risk for environmental justice analysis', *Social Science Quarterly*, vol 83, no 1, pp281–297

Mennis, J. L. and Jordan, L. (2005) 'The distribution of environmental equity: Exploring the spatial nonstationarity in multivariate models of air toxic releases', *Annals of the Association of American Geographers*, vol 95, no 2, pp249–268

Mohai, P. and Bryant, B. (1992) 'Environmental racism: Reviewing the evidence', in Bryant, B. and Mohai, P. (eds) *Race and the Incidence of Environmental Hazards: A Time for Discourse*, Westview Press, Boulder, CO

Oakes, J. M., Anderton, D. L. and Anderson, A. B. (1996) 'A longitudinal analysis of environmental equity in communities with hazardous waste facilities', *Social Science Research*, vol 25, pp125–148

OECD (1993) 'OECD core set of indicators for environmental performance reviews', *OECD Environment Monographs*, OECD, Paris, no 83

Pulido, L. (2000) 'Rethinking environmental racism: White privilege and urban development in southern California', *Annals of the Association of American Geographers*, vol 90, no 1, pp12–40

Pulido, L., Sidawi, S. and Vos, R. O. (1996) 'An archaeology of environmental racism in Los Angeles', *Urban Geography*, vol 17, no 5, pp419–439

Schwartz, N. (2010) 'EPA to visit Kettleman City and its birth defect cluster', www. bakersfieldnow.com/news/local/82824862.html

UCC (United Church of Christ) Commission for Racial Justice (1987) 'Toxic Waste and Race in the United States: A National Report on the Racial and Socio-economic Characteristics of Communities with Hazardous Waste Sites', United Church of Christ, New York

USEPA (2009) *Environmental Justice*, United States Environmental Protection Agency, Washington, DC, www.epa.gov/environmentaljustice/, accessed 26 January 2010

US Government Accountability Office (1983) 'Siting of hazardous waste landfills and their correlation with racial and economic status of surrounding communities', Government Printing Office, Washington, DC

Walsh, E., Warland, R. and Smith, D. C. (1993) 'Backyards, NIMBYs, and incinerator sitings: Implications for social movement theory', *Social Problems*, vol 40, no 1, pp25–38

Yandle, T. and Burton, D. (1996) 'Reexamining environmental justice: A statistical analysis of hazardous waste landfill siting patterns in metropolitan Texas', *Social Science Quarterly*, vol 77, no 3, pp477–492

10
Global Geographies, Environmental Injustice and Health Inequities

Introduction

Since the initiation of the environmental justice (EJ) movement in the United States, studies of environmental justice and equity have evolved beyond concerns about toxic contamination in minority communities to include many forms of injustices among diverse population groups and communities around the world. EJ concerns today are increasingly global in scope and multitudinous in nature, ranging from oil, gas and mineral resource exploitation, to deforestation and use of harmful pesticides by agribusinesses, hazardous waste shipments, and threats to communal property rights, land use and traditional lifestyles in indigenous communities (Gophalan, 2003; Banza et al, 2009; Steady, 2009; Westra and Lawson, 2001).

In a recent study, Myers (2008) noted that the emerging EJ movement, and the scholarship around it, has not only become global in scope but locally nuanced as well (p5). Along these lines, he pointed out many questions that have come up in the literature: (a) How applicable is the US EJ framework to these other geographic contexts? (b) What differences exist between environmental justice and the broader mission of social justice? (c) How does the US-led globalization impact the poor communities in the developing world? (d) How can we move past quantifying and cataloguing injustice toward action to eliminate injustices? Some of these questions have already been addressed in the literature, including the preceding chapters of this book. For example, the presentation of the environmental equity (EE) framework in Chapter 9 was an effort to get past the recording of the environmental health impacts of EJ, to move towards response equity. But several other questions remain, and many EJ investigations continue to be conducted in the developed countries. Many scholars now advocate the need to confront these challenges in developing countries.

This chapter examines the global geographies of EJ with emphasis on the linkages between globalization, transnational pollution and the illegal shipments of hazardous wastes in developing countries. The chapter is divided into three parts. The first section presents an overview of EJ challenges in developing countries. In the second section, hazardous waste shipments are discussed along with a conceptualization of the push and pull factors that account for these flows. This is followed by a case study involving the illegal shipment and dumping of hazardous wastes along the coast of Abidjan, Cote d'Ivoire.

Environmental justice issues in the global South

As noted above, concerns about environmental injustice and inequity are no longer limited to disadvantaged communities in the United States. Rather, there is a global dimension that is manifested in other countries, and increasingly so in the developing world. EJ challenges in the developing countries are wide ranging, from mining and other extractive industries in the impoverished areas, to transnational pollution and illegal shipments of hazardous wastes. Globally, many examples of environmental injustice abound, from the Maquiladoras in Mexico (Grineski and Collins, 2008), Vieques in Puerto Rico (McCaffrey, 2008), the Niger Delta region in Nigeria (Adeola, 2009), the Bantustans of South Africa, the Favelas of Brazil (Steady, 2009) and other marginalized communities in Latin America, Asia and sub-Saharan Africa.

In most of these situations, scholars have noted a direct connection between the environmental threats and the emerging global and financial markets. The living environments of the poor, minority and indigenous groups are increasingly the hosts of noxious chemical and industrial plants, extractive facilities (oil and mining), and other destructive land-use activities that are owned or managed by multinational corporations and other foreign entities.

Nearly a decade ago, Stavenhagen (1999) warned against the tendencies of globalization and the potential impacts on marginalized communities. Among the trends that he identified then are the changing policies and practices of transnational corporations. These companies are systematically moving their operations and several aspects of their production chains to the developing nations because of the hurdles and regulatory constraints that hinder their operation in the industrial countries in which their corporate headquarters are located (Stavenhagen, 1999).

Hazardous waste trade flows

One of the environmental health threats associated with these global activities is the increasing exposure of developing world residents to chemicals and hazardous substances that originate from the developed countries. Each year, estimates show that approximately 300 to 500 million tons of hazardous wastes are generated globally and nearly 90 per cent of these wastes originate from the wealthy industrialized countries. Though most of these wastes are handled internally within the developed countries, about 2 per cent is exported. Between 1993 and 2001, transnational shipments of wastes increased from 2 million tons to more than 8.5 million tons (UNEP, 2006). The bulk of the waste is normally traded between the developed countries; however, since the early 1980s, increasingly large amounts of the wastes are being sent to the poorer nations for reuse, recycling and in some cases illegal dumping. India, China and many African countries have been actively involved in the importation of these wastes (Asante-Duah et al, 1992; Clapp, 2001; Gbadegesin, 2001).

Increasingly, e-wastes account for a significant portion of these international shipments. These are waste products consisting of electronic appliances that may be recycled and re-used. By all accounts, however, most of these electronic products that are imported into these countries are completely unusable and end up being toxic wastes. Many of these countries lack the appropriate technologies and expertise to properly handle these materials, so they are dumped in an uncontrolled manner, along roadsides or in open access areas, or simply burnt at the municipal waste sites, thus endangering the lives of the residents and ecosystems (Schmidt, 2004; Kimani, 2007). In Lagos, Nigeria, more than 400,000 second-hand computers are reportedly imported every month and only one-quarter of these products that are shipped are re-usable (UNEP, 2006). In Ghana, e-wastes and other hazardous wastes have been found in the municipal waste sites such as the Abgboboshie dump (McConnell, 2009). In a pilot study of the Dandora waste dump in Nairobi, Kenya, soil samples collected from locations adjacent to the site showed excessive levels of lead, mercury, cadmium, copper and other heavy metals. Among 328 school-aged children residing in communities proximal to this site, the study found respiratory illnesses impacting 46.9 per cent, dermatological disorders (14.5 per cent), gastrointestinal illnesses (17.9 per cent), diseases impacting the skeletal and central nervous systems (4.5 per cent) and a host of other adverse health conditions (Kimani, 2007). Figure 10.1 summarizes the flowchart generated from this study, and other recent findings illustrating the linkages between the toxic chemicals at the hazardous waste sites, the routes of exposure and health effects observed among residents in the host communities.

Concerns about the emergent health risks associated with the international transfer of hazardous substances have led to a number of multilateral environmental agreements (MEAs). The Basel Convention on the Control of Transboundary Movements of Hazardous Wastes and their Disposal was first proposed in 1989 (Basel) and later ratified in 1992. This agreement was designed to regulate the hazardous waste trade (or the so-called 'silent trade') between countries. It is now recognized by 170 countries, 46 of which are within the African continent. To ensure greater protection of African countries, the Bamako Convention on the Ban of the Import into Africa and the Control of Transboundary Movement and Management of Hazardous Wastes within Africa was proposed by the Organization of African Unity (OAU) in 1991 (Bamako) and later ratified in 1998. To date, this convention has been ratified by only 21 African countries.

While these international treaties are commendable they have not fully succeeded in curbing the flow of illicit shipments and disposal of wastes in these poor countries. They have assisted in tracking the legal shipments of hazardous materials but even reports of these legal activities are incomplete. The characteristics, sources and destinations of the wastes are not always accurate. The official figures are at best conservative estimates that

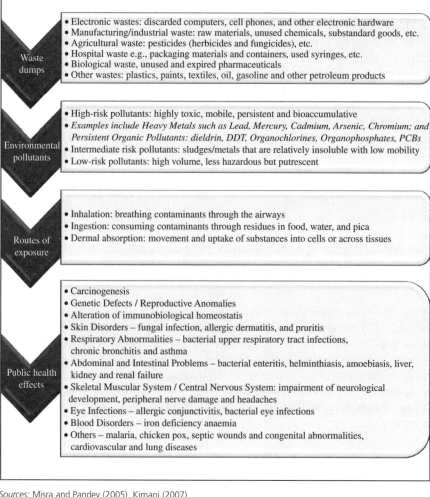

Sources: Misra and Pandey (2005), Kimani (2007)

Figure 10.1 *Health effects on populations exposed to hazardous substances from waste disposal sites*

underrepresent the true contents and hazardousness of the material flows between the countries.

The driving forces of hazardous waste flows

In line with the EE framework presented earlier in Chapter 9, there are many driving forces and mechanisms that account for the transboundary shipment of hazardous materials into developing countries. Drawing on the comprehensive reports and findings of previous studies (Adeola, 2001; Asante-Duah and Nagy, 2001; Gbadegesin, 2001; McCurdy, 2001; Lipman, 2002), Table 10.1 identifies the primary forces that account for hazardous waste flows, noted here as the push and pull factors.

Table 10.1 *Factors that contribute to hazardous waste flows between industrialized and developing countries*

Push factors and characteristics of source regions in the global North	Pull factors and characteristics of the destination areas in the global South
• Industrialized countries with large volume of wastes produced annually	• Developing countries with fewer industrial/ manufacturing activities and therefore lower volume of waste production
	• Market opportunities for materials that can be recovered, reclaimed, recycled from wastes otherwise destined for final disposal
• Increasingly stringent antipollution/ environmental laws	• Lax environmental laws and few regulatory/ monitoring mechanisms in place
• Higher excise taxes and rising costs of waste disposal	• Lower costs of disposal
• Potential future liability for damage caused by wastes disposed of domestically	• Open spaces; pristine landscapes; limited competition for space
• Urban sprawl and housing construction diminishing space and domestic capacity for disposal of certain types of wastes	• Limited opposition from internal groups
• Mounting pressure from environmental groups; NIMBY and NIABY syndrome	• Political instability
• Full disclosure, labelling and annual reporting of all hazardous operations	• Lack of knowledge of toxicity of the imported materials or full disclosure of the contents

Note: Modified after Asante-Duah and Nagy (2001)

Push factors of hazardous waste flows

The push factors are affiliated with the source regions or origins of the hazardous materials and e-wastes. Industries in the developed countries produce nearly all of the hazardous wastes but are faced with increasingly stringent environmental laws that prohibit the disposal of the chemicals in these source countries. This is happening amid growing concerns about the increasing excise taxes on their operations, and their future liability or compensatory charges for environmental pollution. A good case in point is Thor Chemical, which had its base operations in the United Kingdom with a subsidiary in South Africa. Due to its poor history of mercury incineration, air quality contamination and poisoning of its workers, the stricter environmental laws and stiff penalties forced this company to relocate to South Africa, a country with less stringent environmental regulations. There, it operated under the guise of a recycling plant, illicitly shipping mercury waste, contaminating communities and poisoning workers in the Eastern Province of Kwa Zulu Natal. Following discovery of these operations, subsequent protests from environmental groups led to the shutting down of operations, unfortunately there are still reports of stockpiles of mercury wastes and contamination of ground-water and nearby streams in the area (Phalane and Steady, 2009).

Aside from strict environmental laws in the developed countries, suburbanization and the housing construction boom in recent decades have significantly reduced their options for facility siting and the open space available for their operations. Further, mounting pressure from environmental activists, the greater awareness of EJ among residents in these countries, and the 'not in my back yard' (NIMBY) or 'not in anyone's back yard'(NIABY) syndromes have forced these waste producers to look beyond their borders for disposal sites.

Pull factors of hazardous waste flows

The easiest targets for hazardous waste flows are the developing countries. Given the economic plight of several of these countries, governments and residents are desperately searching for new market opportunities, and so they turn to the foreign companies and in particular the shipping and electronic industry for materials recovery, reclamation and recycling. These countries are therefore attractive destination points for the waste handlers. Some countries are enticed into accepting the hazardous wastes in return for jobs, foreign investments and other economic opportunities. The situation in African countries is enhanced further by the wide open spaces and lack of formal regulatory mechanisms, resulting in low costs of waste disposal. The cost of waste disposal in West Africa, for example, was previously estimated by Gbadegesin (2001) as a $12 billion a year business. While treating or disposing of a hazardous waste material in a wealthy industrialized country would cost an average of $2000 to $3000 per ton, through illicit negotiations, the cost can be a meagre $2.50 a ton for the same hazardous waste material in an African country (Gbadegesin, 2001, p195). The study cited many instances of toxic dumping throughout Africa including shiploads of radioactive waste in Benin (from France), pesticide sludge and chemical waste in Congo (from the United States), uranium tailing wastes in Gabon (from the United States), garbage and incinerator ash in Guinea (from Norway and the United States) and many more.

Political instability of destination countries has also been one of the most important factors governing the importation of hazardous materials. For instance, in 1992, Italy signed a contract with an unrecognized government in Somalia for the disposal of their hazardous wastes for 20 years in exchange for financial support (Hussein, 2001). Prior to this agreement, Somalia was in shambles with constant civil wars, no government and an invisible national police. In another situation, Guinea-Bissau was unstable politically and economically in the 1980s, a period during which the government was offered four times the value of its GNP to accept 15 million tons of toxic wastes for 15 years (Clapp, 2001). With the lack of investments and funds coming in, Guinea-Bissau agreed at first, but with pressure from neighbouring countries, they withdrew from the initial contract. All of these examples show that collectively, foreign companies and governments take advantage of the economic and political plight of low-income countries, the situations in which they are likely to face limited resistance, limited public opposition and least expense in their negotiations to dispose of hazardous wastes.

Finally, as noted in Table 10.1, many of the hazardous wastes transactions involve the lack of full disclosure of the true content of the wastes. The receiving countries may not be fully aware of the toxicological properties of the wastes that are being imported either because the transactions are made between unscrupulous individuals or the wastes are mislabelled to disguise the true contents. The receiving countries may not have the waste handling facilities or the technical expertise to evaluate the contents of the waste shipment. Without the right equipment and technical expertise to properly handle, recycle, treat or dispose of these wastes, the end result is storage in leaking barrels, open burning or disposal in open dumpsites next to residential communities.

A geographic case study of illegal dumping of hazardous wastes in Cote d'Ivoire

The Cote d'Ivoire study offers a great example of the circumstances outlined above that often lead to the illegal shipment and dumping of hazardous materials in developing countries with devastating impacts on local residents. This preliminary study by Margai and Barry (2008) involved the use of atmospheric dispersion models to delineate the toxic plume footprints of the most dangerous chemicals dumped in 17 locations across the city in August 2006. The footprints were then linked to the community attributes to create a demographic profile of the residents who were most vulnerable to the environmental health consequences of this incident. Following below is a detailed description of the study area, the analytical procedures and findings.

Study area: Physical setting and political circumstances leading up to the incident

Geographically, Cote d'Ivoire is located along the Gulf of Guinea in West Africa. The coastal lowland in the south is lined by pristine beaches while the northern plateau consists of mostly forest areas. The spatial extent of this country is relatively similar to New Mexico, US with an area of approximately 125,000 square miles. The country was colonized by France from 1647 till 1960 when it gained independence. Thereafter, the country went through periods of relative stability under the leadership of Felix Houphouet-Boigny, their first president. Unlike other African countries in the area, Houphouet-Boigny requested that France maintain its presence to assist in the economic development of the country. The country had a booming economy with most of its funds coming from the agricultural production of crops such as cocoa, coffee, mangoes, avocados and pineapples. Economic stability in Cote d'Ivoire attracted a large number of immigrants from neighbouring countries to take advantage of the job opportunities. The country subsequently grew rapidly from roughly 3 million residents in 1960 to nearly 18 million inhabitants by 2006, primarily because of high fertility rates and immigration from neighbouring countries. The large influx of immigrants later became a source of discontent, violence and xenophobia among Ivorian nationals.

The period of relative stability and economic growth of Cote d'Ivoire ended with the death of Houphouet-Boigny in 1993. Successive presidents were deemed corrupt, and inept in the management of government operations. Their governments were destabilized by the formation of rebel factions and many coup attempts, most notably in 1999 and 2002. Further, the question of 'ivoirite' or 'ivorianness' was raised on many occasions because of the ongoing influx of immigrants from war-torn countries in the West African region. In 2006, proof of citizenship became a major issue. There were 3.5 million individuals without ID cards proving their status either as immigrants or Ivorian citizens (Skogseth, 2006). Some individuals believed that citizenship came about through birth in the country while others believed that parental lineage should be the primary basis of citizenship. The courts were ordered to examine this issue but the proceedings were contentious because many groups opposed the hearings. Violence ensued and created the threat of another coup d'etat.

The hazardous waste incident

It was against the backdrop of immigrant xenophobia, political and economic instability that the hazardous waste incident occurred in Cote d'Ivoire. On 19 August 2006, the Probo Koala, a Panamanian registered ship coming from Amsterdam (Netherlands) arrived at the Abidjan port. The firm that handled the 528 tons of toxic wastes stated that the materials were inspected by health services and customs officials and no abnormalities were found (Bosire, 2006). Trafigura, the Dutch company that chartered the ship, stated that they had advised the Ivorian officials of the hazardousness of the wastes and insisted that special treatment was needed prior to disposal. Although Trafigura acknowledged the toxicity of the wastes, the company violated the Basel Convention by hiring an incompetent and incapable contractor.

At 7 p.m. on 19 August 2006, tanker trucks from the Probo Koala made their first trip to dispose of the toxic wastes at the Akouedo dumpsite (Bosire, 2006). Knowing of the dangers of the toxic material, workers at the dumpsite closed two hours earlier than the regular closing time. Over the course of the next two days, the tankers discreetly disposed of the wastes across 17 sites around Abidjan. These included the following locations; Abattoir municipal d'Abobo, Route d'Alepe, Abobo Anador, Decharge d'Akouedo, Abobo Foret du Banco, Foret du Banco-Cote MACA, Vridi Canal, Tri postal Vridi and Route de Anyama. Most of the toxic wastes were disposed of in open areas such as dumping areas, along roadsides, residents' backyards and woody areas.

Data sources

Demographic data: To evaluate the health risks of exposure to the hazardous waste, information regarding the demographics of Cote d'Ivoire was acquired through Demographic and Health Surveys (DHS). The large national database acquired for Cote d'Ivoire consisted of 9686 records of individuals (women of reproductive ages 15–49 and men aged 15–59 years) interviewed during the 2005 survey. The data, collected from 253 population clusters across the country, consisted of several variables of value to this study including the ethnic distribution, religiosity, age distribution, employment rates, urbanization and access to basic services and amenities. A proxy measure of the socio-economic status (SES) of residents was based on the Wealth Index. Cote d'Ivoire is an ethnically diverse country with more than 60 ethnic groups. Based on their linguistic families, these groups may be organized into four major categories: Mande, Gour, Krou and the Kwa. The Akan group, which is part of the Kwa cluster, represents over 40 per cent of the Ivorian population (Skogseth, 2006). The Krous represent about 11 per cent of the population. To evaluate the ethnic composition and the majority–minority attributes of the residents in this study, we grouped the Ajoukrou, Abbey, Aboure, Alladian, Abidji, Abron and Agni into the Kwa cluster and classified these as the major ethnic group. The Ahizi ethnic group was used as a proxy for the Krous, the minority ethnic group.

Hazardous waste data: The details regarding the hazardous waste incident were provided by contacting officials in the United Nations Institute for Training and Research (UNITAR) Operational Satellite Applications Programme (UNOSAT), who were the lead coordinators in the emergency response to the situation in collaboration with other governmental entities. The data garnered from these entities included information regarding the hazardous waste, the amount of chemicals released, geographic coordinates of the disposal sites and official injury statistics. The United Nations Disaster Assessment and Coordination (UNDAC) team was specifically in charge of investigating the causes and effects of the hazardous disposal (UNEP, 2006). They confirmed that over 500 tons of hazardous wastes were dispensed from the ship. The dump sites included the primary landfill, called Akuedo, but additional sites were dispersed around the city, along roads, water bodies, in forested areas, sewage systems and lagoons.

The following chemicals were found in the hazardous wastes: hydrogen sulphide, mercaptans, phenols and hydrocarbons (a mixture of olefins, naphtenes, paraffins and aromatics) and were all categorized to be harmful to human health (UNEP, 2006). According to the UNDAC report, groundwater wells were distant from the polluted sites and therefore no immediate health risks were expected from the drinking water sources. The primary concern was with atmospheric dispersal of the pollutants and contamination through inhalation.

The incident resulted in several injuries and fatalities among local residents. By 18 September, health care professionals had treated over 44,000 people, 66 of whom were sent for further testing (UNEP, 2006). A total of 15 were believed to have died shortly after exposure to the contaminants (Agence France-Presse, 2007). UNDAC reported that future health problems should not be expected because the chemicals found in the wastes generally had short periods of toxicity, and were less likely to be persistent or bioaccumulative.

Analytical procedures and results

Our main goal in this case study was to evaluate the geographical distribution of the dump sites and determine population vulnerability to the exposure risks based on their demographic and socio-economic attributes. From an EJ perspective, one could argue that the entire country was deliberately targeted and treated unfairly by the illicit corporate activities. However, we were primarily interested in learning more about the residents that were most impacted by this incident. Were they likely to be migrant families, or long-term residents from religious or ethnic minority groups? Were they likely to be less educated, with low income levels and residing in impoverished neighbourhoods?

Location of 2006 illegal hazardous dumpsites in Abidjan
relative to population settlements and waterways

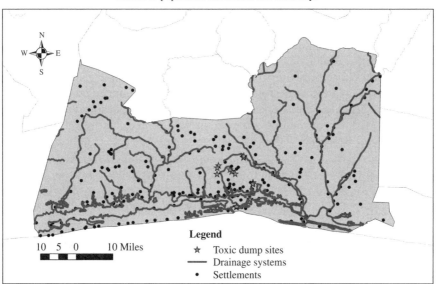

Figure 10.2 *Location of the illegal dumpsites in Abidjan*

Was their profile consistent with what we have learned about residents in other vulnerable EJ communities in the developed world? Addressing these questions was beneficial not only for identifying target populations with significant exposures, but also planning for a more extensive environmental epidemiological study.

Data analysis was performed in a sequence of four major steps. The first involved the analysis of the demographic data to obtain a national profile of the population. The DHS data, as noted before, were garnered across the 253 population clusters across the country. Using the SPSS (Statistical Package for the Social Sciences) software, we obtained frequency distributions, and mean estimates for the variables of interest: Muslims (the major religious group), Kwa ethnic group (a majority), Krou ethnic Group (a minority), urbanization, age, educational attainment, housing tenure (length of stay) and a socio-economic index. Information on these variables was then integrated into ArcGIS. Since the data were based on sampling points across the country, the kriging approach was used to estimate the unknown values based on the sampled locations, and generate prediction maps for each of the demographic indicators (see sample Figures 10.3a and b).

Demographic analysis was also performed for Abidjan, the city where the incident occurred. Sixty-six of the 253 population clusters fell within the city boundaries. The data contained within these 66 clusters were culled and retained for further analysis.

The second step involved the delineation of impact zones or 'footprints' of the dumpsites using a dispersion-based modelling approach that incorporates

Educational status of residents in Côte d'Ivoire relative to high-impact areas during the hazardous disposal incident

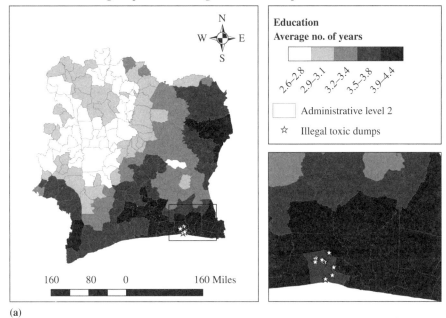

(a)

Religious patterns in Côte d'Ivoire relative to high-impact areas during the hazardous disposal incident

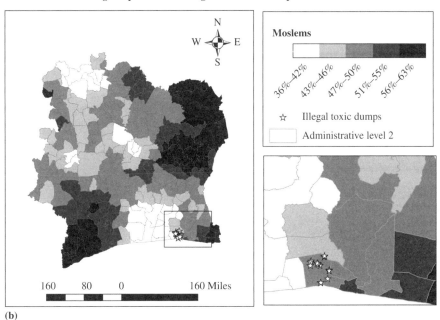

(b)

Figure 10.3a–b *Predictive maps of selected demographic indicators in Cote d'Ivoire*

the toxicological properties of the chemical, the amount and location of release, and the atmospheric conditions during the event. Using a Gaussian modelling approach, a risk zone was delineated over which residents were most likely to be exposed to the contaminants with potentially adverse health consequences. Based on the toxicological information supplied by UNDAC, the 17 locations of the dumpsites were spatially referenced in the GIS. The ALOHA (Areal Location of Hazardous Atmospheres) program was used to delineate the plume, or footprint, over which residents were at most risk of suffering adverse health consequences from the environmental releases of the contaminants (see figures 10a and b).

Four major chemicals were detected at the disposal sites: methyl mercaptans, hydrogen sulphide, phenols and polycyclic aromatic hydrocarbons (PAH). Hydrogen sulphide and methyl mercaptans were the most volatile chemicals in the wastes (UNEP, 2006) and for that reason we chose to model

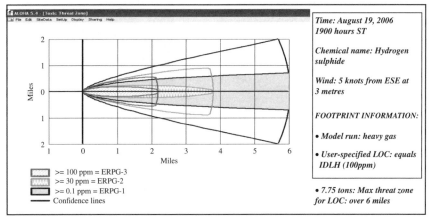

(a) Footprint of the Hydrogen Sulphide gas release

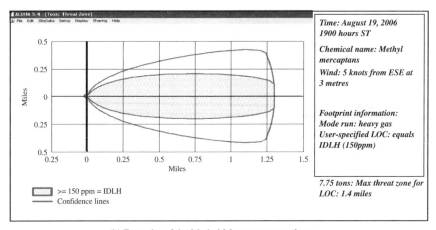

(b) Footprint of the Methyl Mercaptan gas release

Figure 10.4a−b *Footprints of hazardous chemicals released during the 2006 incident in Abidjan*

these two chemicals. Based on an estimated truckload of 7.75 tons of deposited chemicals per site, there was a 2.2-mile radius of excess risk associated with the release of hydrogen sulphides and an overall risk zone stretched over six miles (see Figure 10.4a). According to the Agency for Toxic Substances and Disease Registry database (ATSDR, 2006a) inhaling or ingesting hydrogen sulphide at such high levels may cause death. Lower concentrations may cause irritation to the throat, nose and eyes and may cause breathing problems for asthmatics. For the methyl mercaptans, we used an estimated truckload of 7.75 tons per site, and this produced a 1.4 mile zone of excess risk (see Figure 10.4b).

We found very little information in the chemical library on the toxicological effects of methyl mercaptans. However, the ATSDR (2006b) database does suggest the possibility of coma and death following high levels of exposure to these substances. Based on the results obtained from the dispersion modelling, we chose to work with a 2.2-mile zone of excessive risk, the maximum distance over which the atmospheric effects of the toxic contaminants were excessive and likely to lead to adverse health impacts.

The third stage of the analysis involved the integration of the footprints into the GIS environment followed by a detailed evaluation of the dump sites in relation to the communities that were proximal to the impact zones. Figure 10.5 illustrates this procedure using one of the dump sites. Overall, a generalized risk zone of 2.2 miles was established around each of the 17 sites, and the proximal

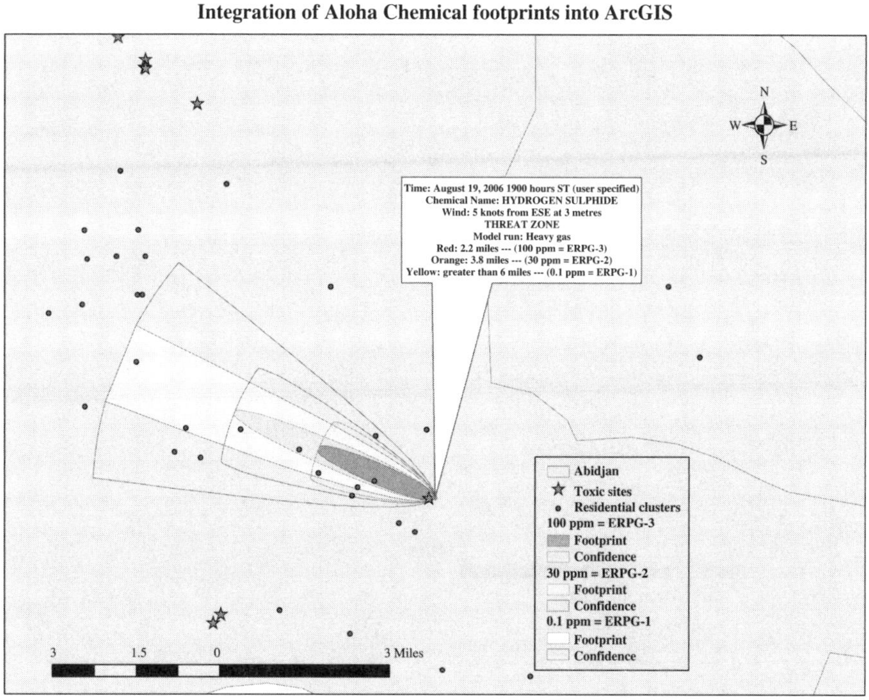

Integration of Aloha Chemical footprints into ArcGIS

Figure 10.5 *Integrating Aloha Chemical footprints into ArcGIS*

relationships between the impact zones and selected demographic variables mapped in the city of Abidjan. In order to isolate the demographic profile of the risk zones, a spatial query was performed to identify all residential clusters that fell within or part of the risk zone of each dump site. Nineteen of the city's 66 residential clusters in the sampled database fell into this buffer (Figure 10.6). These areas were designated as high-impact areas and all others were characterized as low-impact areas. Within the DHS database, there were 912 individuals in the 47 clusters identified as low-impact zones, and 796 individuals residing in the 19 clusters identified as high-impact areas. The population characteristics (religiosity, education, housing tenure, age and ethnic composition) of these zones were then extracted and exported into SPSS for statistical analysis.

The final step in the analysis involved the computation of descriptive statistics, a toxic demographic difference index, and a more advanced analysis using stepwise logistic regression. The descriptive statistics obtained for the entire sample, revealed that the majority of the residents were Kwa, and no foreigners were included in the database (Table 10.2). This was surprising given the large influx of immigrants into this country, as documented earlier. It is possible that these immigrants failed to disclose their status to avoid the xenophobic sentiments alluded to earlier. About 42 per cent of the respondents in the sample had no formal education and about a third fell into the middle and

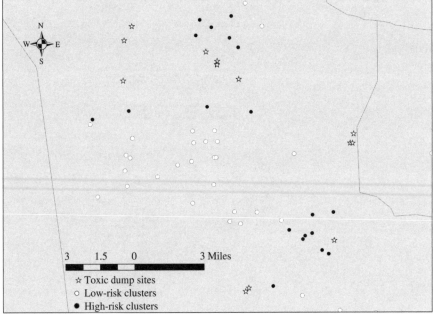

Population clusters within chemical footprint zones in Abidjan

☆ Toxic dump sites
○ Low-risk clusters
● High-risk clusters

Figure 10.6 *Location of the population clusters within the areas of excessive risk in Abidjan*

Table 10.2 *Frequency distribution of selected demographic characteristics of residents in Abidjan*

Categorical variable	N = 1708%
Hazardous risk zones	
Low	53.4
High	46.6
Kwa ethnic group	80.9
Ahizi ethnic group	19.0
Foreigners	0
Employed	65.7
Religion	
Christians	44.4
Moslems	42.9
Other	12.8
Education	
No education	41.9
Incomplete primary	19.2
Complete primary	3.3
Incomplete secondary	26.0
Complete secondary	1.3
Higher	8.4
Wealth index	
Poorest	10.7
Poorer	11.2
Middle	13.5
Richer	24.2
Richest	40.3

lower rankings of the wealth index. The proportion of Christians and Moslems was fairly even in the sample taken in Abidjan and appeared to be nationally representative. The average age of respondents was 27.8 years, and they had an average of eight members in their households, both characteristics fairly typical of many African countries.

A TDDI showed that those who faced the greatest risk of exposure to the chemical hazard have lived in the community for an average of 17 years, and therefore less likely to be immigrants (Table 10.3). They were more likely to be employed. A greater proportion of the residents in the high-impact zones were Moslems and were less likely to have access to piped water, electricity and other basic amenities. When compared to the low-risk zones, the household sizes in the high-impact areas were larger, and also likely to have more children under the age of five.

Further analysis using the stepwise logistic regression method involved the risk zone as a binary outcome (dependent variable). The odds of being exposed to the hazardous chemicals released during the 2006 incident were expressed as a function of the following independent variables: wealth index, educational attainment, religiosity, ethnicity, employment status, access to piped water, flush toilet and electricity, and length of stay in the community (see Table 10.4). The

Table 10.3 *Toxic demographic difference indices for risk zones during the Abidjan incident*

	Risk zone	N	Mean	Std deviation	T test	TDDI (1 − p)
Current age – respondent	Low risk	912	27.55	8.637	− 1.306	0.806
	High risk	796	28.12	9.404		
Length of stay (years)	Low risk	874	9.2197	11.03404	− 12.131	1.00
	High risk	740	17.6662	15.99013	***	
KWA %	Low risk	912	81.14	.39140	.255	0.202
	High risk	796	80.65	.39526		
AHIZI %	Low risk	912	18.86	.39140	− .124	0.099
	High risk	796	19.10	.39330		
WORKING %	Low risk	912	60.09	.48999	− 5.351	1.00
	High risk	796	72.24	.44812	***	
MOSLEM %	Low risk	912	34.43	.47540	− 7.631	1.00
	High risk	796	52.51	.49968		
Access to PPWATER %	Low risk	912	91.67	.27654	18.255	1.00
	High risk	796	55.40	.49739	***	
Access to ELECTRIC %	Low risk	912	89.14	.31125	21.355	1.00
	High risk	796	45.48	.49826	***	
No of household members	Low risk	912	7.93	4.664	− 4.154	1.00
	High risk	796	8.97	5.498	***	
No of children 5 and under	Low risk	912	.99	1.071	− 7.211	1.00
	High risk	796	1.48	1.672	***	

***significant at $p < 0.01$

use of the stepwise procedure reduced the likelihood of multicollinearity among the variables. The model derived at the end of the iterative procedure consisted of six variables: education, wealth, access to piped water, flush toilet, household size, ethnicity and length of stay in the community. The model was highly significant with a Nagelkerke R square of 0.584 suggesting that at least 58% of the variability in hazardous exposure risk can be explained by these demographic attributes. The strongest variable was the wealth index. Those who were poor in the city faced the greatest risk of exposure to this chemical. The odds ratio also showed that residents with little or no formal education were twice as likely to be exposed to the chemical. The odds declined with increasing education but education remained significant. Those without the basic amenities such as piped water and modern sanitation facilities were the most likely to suffer from this tragedy. The odds were slightly higher (only 4 per cent) for those who had lived here longer and lived in larger household units. Finally, the Kwa majority group faced a slightly lower risk of exposure to the toxic chemicals when compared to the minority group.

Overall, the analytical methods used in this study were very helpful in evaluating vulnerability to toxic wastes dumpsites. Though race was not used in this study, the results based on the other demographic indicators supported the pattern of environmental inequities identified in the developed world. The poor, working class and, in this case, the ethnic minorities, residing in crowded households that lack basic amenities were the most susceptible to the chemical hazards.

Table 10.4 *Stepwise logistic regression of exposure risk to hazardous chemical releases during the Abidjan incident*

Variables in the equation	B	S.E.	Wald	df	Sig.	Exp(B)
Education			8.830	3	.032	
Higher educ (reference)						
No education	.702	.243	8.320	1	.004	2.017
Primary	.606	.248	5.958	1	.015	1.833
Secondary	.440	.233	3.559	1	.059	1.553
No of house members	.043	.013	10.996	1	.001	1.044
Access to piped water	− 1.914	.191	100.254	1	.000	.147
Access to flush toilet	− 1.162	.177	43.197	1	.000	.313
Wealth index *Richest*			61.716	4	.000	
group (reference)						
Poorest	21.151	2777.017	.000	1	.994	1.533E9
Poorer	2.879	.373	59.677	1	.000	17.805
Middle	.304	.212	2.047	1	.153	1.355
Richer	.169	.174	.940	1	.332	1.184
Length of stay	.036	.006	41.269	1	.000	1.037
KWA ethnic group	− .904	.200	20.425	1	.000	.405

Model summary						
Final step	− 2 Log likelihood		Cox & Snell R Square		Nagelkerke R Square	
	1308.431		.438		.584	

Given the illicit nature of the disposal incident, the results obtained in this study are conservative, representing perhaps a lower estimate of the chemical exposure levels incurred by these residents. More detailed environmental and epidemiological investigations are required to secure baseline data and monitor their long-term health status. This study provides a first step toward the selection of the risk areas and prioritization of resources for a more detailed epidemiological investigation.

Chapter summary

The EJ movement which started in the United States three decades ago now has a global dimension with similar exposure risks and population group vulnerabilities in other countries. As minority and working-class communities in the developed world become more vigilant and adept in fighting environmental injustices, the burden of exposure is gradually shifting to new environments in the developing world. The case of hazardous dumping in the Cote d'Ivoire shows that the frontline for EJ continues to evolve. The risks are greater in low-income communities around the world as corporate tactics change and institutions shift their operations to new locations with limited knowledge of the dangers at hand, hence limited resistance and opposition. As a global community, societal awareness and response to these environmentally unjust acts remain crucial in protecting the health of residents. The approaches used in this chapter illustrate how geographic perspectives and tools can be used to assist with these efforts by pinpointing the risk zones, and creating a profile of the most vulnerable areas for environmental remediation and long-term biomonitoring of the victims.

References

Adeola, F. O. (2001) 'Environmental injustice and human rights abuse: The states, MNCs, and repression of minority groups in the world system', *Human Ecology Review*, vol 8, no 1, pp39–59

Adeola, F. O. (2009) 'From colonialism to internal colonialism and crude socio-environmental injustice: Anatomy of violent conflicts in the Niger delta of Nigeria', in Steady, F. C. (ed) *Environmental Justice in the New Millennium: Global Perspectives on Race, Ethnicity and Human Rights*, Palgrave Macmillan, New York

Agence France-Presse (2007, 17 February) *Death Toll from ICoast Pollution Rises to 15*, www.reliefweb.int/rw/RWB.NSF/db900SID/YAOI-6YK47K?OpenDocument &rc=1&emid=AC-2006-000134-CIV, accessed 7 July 2007

Agency for Toxic Substances and Disease Registry (2006a, July) *Toxicological Profile: Hydrogen Sulfide*, www.atsdr.cdc.gov/toxprofiles/tp114.html, accessed 10 July 2007

Agency for Toxic Substances and Disease Registry (2006b, July) *Toxicological Profile: Methyl Mercaptans*, www.atsdr.cdc.gov/toxprofiles/tp139.html, accessed 10 July 2007

Asante-Duah, D. and Nagy, I. V. (2001) 'A paradigm of international environmental law: The case for controlling the transboundary movements of hazardous wastes', *Environmental Management*, vol 27, no 6, pp779–786

Asante-Duah, D., Kofi, D., Saccomanno, F. F. and Shortreed, J. H. (1992) 'The hazardous waste trade: Can it be controlled?', *Environmental Science and Technology*, vol 26, pp1684–1693

Banza, C. L. N., Nawrot, T. S., Haufroid, V., Decrée, S., DePutter, T., Smolders, E. et al (2009) 'High human exposure to cobalt and other metals in Katanga, a mining area of the Democratic Republic of Congo', *Environmental Research*, vol 109, no 6, pp745–752

Bosire, B. (2006) 'UN Seeks Help To Clean Up Deadly Ivorian Toxic Waste Dumps' www.terradaily.com/reports/UN_Seeks_Help_To_Clean_Up_Deadly_Ivorian_Toxic-Waste_Dumps_999.html, accessed 7 July 2007

Clapp, J. (2001) *Toxic Exports: The Transfer of Hazardous Wastes from Rich to Poor Countries*, Cornell University Press, Ithaca, NY

Clay, R. (1994) 'A continent in chaos: Africa's environmental issues', *EnviroNews*, vol 112, no 12, pp1018–1023

Demographic and Health Surveys (2005) 'Cote d'Ivoire: MEASURE DHS', ICF Macro, Calverton, MD

Gbadegesin, S. (2001) 'Multinational corporations, developed nations, and environmental racism: Toxic waste, exploration, and eco-catastrophe', in Westra, L. and Lawson, B. E. (eds) *Faces of Environmental Racism: Confronting Issues of Global Justice*, 2nd Edition, Rowman & Littlefield Publishers, Inc, Lanham, MD, pp187–202

Gophalan, H. N. (2003) 'Environmental health in developing countries: An overview of the problems and practices', *Environmental Health Perspectives*, vol 111, ppA446–A447

Grineski, S. E. and Collins, T. (2008) 'Exploring patterns of environmental injustice in the global South: Maquiladoras in Ciudad Jua'rez, Mexico', *Population and Environment*, vol 29, pp247–270

Hussein, A. M. (2001) 'Environmental degradation and environmental racism', in Westra, L. and Lawson, B. (eds) *Faces of Environmental Racism: Confronting Issues of Global Justice*, Rowman & Littlefield Publishers, Inc, Oxford, pp203–227

Kimani, N. G. (2007) *Environmental Pollution and Impacts on Public Health: Implications for the Dandora Municipal Dumping Site in Nairobi, Kenya*, in cooperation with the United Nations Environment Programme (UNEP) and St Johns Catholic Church, Kogocho, Kenya, p14

Lipman, Z. (2002) 'A dirty dilemma: Hazardous waste trade', *Harvard International Review*, vol 23, no 4, pp67–71

Margai, F. L. (2001) 'Health risks and environmental inequity: A geographical analysis of accidental releases of hazardous materials', *The Professional Geographer*, vol 53, no 3, pp422–434

Margai, F. M. (2007) 'Geographic targeting of risk zones for childhood stunting and related outcomes in Burkina Faso', *Journal of World Health and Population*, June, pp1–19

Margai, F. M. and Barry, F. (2008) 'Emerging risks and health consequences of global environmental inequities: The case in illegal hazardous waste dumping in Cote d'Ivoire', Paper presented at the Association of American Geographer's Conference, Boston, MA, 27 March

McCaffrey, K. T. (2008) 'The struggle for environmental justice in Vieques, Puerto Rico', in Carruthers, D. V. (ed) *Environmental Justice in Latin America: Problems, Promise and Practice*, The MIT Press, Cambridge, MA

McConnell, A. (2009) 'Toxic technology, a photostory of e-wastes in Ghana', *Geographical*, the magazine of the The Royal Geographical Society, July, pp22–29, www.geographical.co.uk

McCurdy, H. (2001) 'Africville: Environmental racism', in Westra, L. and Lawson, B. (eds) *Faces of Environmental Racism: Confronting Issues of Global Justice*, Rowman & Littlefield Publishers, Inc, Oxford, pp95–112

Misra, V. and Pandey, S. D. (2005) 'Hazardous waste: Impact on health and the environment for development of better waste management strategies in future in India', *Environment International*, vol 31, pp417–431

Myers, G. A. (2008) 'Sustainable development and environmental justice in African cities', *Geography Compass*, vol 2, pp1–14

Phalane, M. E. and Steady, F. C. (2009) 'Nuclear energy, hazardous waste, health and environmental justice in South Africa', in Steady, F. C. (ed) *Environmental Justice in the New Millennium: Global Perspectives on Race, Ethnicity and Human Rights*, Palgrave Macmillan, New York

Schmidt, C. W. (2004) 'Crimes: Earth's expense', *Environmental Health Perspectives*, vol 112, ppA97–A103

Skogseth, G. (2006) 'Cote d'Ivoire: Ethnicity, Ivoirite and conflict', *LandInfo*, vol 2, pp1–35

Stavenhagen, R. (1999) 'Structural racism and trends in the global economy', Consultation on Racism and Human Rights, International Council on Human Rights Policy, Geneva, 3–4 December

Steady, F. C. (2009) 'Environmental justice cross culturally: Theory and praxis in the African Diaspora and in Africa', in Steady, F. C. (ed) *Environmental Justice in the New Millennium: Global Perspectives on Race, Ethnicity and Human Rights*, Palgrave Macmillan, New York

The Basel Convention on the Control of Transboundary Movements of Hazardous Wastes and their Disposal, www.basel.int/text/documents.html, accessed 1 September 2010

The Basel Action Network (2007) 'E-Waste Nigeria', www.ban.org/ban_news/2006/0612_dirty_business.html, accessed 7 July 2007

UNEP (2006) *United Nations Disaster and Coordination Report*, www.loe.org/images/070223/undac_civ_11sep.pdf, accessed 7 July 2007

Westra, L. and Lawson, B. (eds) (2001) *Faces of Environmental Racism: Confronting Issues of Global Justice*, Rowman & Littlefield Publishers, Inc, Oxford, pp95–112

11
Population Disparities in Water Access, Sanitation and Health Implications

Introduction

Securing access to safe drinking water and adequate sanitation facilities for all people irrespective of their social background or economic status remains an elusive goal for many governments despite the numerous global initiatives to address these challenges. The United Nations first declared 1981–1990 as the International Drinking Water Supply and Sanitation Decade. Further commitment to address water-related disparities came in a collective decision to make water supply, sanitation and hygiene one of the targeted areas in the Millennium Development Goals (MDGs). More recently, the time period 2005–2015 has been declared the 'Water for Life' International Decade for Action. These efforts, while successful in shining the global spotlight on water, have unfortunately not fully succeeded in providing universal coverage across and within countries.

More than 1.1 billion of the world's population (or approximately 17 per cent) still lack access to clean water, and about 2.5 billion reside in communities without basic sanitation facilities (Krisberg, 2009). Significant strides have been made in some regions, such as eastern and southern Asia, where coverage has increased by 20 per cent since the 1990s. But in other developing regions, such as sub-Saharan Africa, few countries are on track to meet the targeted goals for 2015. There are still many unserved and underserved communities around the world, and water and sanitation-related diseases continue to pose serious health challenges among these vulnerable populations, particularly children.

While the international efforts to improve the standards have been primarily in the developing countries, developed countries are not entirely immune from waterborne health hazards. They too are faced with ongoing challenges of water scarcity, disparities in water pricing and affordability, and pollution and health problems associated with biological, chemical and physical contaminants in drinking and recreational water.

This chapter will examine the global challenges and population inequities in water and sanitation access. We start with an overview of the distribution of the Earth's freshwater sources and the critical role of water in the study of human health and welfare. Disparities in access and use of these water resources are discussed, including the adverse health consequences observed in poverty-stricken regions. The definition of water access and thresholds adopted to evaluate access remain inconsistent across countries. We shall discuss these definitional issues and then offer a multidimensional evaluation of water access based on the Penchansky and Thomas (1981) Model of Access. The chapter concludes with a discussion of geographic information systems (GIS) and geostatistical approaches that are used in evaluating access and identifying water poor areas and communities at risk of water contamination.

Water: An indicator of environmental health and group inequities

The importance of water in the study of environmental health hazards and health disparities cannot be overstated. Water is essential for all forms of life on Earth and therefore a prime indicator of the overall state and quality of the physical environment. The hydrological cycle, a natural though anthropogenic-ally altered process, is largely responsible for circulating, conserving, recycling, cleansing and redistributing water in its many varied forms around the Earth. Nearly 70 per cent of the Earth's surface is covered with water. Though this figure appears abundant, about 97.5 per cent of this earthly water is saline and therefore not readily usable. Of the remaining 2.5 per cent, about 70 per cent is locked up in glaciers and 30 per cent in soils, leaving less than 1 per cent (or .007 per cent of the total Earth water) readily accessible for human use (Gleick, 2000). In addition to the globally limited supplies of freshwater, the prime sources are unevenly and irregularly distributed among the world's regions and populations. Access and use of these water resources have historically been, and remain, the key source of group inequities and conflicts among various ethnicities, economic groups and countries around the world. Also anticipated are changes in global climate that are likely to have profound impacts on the hydrological cycle. Long-term changes are projected in the quantity and quality of freshwater sources, further compounding the effects of the observed regional and group disparities (Rose et al, 2001; Cooley et al, 2009).

Studying the water-related health disparities also requires recognition of the critical role of water in the human body and overall well-being. Water is the principal constituent of the human body, accounting for about 55 per cent of the body weight of adult females and 65 per cent of males. This total body water is distributed among different fluid compartments, within, outside and between the body cells, in the gastrointestinal, urinary and respiratory tracts. All other important functions, including the brain and bodily organs, collectively operate within a fluid-rich environment. As with the hydrological cycle, water lost through normal human physiological functions such as respiration, perspiration and urination must be promptly replaced to ensure the proper water balance in the human body. One begins to feel thirsty after losing only 1 per cent of the bodily fluids and continuing loss in excess of 10 per cent or more of this body water is life threatening, resulting in severe dehydration, electrolyte imbalance and changes in body chemistry, kidney failure and eventually death.

The basic physiological requirement is that individuals consume at least 2 litres a day, and a total daily supply of at least 50 litres per capita is considered adequate to meet the basic personal and hygienic needs. These recommended requirements do not match the consumptive needs and actual patterns of water use however. Water use patterns vary around the world depending on the physiological status of individuals, their daily regimen, temperature and humidity of the physical environments in which they reside, their cultural behaviours and rituals. For example, due to the excessive moisture loss in hot environments, water needs are greater in these regions, rising sharply as ambient temperatures exceed 25°C (Gadgil, 1998). An individual in a warm tropical environment, who is involved in strenuous physical activities, will likely require a higher daily intake of water than a sedentary person in a temperate environment.

Water needs also vary across cultural groups. Adherents of the Muslim faith, for example, are required to pray at least five times a day, and must cleanse themselves beforehand. The high demand for water in these communities is usually evident by the buckets or pools of water placed outside the mosques for worshippers, or the small kettles of water that individuals carry for this purpose. Among Christians, water is also symbolic of spiritual purification, as seen in the performance of baptismal rites in the church, or spiritual cleansing rituals of groups in streams and rivers. The association between water and religion is perhaps most visible among the Hindus, for whom all rivers are considered to be sacred with cleansing properties. Rivers are used to attain both physical and spiritual purity and provide the bases for nearly all rites and ceremonies.

The physical, cultural and social contexts of water use must therefore be considered when evaluating the consumptive needs across world regions. Using these parameters, a review of water use across world regions, however, reveals a geographical mismatch with significant inequalities between the tropical environments with greater consumptive needs and the more temperate countries. Globally, the highest levels of water use are in the United States, with an average use of 575 litres per person per day, when compared to 200–300 litres in many European countries. In many tropical countries in Southeast Asia and Africa, where consumptive needs are relatively greater because of the hot environments and manual occupations that residents are typically engaged in, water use is less than 50 litres (HDR (Human Development Report), 2006; Fonseca and Cardone, 2006).

The significance of water as an environmental health indicator is more readily evident today when examining the Global Environmental Burden of Diseases database compiled by the World Health Organization (WHO). An analysis of the disease-adjusted life years (DALYs) in this database shows that water-related diseases, especially diarrhoea, consistently serve as a leading cause of global morbidity and mortality. Nearly 88 per cent of all diarrhoeal-related deaths are caused by the lack of access to safe drinking water, basic sanitation and availability of water for hygienic uses. Diarrhoea is responsible for the deaths of 1.8 million people every year, and 90 per cent of those individuals are children under the age of five (WHO, 2004). Statistically, of the 192 countries examined in the disease burden database, the areas facing the greatest challenges are the countries in the African subregions D and E, and the Middle Eastern subregion D with 30–35 per cent of their population lacking access to safe drinking water, and 45–60 per cent with limited access to improved sanitation services (Figure 11.1).

Access to water and sewer services is also a prime indicator of the prevalence and severity of many neglected diseases that exist among the world's poor and marginalized groups. These are mostly parasitic infections such as ascariasis, dracunculiasis, schistosomiasis, filiariasis and onchocerciasis. They are most prevalent in the developing countries, though there is increasing evidence of their emergence among the poor and immigrant communities in the developed countries. Neglected diseases often lack media attention and visibility because they are localized and do not cause dramatic outbreaks that impact large numbers of people as do pandemics such as SARs and H1N1. Nonetheless, they exact a significant toll on people, resulting in blindness, severe disabilities and other chronic conditions. Nearly 100 per cent of the morbidity and mortality rates from these neglected diseases are attributable to unsafe water and sanitation and these conditions can be considerably reduced by the implementation of simple interventive and cost-effective programmes (Esrey et al, 1991; Hutton and Haller, 2004; Haller et al, 2007). Other vector-borne diseases such as malaria and Japanese encephalitis have also been linked to water-related projects such as dams, reservoirs and irrigation schemes.

Disparities in water access not only result in health inequities, they also contribute to gender inequities. In low-income countries, women and young

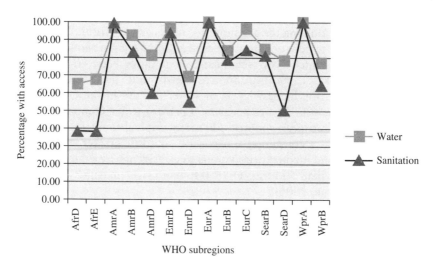

Data source: DHS (2007)

Figure 11.1 *Regional differences in access to improved water and sanitation services*

girls who would otherwise be in school, productively employed or involved in other prominent societal roles spend long hours hauling water for their families. In Africa alone, it is estimated that more than 40 billion work hours are lost each year to the process of securing water for domestic use (Haws, 2006; Aderigbe et al, 2008). For many of the households with limited access to water, 71 per cent of this task is completed by women and girls (WHO, 2004). In evaluating the effects of water access on female poverty, Haws (2006) recounts the often difficult and dangerous task that women face in finding, collecting, carrying and managing water. A typical day starts out at dawn when women venture out to seek water. Upon filling their containers, which could weigh as much as 45 pounds, the journey home is equated to carrying a large airline carry-on bag on the head, for miles at a time. This routine, which includes multiple trips per day, is believed to account for 25 per cent of the women's daily caloric intake. In the long run, the strenuous trips to and from the water points pose serious consequences for the women's health in these communities. Reported impacts include chronic pain in the hips, knees and backs, complications during pregnancies, and a greater risk of contracting water-borne diseases due to the frequent contact with contaminated water (Haws, 2006).

Overall, disparities in water and sanitation access are linked to the broader issues of poverty and social justice. Haw's (2006) fieldwork and many other research activities have established a firm connection between water and socio-economic inequities. The rural poor households are the most vulnerable, but increasingly a growing number of residents in the urban and peri-urban areas face similar challenges. These communities pay the highest prices for water due to the lack of water utilities and infrastructures in the low-income neighbourhoods in which they reside (HDR, 2006). In some countries, water resources have also reportedly been used as a political weapon to penalize or manipulate underrepresented groups, depriving them of a basic human need. These resources have been used to achieve political objectives, including the targeting of infrastructural systems such as pipes, canals and dams during military operations (Cooley et al, 2009).

Finally, as we examine the health challenges that arise from water access, it is important to note that much of the emphasis in the literature is on the consumptive use of water for domestic purposes. Relatively speaking, this constitutes only a small, albeit important fraction of the total water withdrawals. About 70 per cent of the world's water is used for agriculture, 22 per cent for industry and only 8 per cent is for domestic use. But here too, disparities abound when comparing the withdrawal patterns among countries. In low- and middle-income countries, the bulk of their water is devoted to agricultural activities (82 per cent), 10 per cent is used for industry, and only 8 per cent for domestic use. On the contrary, high-income countries use 59 per cent of their water for industry, 30 per cent for agriculture and 11 per cent for domestic use. These withdrawal patterns are likely to change with increasing population growth, urbanization and industrialization in the developing regions, producing even greater scarcity in the limited freshwater supplies.

Evaluating access to water and sanitation services

When examining the spatial patterns of health disparities associated with water and sanitation services, it is instructive to examine the notion of access, a concept that has been widely used in the literature (WHO, 2004; Jimenez and Perez-Foguet, 2008; O'Hara et al, 2008). Several definitions of access have been offered in the past, often focusing on the location, adequacy and safety of the water supply. In the 1990s, access to safe drinking water was assessed by looking at the proportion of people with access to an adequate amount of safe water located within a definable distance from the household. A review of the previous definitions used by developing countries revealed considerable variability in the thresholds used by these countries (see Tables 11.1a/b). Some countries based their criterion on a minimum distance of 50 metres. Others were more generous, using 100 metres, or distances as high as 2000 metres in rural areas. With respect to water supply, many countries chose a quantity of 20 litres, while others preferred the use of 30 to 50 litres or higher as the minimum per capita use per day for rural residents.

In subsequent years, the definition of access has been revised to focus instead on improvements in water and sanitation services relative to the pre-established baseline levels. An *improved* access to water is characterized as one in which residents have access to a household connection, a public stand post/pipe, a borehole, a protected spring, dug well or collected rainwater. Improvement in sanitation is described as access to a public sewer, a septic tank, pour flush latrine or a ventilated improved pit latrine (Table 11.2).

The current definition of access now expands on the preceding criteria by including the notion of sustainability. In a recent report compiled by the UN, the WHO/UNICEF Joint Monitoring Programme for Water Supply and Sanitation (JMP) defines access to drinking water in terms of distance to a source that is less than one kilometre away from its place of use, including the possibility of reliably obtaining at least 20 litres per member of a household per day (WHO/UNICEF, 2009). Basic sanitation is described in terms of the lowest-cost

Table 11.1a *Definition of access based on geographic location of safe drinking water source*

| | Number of countries defining access as 'water source at a distance of less than' | | | | | | | | |
	50 m	100 m	250 m	500 m	1000 m	2000 m	5 min	15 min	30 min
Urban	20	6	3	8	1	–	1	–	1
Rural	10	1	6	17	4	4	–	1	1

Table 11.1b *Definition of access based on water quantities for rural areas*

| | Number of countries defining the minimum quantity per person per day as | | | | |
	15–20 litres	20 litres	20–30 litres	30–50 litres	> 50 litres
Rural	1	19	5	10	3

Source: World Health Organization, 1996

Table 11.2 *Definitions of access based on improved water source, 2000*

Intervention	Improved	Unimproved (either unsafe or costly)
Water supply	• House connection • Standpost/pipe • Borehole • Protected well/spring • Collected rainwater • Water disinfected at the point-of-use	• Unprotected well • Unprotected spring • Vendor-provided water • Bottled water • Water provided by tanker truck
Sanitation	• Sewer connection • Septic tank • Pour flush • Simple pit latrine • Ventilated improved pit latrine	• Service or bucket latrines • Public latrines • Latrines with an open pit

Source: Global Water Supply and Sanitation Report, 2000

technology that ensures the hygienic disposal of faecal waste and a clean and healthful living environment both at home and in the neighbourhood of users. Access to sanitation now includes both safety and privacy in the use of these services.

While the aforementioned definitions provide basic metrics for countries to evaluate access, there some limitations in their use. First, as shown above, they have not been consistent enough to allow for comparison across countries. Further, these inconsistencies do not allow for the accurate monitoring of progress within countries to determine how far or close they are in attaining the targeted goals of the MDGs. In a recent study by Jimenez and Perez-Foguet, (2008), they confirmed that the lack of an internationally consistent definition and measurement methodology of access has caused confusion and uncertainty in the figures that are disseminated worldwide. Finally, it is safe to argue that these definitions do not fully capture all of the primary components of access. Some elements are missing such as the reliability of supply, affordability and acceptability of the water supplied.

A more comprehensive picture of access is proposed in this chapter using the Penchansky and Thomas (1981) Model of Access. This model was first applied to the study of health services, but it readily applies to water as a consumptive resource. Access to water can be described as a multidimensional construct with five components: availability, accessibility, accommodation, affordability and acceptability. Each of these components measures the degree to which individuals are able to benefit from water services in a reliable and sustainable manner (Figure 11.2). Following below is a description of each dimension. Since previous definitions have focused primarily on availability and geographic accessibility, our emphasis will be on the remaining three dimensions. Examples will be drawn from case studies of various communities around the world to illustrate how these components are measured and used to evaluate disparate patterns among population groups.

Availability. All of the previous and current definitions used globally focus on water availability as the primary basis of water access. Availability describes not only the nature and sources of protected water sources but also the degree to

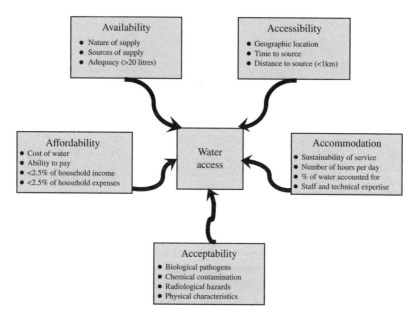

Figure 11.2 *The five dimensions of access to water services*

which residents have an adequate supply of this safe water to meet their personal and domestic needs. Personal needs include the water required to meet their basic physiological needs as well as for bathing and personal hygiene. The domestic needs include the water required for cooking, laundry and other household chores. As noted before, the metric differs across countries; however, the UN guidelines recommend that a reliable supply of at least 20 litres per capita should be the minimum threshold for characterizing access to water.

Accessibility has also been used extensively in the literature to delineate the geographic location of water services. As noted earlier, initial definitions of access focused on the distance (or time) to protected water points for households without pipe water connections. Again following the UN guidelines, a distance of less than one kilometre away from the water point is considered to be a reasonable basis for measuring this dimension of water access. A recent case study of water access in a metropolitan community in Nigeria using this parameter revealed the challenges that some residents face in securing water. Accessibility was measured both in terms of distance and time spent in securing the water (Aderigbe et al, 2008). The researchers found that 37 per cent did not have access to water in the households. Among the households lacking access, about 68 per cent travelled 1–5km daily, and 10.1 per cent more than 5km daily to secure water for domestic use. In terms of time spent on this activity, 50 per cent of the households spent an hour a day, 30 per cent spent about two to three hours and 19 per cent more than three hours. The authors concluded that these observed disparities in geographic access to water are clearly linked to lower productivity, reduction in earning power, and hunger and poverty among these disadvantaged households.

Affordability is a growing area of concern in both developed and developing countries, yet it is comparatively one of the least studied aspects of water access. It describes the costs incurred by residents to secure water, and their ability to pay for a minimum level of this service. One of the measures used to evaluate this dimension is the affordability ratio, which is the share of monthly household income that is spent on water. Some authors contend that it is better to use household expenditures rather than household income, because expenditures are usually more accurate, easier to capture, and more reliable particularly in developing countries where informal sector activities account for a large portion of the household income (Fankhauser and Tepic, 2007).

In an era of dwindling water supplies and growing concerns about water pollution, affordability is an increasingly important dimension of water access. Concerns about water quality require a constant revision of environmental regulations to ensure the safety of water supplies that are managed by utilities. In many developed countries, the rising costs incurred by the utilities when implementing these safety measures are ultimately passed on to the consumers. When looking at the share of these water prices relative to household expenditures, they are inversely related to the income levels of residents (OECD, 2003). Low or fixed income residents are frequently the most likely to be disproportionately impacted by these rising rates even after adjusting for inflation. These groups are also the most likely to reside in old and substandard housing structures with inefficient plumbing fixtures and leakages that contribute further to higher water bills.

To improve affordability among vulnerable population groups (such as the elderly, disabled, unemployed or underemployed), the US federal government, for example, uses a threshold of 2.5 per cent of the median household income. Thus, a total water bill that is greater than 2.5 per cent of the median household income would be considered excessive in a given community. Similar thresholds that range from 2.5 to 5 per cent of either the household income or expenditures are being used in other countries (Fankhauser and Tepic, 2007). The case for using these thresholds is to ensure that household monthly water bills do not impose undue economic hardships on low or fixed income households in a service area. Water rates should be affordable and low enough so that the poor, the elderly and other vulnerable groups do not trade off other essential life saving services (such as food, energy or health care) in order to pay their water bills. Additional measures used by various municipalities to provide water coverage include targeting certain population groups for subsidies, ongoing reduction of the total water bill to an affordable level, payment schedules, forgiveness of payments arrears, financial incentives to install water reduction plumbing devices, and home repairs to eliminate leakages.

In the developing world and other countries seeking transition to more modern economies (such as eastern European and former Soviet Union countries), the total water burden remains high among disadvantaged communities (Frankhauser and Tepic, 2007; Freeman et al, 2009). In most cases, the low-income residents pay more for the same amount of water than those with high income levels. A key challenge to improving these conditions is cost recovery. Many service providers in these countries are unable to generate enough revenues to cover the cost of the services delivered to residents. The use of public/private partnerships, water vendors, prepaid water meters and other initiatives are being put in place to ensure access. Prepaid water meters are used in South Africa, Brazil, Nigeria, Tanzania, Namibia and other countries looking to recover some of the expenses incurred for water delivery. These are often placed in low-income neighbourhoods where residents insert coins or use prepaid cards to get water. Some of these practices have come under intense scrutiny due to the potentially negative impacts on the poor. Research findings so far suggest that these meters cost more than water billed from utilities, forcing families to make trade-offs or resort to the old practices of hauling water from unprotected sources.

Accommodation describes the degree to which the provision of water services is consistent and dependable in meeting the basic needs of residents. This dimension of water access is equivalent to the sustainability of water supply and includes the ability to provide basic and reliable infrastructure for storing, treating and delivering water supplies to the population. In many developing countries, rapid urbanization, the proliferation of slum settlements in peri-urban areas, and obsolete water delivery systems have significantly impacted the ability to provide reliable supplies for the populace. Weak infrastructures and inefficiencies in the system often produce significant disparities in access. The poor neighbourhoods are often the most likely to suffer from these deficiencies and may be forced to purchase water from informal street vendors at a much higher price. Table 11.3 shows the differences in the costs of water (in US$) incurred by residents with household connections versus those that rely on informal vendor prices in selected cities in Asia. Disparities were found in nearly all of these cities, a pattern that is characteristic of many urbanized areas in the developing world. In New Delhi, India, the cost of water from the informal vendors is more than 400 times higher than the water supplied through household connections, a problem due in part to inefficiencies in the water utilities. In a detailed assessment of Indian cities, McKenzie and Ray (2009) found that for utility-managed systems, water was only available for a few hours per day, with irregular pressure and of questionable quality. Intermittent water supply, insufficient pressure and unpredictable services are all identifiable characteristics of a weak accommodation of the basic needs of a population. Following the lead of McKenzie and Ray (2009), the following variables can be adopted as measurable attributes of water accommodation or sustainability: (i) the number of hours per day of water supply; (ii) the percentage of water that is unaccounted for, or percentage of water produced that does not reach the customers; (iii) reports of uncontrolled leakages or illegal connections; (iv) the level of staffing and their technical expertise in coping with the utility-based water storage, treatment and delivery problems.

Acceptability refers to the quality of the water used by residents to meet their daily consumptive needs. Quality is both a measurable indicator of safety, in terms of the microbial, chemical and physical characteristics of the water, as well as its taste, odour or colour as perceived by residents who can then determine whether or not it is acceptable. Many governments either have their

Table 11.3 *Comparing the cost of water among households in selected Asian cities*

City	A: Cost of water for domestic use (house connection: 10 m³/month) in US$/m³	B: Price charged by informal vendors in US$/m³	Ratio (B/A)
Vientiane (Lao PDR)	0.11	14.68	135.92
Faisalabad (Pakistan)	0.11	7.38	68.33
Bandung (Indonesia)	0.12	6.05	50.00
Delhi* (India)	0.01	4.89	489.00
Manila (Philippines)	0.11	4.74	42.32
Phnom Penh (Cambodia)	0.09	1.64	18.02
Bangkok* (Thailand)	0.16	1.62	10.00
Ulaanbaatar (Mongolia)	0.04	1.51	35.12
Hanoi (Viet Nam)	0.11	1.44	13.33
Mumbai* (India)	0.03	1.12	40.00
Ho Chi Minh City (Viet Nam)	0.12	1.08	9.23
Karachi (Pakistan)	0.14	0.81	5.74
Dhaka (Bangladesh)	0.08	0.42	5.12
Jakarta (Indonesia)	0.16	0.31	1.97
Colombo* (Sri Lanka)	0.02	0.10	4.35

* Some water vending, but not common
Source: *Second Water Utilities Data Book*, Asian Development Bank, 1997

own nationally established standards, or follow the guidelines established by the WHO. These international guidelines were first published in the 1980s and have been revised a couple of times. These are not mandatory nor are they universally applicable standards. Rather they provide recommendations for countries to develop their own safety measures based on their local and national contexts (WHO, 2008). Drawing from scientific studies, these guidelines offer what are considered to be maximum acceptable values for at least four kinds of water contaminants: (i) biological agents; (ii) toxic chemicals; (iii) radioactive hazards; and (iv) physical hazards. Much of the emphasis is on the biological hazards since they account for a significant portion of waterborne diseases. These consist of bacterial, viral, protozoan and helminthic organisms that originate primarily from human and animal faecal sources. Without proper protective measures, people are exposed to these infectious agents through bathing, inhalation of water droplets or ingestion of faecally contaminated water. The latter is the most common pathway for disease transmission and requires the implementation of protective measures at all stages of water procurement including protecting the catchment or watershed, the use of appropriate treatment methods and the management of the distribution systems.

When compared to microbial agents, the health concerns associated with chemical hazards are less readily apparent, and only arise after prolonged periods of exposure. These risks nonetheless are widespread especially from non-point sources and produce serious life-threatening illnesses. Table 11.4 shows the four major risk sources of chemical hazards in drinking water. Given the variety of chemical hazards, the WHO recommends a prioritization of risks,

Table 11.4 *Risk sources of chemical contamination of drinking water*

Source	Examples	Examples of Chemicals of concern
Naturally occurring chemicals (including naturally occurring algal toxins)	Rocks, soils, cyanobacteria in surface water	Arsenic, Fluoride, Selenium
Chemicals from Agricultural Activities	Application of manure, fertilizers and pesticides; intensive animal production practices	Nitrates, Nitrites, Ammonia, pesticides
Chemicals from Human settlements including those used for public health purposes	Sewage and waste disposal, urban run-off, fuel leakage	Nitrates, organic chemicals
Chemicals from industrial activities	Manufacturing, processing, mining	TrichloroEthylene (TCE) Arsenic, cadmium,
Chemicals from water treatment and distribution	Water treatment chemicals, corrosion and leaching from storage tanks and pipes	Lead, copper, chlorine

Source: WHO (2008). *Guidelines for Drinking Water Quality,* 3rd Edition

with emphasis on chemicals that are more global in scope, and pose the most serious risks to human health. For example, arsenic, a naturally occurring chemical, has been reported in many countries, most notably Bangladesh, China, India, Thailand, Mexico, Argentina and the United States. Bangladesh has been at the forefront of the health crisis caused by excessive exposure to this chemical. More than 35 million people have been exposed to elevated levels through drinking water from tube wells. Roughly 1.5 million of these residents have developed arsenicosis, a health condition that produces lesions on the skin. Other chemicals of concern that are being closely monitored in many countries include fluoride, selenium, nitrates and lead. The risk of radionuclides in drinking water also exists, but to a far lesser extent than the microbial and chemical hazards.

Finally, the physical properties of drinking water such as the hardness, pH and total dissolved solids are worthy of consideration when examining acceptability as a measure of water access. Many studies have also shown that the physical attributes of water such as appearance, taste and odour, though subjective, are relevant measures. These characteristics do not necessarily have a direct effect on health, yet they impact the perception and attitudes of residents toward their drinking water sources. A utility-based water that has an unpleasant taste or odour, or is turbid, affects consumer confidence. This in turn may force residents to abandon the water source and resort to others that are not only more expensive but also less safe (WHO, 2008).

The acceptability of the water supply therefore goes beyond the definitive and measurable levels of microbial and chemical agents to include the more subtle, subjective aspects that may hinder the use of the water. The poor physical characteristics are caused by the presence of natural inorganic or organic chemical contaminants, synthetic chemicals, biological contaminants, corrosion of pipes, the treatment methods used or the storage systems. For example, in freshwater sources containing ferrous salts, oxidation may produce rust coloured deposits in the water. Hardness of the water may be caused by higher calcium and magnesium levels, and the taste may be affected by copper leaching or corroding from copper pipes in old dwelling structures. Residential perception of these characteristics could therefore serve as indicators of quality and acceptability of the water supply, sometimes requiring further investigation to uncover the source of the problems and potential health risks. In many developing countries, the water is not tested regularly for biological or chemical contaminants, so utilities and residents rely primarily on the taste, odour or colour of the water to determine whether it is of acceptable quality or not.

Application of geospatial technologies in evaluating water access and quality

Access to water is inherently a geographical problem that is amenable to many of the analytical approaches used in the discipline. As demonstrated in this chapter, inequities in the regional distribution and use of water abound, and more importantly, these disparities in coverage have profound impacts on human health. Though countless studies of the impacts of water access and quality on population have been completed, the most recent efforts involving the use of geospatial methodologies have been targeted at three areas: (i) using GIS and GPS tools to develop a water point mapping (WPM) system; (ii) exploring relationships between water access, and social justice; and (iii) using advanced geostatistical modelling to assess the health risks of water pollution and identify vulnerable populations. Examples of the research topics are provided below.

(i) Mapping water access

The use of the water point mapping approach has been offered as a more reliable option for establishing water access indicators and monitoring progress. The approach relies on the use of global positioning systems (GPS) to pinpoint the location of all improved water points in an area, and measure the five dimensions of access discussed earlier, including the quantity, quality, reliability, management and technical information regarding each site. This information is then entered into a GIS environment for subsequent integration with relevant data on the physical, demographic and administrative characteristics of the area. Collectively, the data layers would be used to evaluate the patterns of water access as a multidimensional, multifactorial attribute that is mappable at the community, administrative, regional and national levels. Jiminez and Perez-Foguet (2008) have been strong advocates of this methodology which they believe would greatly assist in the identification of unserved or underserved areas and improve planning. Using Tanzania as a case study, the authors use the acronym EASSY to describe the advantages of the WPM approach: *Easy* to get data at the local level; *Accurately* defined; *Standardized* and internationally applicable; *Scalable* at administrative levels; and *Yearly* updatable. They note, however, that securing the data at the baseline level might be expensive for some countries (approximately $12–15 per site) along with the data treatment and management requirements. Nonetheless, they argue that in the long run, the implementation of such a system will be cost-effective and will provide a reliable system for monitoring progress in reaching vulnerable communities.

The approach is potentially a great way to capture data on water access at the community level rather than the aggregated information that is often disseminated by governments and international organizations. For now, however, since few countries are willing to commit the necessary resources to capture this information, one can utilize the data compiled by the Demographic Health Surveys to map the patterns of water access at the settlement (cluster) or administrative levels within countries.

(ii) Exploring relationships between water access and social justice

This application of geospatial methods to evaluate the demographic and health status of residents in developing countries has been illustrated in some of the preceding chapters of this book. In this chapter, we chose to apply similar methodologies to the 2007 DHS data for Tanzania to visualize the associations between water access and the socio-economic status of residents. Data for water access and poverty were secured at the household level within clusters. There were 8497 records of households interviewed during the 2007 survey. Using the SPSS software package, the following variables were extracted, and aggregated to the cluster level: urbanization; altitude; poverty; access to improved water sources; time to water source; and access to improved sanitation services. The univariate statistics of these variables were calculated along with the computation of the relevant rates and ratios. These measures were then exported into the ArcGIS software for geostatistical analysis and mapping. Since the data were presented at the sampled points, ordinary kriging was performed based on the variable properties and distribution to create the predictive maps of the variables (see Figure 11.3). The maps confirmed that the most disadvantaged communities were in the northeastern and central parts of the country, particularly in the Shinyanga and Tabora regions. These were also the least urbanized regions. Poverty levels were highest in these regions and, not surprisingly, residents in these areas also had very limited access to improved water and sanitation services. The northeastern quadrant also emerged as the most isolated and mountainous region of the country. Time to water source in this region averaged up to nearly two hours, and as noted earlier in the chapter, this creates a significant burden for women and girls who are likely to take on the task of providing water for household members. Time to water source was found to be highly correlated with poverty ($r = .725$; $p < 0.001$) and altitude ($r = .701$; $p < 0.001$). The relationship with urbanization was low but yet positive and significant ($r = .329$; $p < 0.001$) suggesting that to some degree residents in the urban areas may also be facing similar challenges in securing access to improved water sources.

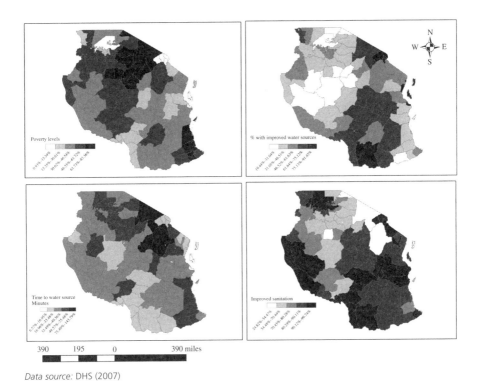

Data source: DHS (2007)

Figure 11.3 *Tanzania: Regional patterns of poverty and access to improved water and sanitation services*

(iii) Generating water pollution risk maps

Another area of significant growth in recent years has been the use of geostatistical methods to evaluate the environmental health risks of water pollution. One such example can be drawn from a study of rural drinking water quality in the western part of Sichuan province, China (Ni et al, 2009). As reported earlier, China has been hard hit with pollution from both point and non-point sources, particularly factory wastes, municipal sewage and agricultural run-off. In addition to biological contaminants, excessive levels of fluoride, arsenic and other toxic chemicals have been reported along the waterways, causing grave concerns for population health, and dramatically reducing international confidence in their seafood and agricultural products (Lall et al, 2008). The study by Ni et al (2009) involved the collection of 221 water samples in the study area. The samples were tested for 21 parameters including bacteriology (faecal and total coliforms), toxicology (iron, manganese, fluoride, mercury, arsenic, cadmium, chromium, lead and nitrates), hydrochemical characteristics (pH, COD, total hardness, total dissolved solids, chloride and sulphate) and physical quality (colour, turbidity, odour and visible materials). The data for these parameters were obtained from the sampled points and not the entire study area. So, following the procedures outlined in the previous section, the sampled data were integrated into a GIS, and a universal kriging approach was used to predict the overall risks of water quality in the study area. The carcinogenic and non-carcinogenic risks of these hazards were also assessed and used to produce single-factor risk maps, and a total risk map of water quality. The data layers were later linked to the physical and demographic layers of the study area to delineate the risk sources and the vulnerable areas. The authors found the approach valuable for assessing the health risks of water quality. Future studies, they argued, will require more accurate data, more samples and an evaluation of exposure risks using other transmission routes and pathways beyond just drinking water.

All of the studies described above collectively demonstrate how geographic tools are being put to use to evaluate water as an index of environmental health and health disparities. The results also provide the basis for generating new strategies to provide coverage in the unserved and underserved areas.

Conclusion

The disparities in the distribution and access to freshwater sources are responsible for a host of environmental health outcomes in many countries. Even as governments and non-governmental entities strive toward minimizing these disparities, there is still some disagreement in the international arena over the proper means of measuring access. This chapter offers a broader characterization of this concept that includes not just the availability, location and adequacy of supply, but the degree to which this supply is affordable, reliable and acceptable to the populations in need. Geographic methodologies can be effectively used to map out these different dimensions and identify the areas where people lack coverage or face adverse health risks because of exposure to excessive levels of bacterial, chemical or physical contaminants.

References

Aderibigbe, S. A., Awoyemi, A. O. and Osagbemi, G. K. (2008) 'Availability, adequacy and quality of water supply in Illorin Metropolis, Nigeria', *European Journal of Scientific Research*, vol 23, no 4, pp528–536

Cooley, H., Christian-Smith, J., Gleick, P. H., Allen, L. and Cohen, M. (2009) 'Understanding and reducing the risks of climate change for transboundary waters', www.pacinst.org/reports/transboundary_waters/transboundary_water_and_climate_report.pdf, accessed 10 June 2010

Esrey, S. A., Potash, J. B., Roberts, L. and Shiff, C. (1991) 'Effects of improved water supply and sanitation on ascariasis, diarrhea, dracunculiasis, hookworm infection, schistomiasis and trachoma', *Bulletin of the World Health Organization*, vol 69, no 5, pp609–621

Fankhauser, S. and Tepic, S. (2007) 'Can poor consumers pay for energy and water? An affordability analysis for transition countries', *Energy Policy*, vol 35, pp1038–1049

Fonseca, C. and Cardone, R. (2006) *Cost Estimates, Budgets, Aid and the Water Sector: What's Going On?: An analysis illustrated with data from 12 sub-Saharan African countries*, IRC International Water and Sanitation Centre, Delft, The Netherlands, www.irc.nl/page/33109, accessed 5 March 2010

Freeman, M. C., Quick, R. E., Abbott, D. P., Ogutu, P. and Rheingans, R. (2009) 'Increasing equity of access to point-of-use water treatment products through social marketing and entrepreneurship: A case study in western Kenya', *Journal of Water & Health*, vol 7, no 3, pp527–534

Gadgil, A. (1998) 'Drinking water in developing countries', *Annual Review of Energy and the Environment*, vol 23, pp253–286

Gleick, P. H. (2000) *The World's Water 2000–2001: The Biennial Report on Freshwater Resources*, Island Press, Washington, DC

Haller, L., Hutton, G. and Bartram, J. (2007) 'Estimating the costs and health benefits of water and sanitation improvements at global level', *Journal of Water & Health*, vol 5, no 4, pp476–480

Haws, N. J. (2006) 'Access to safe water and sanitation: The first step in removing the female face of poverty', *Women's Policy Journal*, vol 3, pp41–46

HDR (Human Development Report) (2006) *Ending the Crisis in Water and Sanitation*, United Nations Development Programme, New York

Hutton, G. and Haller, L. (2004) *Evaluation of the Costs and Benefits of Water and Sanitation Improvements at the Global Level*, World Health Organization, Geneva, Switzerland, WHO/SDE/WSH/04.04

Jimenez, A. and Perez-Foguet, A. (2008) 'Improving water access indicators in developing countries: A proposal using water point mapping methodology', *Water Science and Technology*, vol 8, no 3, pp279–287

Krisberg, K. (2009) 'Access to safe water a growing concern around the globe', *Nation's Health*, vol 39, no 8, pp1–14

Lall, U., Heikkila, T., Brown, C. and Siegfried, T. (2008) 'Water in the 21st century: Defining the elements of global crises and potential solutions', *Journal of International Affairs*, vol 61, no 2, pp1–17

McKenzie, D. and Ray, I. (2009) 'Urban water supply in India: Status, reform options and possible lessons', *Water Policy*, vol 11, pp442–460

Ni, F., Liu, G., Ye, J., Ren, H. and Yang, S. (2009) 'ArcGIS-based rural drinking water quality health risk assessment', *Journal of Water Resource and Protection*, vol 1, pp315–361

OECD (2003) *Social Issues in the Provision and Pricing of Water Services*, Organisation for Economic Co-operation and Development, Paris

O'Hara, S., Hannan, T. and Genina, M. (2008) 'Assessing access to safe water and monitoring progress on MDG7 target 10 (access to safe water and basic sanitation): Lessons from Kazakhstan', *Water Policy*, vol 10, pp1–24

Penchansky, R. and Thomas, J. W. (1981) 'The concept of access: Definition and relationships to consumer satisfaction', *Medical Care*, vol 19, no 2, pp127–140

Rose, J. B., ₋pstein, P. R., Lipp, E. K., Sherman, B. H., Bernard, S. and Patz, J. A. (2001) 'Climate variability and change in the United States: Potential impacts on water and foodborne diseases caused by microbiologic agents', *Environmental Health Perspectives*, vol 109, no 2, pp211–220

WHO (2004) *Health Through Safe Drinking Water and Basic Sanitation*, WHO Press, World Health Organization, Geneva, Switzerland, www.who.int/water_sanitation_health/mdg1/en/index.html, accessed 12 February 2010

WHO (2008) *Guidelines for Drinking Water Quality*, 3rd Edition, incorporating first and second addenda, WHO Press, World Health Organization, Geneva, Switzerland, www.who.int/water_sanitation_health/dwq/fulltext.pdf, accessed 12 February 2010

WHO/UNICEF (2009) *Refining the Definitions: An Ongoing Process and the Ladder Concept*, Joint Monitoring Programme (JMP) for Water Supply and Sanitation, www.wssinfo.org/definitions/introduction.html, accessed 10 June 2010

12
Food Justice, Nutritional Security and Paediatric Health Outcomes

Introduction

During the last five decades, the global food industry has been radically transformed by the modernization of agriculture and changing patterns in the food processing and retailing industry. With increasing mechanization of farming practices, we have witnessed a steady expansion of the total area under cultivation. Agro-technology companies have invested heavily in research and development of innovative farming technologies, agrochemicals and genetically modified crop varieties, with beneficial returns in crop quality and yield, drought tolerance and resistance to disease pathogens. Livestock farmers have also found efficient ways to increase the production of meat and dairy products from grain-fed animals while using advances in veterinary medicine to enhance animal growth and control disease outbreaks. All of these efforts have collectively contributed to a steady increase in global food productivity at a rate that outpaces the burgeoning world population.

The noted achievements in the agricultural sector, unfortunately, have been countered by a host of challenges in food processing, marketing and distribution to consumers. In recent years, the industry has been beset with a litany of scandals from tainted meat, milk and produce to consumer fears over biological contaminants and chemical additives used in the industry. Public health threats emerging from infectious diseases have been rampant. Instances of biological pathogens jumping from animal herds/flocks to humans such as Mad Cow disease, Foot and Mouth disease, SARs and H1N1 have heightened public concerns about food safety. Additional issues revolving around the excessive inputs of agrochemicals, the conversion of food crops to biofuels, and rising food prices have been worrisome as farmers brace for the impacts of global climate change.

Amidst all of these changes have been the perennial claims of inequities between the giant multinational corporations and individual farmers, and the disparities in food access and availability among consumers. Terms such as food justice, fair trade, food insecurity and food deserts are now being used within the context of social and environmental justice to bring attention to food-related disparities. Grassroots organizations are using the term food justice to describe their efforts to eliminate spatial, racial/ethnic and class disparities that exist in global and national food systems, to improve access to arable land and agricultural technologies, and reduce inequities in the distributional networks. The fair trade movement, which began in the Netherlands in the 1980s, is now a worldwide pressure group that seeks fairness in the global marketplace for small food producers to ensure that they receive a guaranteed and favourable price for their products (Millstone and Lang, 2008).

While there are many producer-related disparities that impact the quality and affordability of food commodities, this chapter will focus on consumer-related disparities. Emphasis will be on the social and economic inequities in food access and security, and the nutritional health outcomes particularly among children. We shall examine the multidimensional causes of food insecurity, analyse the relationships between food insufficiency and paediatric health, and identify the demographic, socio-economic and environmental correlates of these conditions. We start with a discussion of food security and access in the developing countries, using the West African country, Burkina Faso, as an example. This will be followed by a discussion of food deserts in the developed countries. Previous studies of food deserts in the developed world have confirmed their existence in the United States; therefore we shall base our discussion of these conditions in the United States.

Food insecurity and childhood vulnerability in developing countries

In a world of abundant food supply with enough to go around many times over, about 1.02 billion people (or 15 per cent of the world's population), still suffer from persistent hunger and malnutrition (FAO, 2009). The rate of hunger has increased at a faster pace during the first decade of the 21st century. Higher domestic food prices, higher unemployment levels and lower household earnings resulting from the recent global economic crisis have contributed to these trends. A map of hunger prevalence levels reveals significant disparities, with high rates in South Asia, Central America and sub-Saharan Africa (Figure 12.1). Though the Asian region has the largest number of people that are undernourished (about 640 million), hunger prevalence levels are greatest in sub-Saharan Africa where about 32 per cent of the residents are affected. In some of the war-torn countries such as the Democratic Republic of Congo, hunger prevalence levels are as high as 75 per cent.

Food insecurity conditions are said to exist when individuals or households lack access to nutritionally adequate foods (in terms of quality, quantity, safety and cultural acceptability), or their ability to obtain these foods is limited, at risk or uncertain (Frongillo, 1999; Smith et al, 2000; Nnakwe and Yegammia, 2002; Margai, 2007). Further evaluation of food insecurity conditions show that these problems extend beyond the nutritional needs of individuals. Other factors at play include: (i) the livelihoods of the population groups; (ii) their perceptions, responses and coping mechanisms; (iii) the trade-offs made between acquiring food versus other basic necessities such as health care,

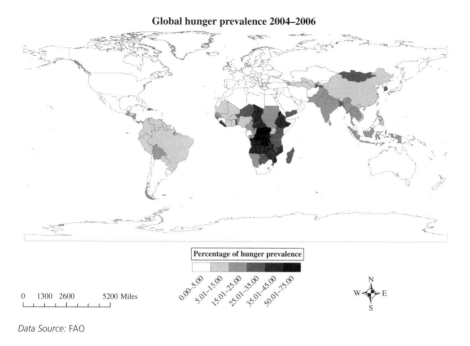

Data Source: FAO

Figure 12.1 *Global hunger prevalence levels*

education, housing or selling off livestock and other productive assets; and (iv) the degree of vulnerability associated with those conditions (Maxwell et al, 1999; Goldberg and Frongillo, 2001).

Health effects of food insecurity

For studies evaluating differential levels of vulnerability to hunger, the general consensus is that children are among the most susceptible population group. In developing countries, anthropometric indicators such as stunting and wasting have been identified as the most direct nutritional consequences of food insecurity (Campbell, 1991; WHO, 1995). Children undergoing long-term nutritional deficiencies are vulnerable to growth retardation, stunting and impaired physical development. Other harmful effects include the cognitive impairment of children, limiting their ability to concentrate and perform complex tasks. Undernutrition has been linked to childhood cognition through iron deficiency anaemia, a prevalent nutritional disorder that influences the child's attention span, memory and overall ability to learn (Skalicky et al, 2000; Weinreb et al, 2002).

Nutritionally deprived children are also prone to common infectious and potentially fatal diseases such as malaria, acute respiratory illness and measles. These conditions are exacerbated when sick children have poor appetites and are unable to eat well, leaving them with fewer of the nutrients required for their cognitive and physical development (Olson, 1999; Smith et al, 2000). In food-poor countries, malnutrition is the leading cause of childhood mortality and explains why one in seven children in these countries is likely to die before reaching the age of five (FAO, 2002).

Causes of food insecurity

Extensive research has shown that food insecurity conditions are triggered, and in some instances exacerbated by events at different spatial scales including the household, community, regional, national and international levels (Smith et al, 2000; Goldberg and Frongillo, 2001; FAO, 2002; Girma and Genebo, 2002). Figure 12.2 illustrates the causative linkages between these factors in explaining the nutritional status and health of children. This conceptualization is based on the comprehensive framework first posited by the United Nations Children's Fund (UNICEF, 1990), identifying the causes of childhood malnutrition as immediate, underlying or basic in nature.

The immediate causes are associated with the personal characteristics of the individual child such as the birth weight, age, birth order, birth interval and diet, all of which have been shown to be positively associated with nutritional health outcomes (Garret and Ruel, 1999; Girma and Genebo, 2002). The underlying causes are manifested at the household level. These are directly related to the care-giving practices and maternal characteristics such as the nutritional status, age, marital status, educational attainment and occupational status. Healthy mothers with moderate to high educational attainment, good occupational

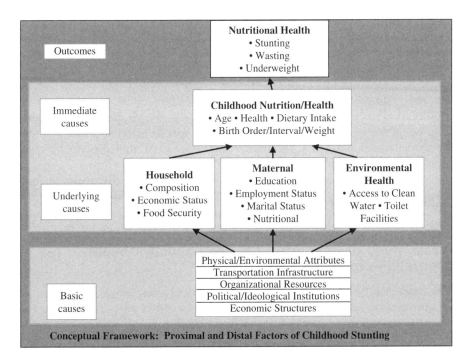

Figure 12.2 *A three-tiered framework for understanding childhood malnutrition*

status, and equal or greater control over household income and decision making are more likely to have nutritionally healthy children. With respect to age, some studies have found that food-secure households are more likely to have mothers in their productive years (ages 20–45), rather than those in the younger or older age groups. The marital status has also been shown to influence household food insecurity, with more vulnerable conditions found among unmarried rural and divorced/separated urban women (Girma and Genebo, 2002). Other household characteristics that impact a child's nutritional status and well-being include access to health services and the hygienic state of the household environment. Limited access to health care facilities, the failure to immunize the child and unsanitary household environments heighten a child's susceptibility to infectious diseases and indirectly influence their overall well-being.

At the third level of the conceptualization are the basic causes of food insecurity. These are manifested at larger spatial scales with variability at the community, regional or national levels. The regional or political subdivision of communities, the presence of environmental hazards (droughts, land degradation, floods, pests), economic/developmental challenges (trade imbalances, currency devaluations and market failures), structural adjustment policies, poor transportation networks and armed conflicts (rebel incursions, civil strife, wars) serve as basic causes of food insecurity in developing countries. In some parts of sub-Saharan Africa, these conditions have been compounded by the HIV/AIDS epidemic that has devastated the workforce leaving behind a less productive population of old adults and orphaned children.

Overall, as shown in Figure 12.2, the three-tiered framework offers a comprehensive way of looking at the direct and indirect linkages between food insecurity and childhood nutritional health. The first application of this framework was completed using geospatial data acquired for Burkina Faso (Margai, 2007). For this book, the research approach was reformulated using the most up-to-date statistics acquired in 2003, and more advanced geostatistical methodologies. The key objectives of this latest study were: (i) to use geostatistical methods to evaluate the spatial patterning of childhood nutritional health outcomes, specifically stunting; and (ii) then proceed by using multilevel modelling to identify the individual, familial risk factors, as well as the contextual risk factors that account for the geographic disparities in food access, and the poor nutritional health outcomes. Summarized below is a discussion of this study and the salient findings.

A case study of food insecurity and paediatric health geographies in Burkina Faso

The food insecurity conditions in Burkina Faso mirror similar situations in other African countries. As noted earlier, the basic causes are multifactorial and originate from a series of physical, environmental, political and social factors. In Burkina Faso, these basic factors include: (i) the country's landlocked location with limited infrastructure and accessibility to external markets; (ii) a multi-ethnic society characterized by diverse groups, with distinct livelihood strategies and behavioural adaptations in different ecological zones; (iii) the prevalence of recurring hazards in a marginal environment; and (iv) a turbulent political past and ongoing struggle to establish a democratic state. In 2003, the country was ranked 173rd out of 175 countries in the Human Development Report (United Nations Development Programme, 2003). Roughly half of the residents were children, below 15 years of age. Hunger levels were persistently higher with childhood malnutrition rates reportedly exceeding the maximum acceptable standards set by the World Health Organization (WHO, 2006).

Data sources and preprocessing

The 2003 Demographic and Health Survey (DHS) data used in this study consisted of 10,645 records of children, their health and nutritional status, the maternal characteristics including their reproductive histories, and the socio-economic and hygienic characteristics of the households. Following the application of sampling weights, the preprocessing of this dataset began by querying to remove all of the children aged three months or lower since the weight and other anthropometric measures of these children are influenced largely by prenatal conditions and maternal risk factors. The remaining childhood data file, consisting of 8593 records, was used to evaluate the nutritional outcomes.

This study focused on stunting (short stature), an indicator of the long-term cumulative effects of food insecurity in which the child's height-for-age is below two standard deviations of the median height-for-age of the standard reference population (WHO, 1995). Using this classification, a binary variable was created for stunting, by assigning a value of 1 to all cases in which the nutritional health outcome of stunting was evident and a value of 0 to those in which the outcome was absent.

Additional variables deemed relevant to the analysis were also secured from the DHS survey. The age, gender and current nutritional and health status of each child were garnered. The maternal attributes including educational achievement, age, marital status, occupation and body mass index were also secured. Among the household and community characteristics, the regional location (administrative subdivision), ethnicity, wealth index, type of residence (rural/urban) and the total number of children under five years were integrated into the data file. The environmental health attributes were based on two proxies – household access to piped drinking water, and the type of toilet facilities.

The other major sources of data used in this study consisted of food balance sheets including per capita food production, non-food crop production and general population statistics, and were derived from the United Nations Food and Agricultural Organization's database. Digital spatial data layers were also secured from the African Data Dissemination Service. These provided information on transportation infrastructure, cropland use intensity, agro-climatic conditions and administrative boundary files at four levels. Using the transportation infrastructure, geographic accessibility of each household within a cluster sampling unit was assessed. First, a query was performed to identify all the primary and secondary roads with year-round access. Seasonal roads were excluded from the analysis. Next, the distance analysis function in ArcGIS was performed and the results categorized based on proximity to these major roads.

Year-round access to transportation lines is deemed relevant for the swift and efficient delivery of resources to various parts of the country. Therefore, communities or households within a proximal distance to these major transportation lines were deemed to be more food secure than others. The distance of each household from the major roads was computed and integrated into the childhood-based file for subsequent analysis.

Data portraying the agro-climatic conditions across the country were also included in the analysis, with each zone reflecting the biophysical conditions that are conducive to cereal production. The intensity of cropland use was also integrated into the statistical analysis. When examining the map of cropland use, limited crop productivity was observed in the drier northern parts of the country where residents have far less favourable conditions for growing cereals than those in the wetter regions in the central and western parts of the country. It was also observed that the eastern region faces constraints in crop productivity due to poor soil conditions. Children residing in these areas are therefore expected to be more susceptible to food insecurity than their counterparts in the central and western regions.

The final comprehensive database consisted of several data layers for use in mapping and statistical validation to discern the spatial characteristics of childhood stunting in Burkina Faso. Figure 12.3 provides some of the data layers and preliminary maps of the physical environmental and socio-economic patterns of the study area generated within the GIS. Data values from all of

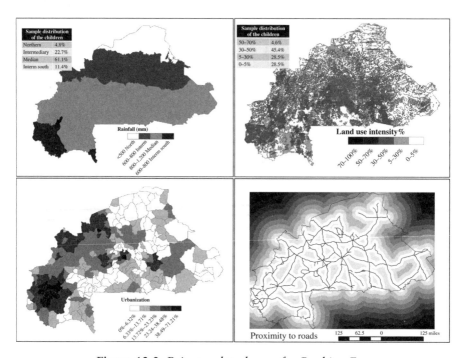

Figure 12.3 *Primary data layers for Burkina Faso*

these files were added to the childhood-based file by performing spatial queries using the cluster-based identification number of each childhood residence.

Mapping the prevalence of childhood stunting

Based on the sample data and the WHO guidelines, the average rate of stunting observed in Burkina Faso was nearly 40 per cent. This national rate was significantly higher than the rate of 28 per cent observed in the earlier study involving the 1999 data (Margai, 2007). Figure 12.4 shows the distributional pattern of the stunting levels from the sampled locations including the variable histogram, normal Q-Q plot, and semivariogram obtained prior to predictive risk mapping. The national risk map was derived using the ordinary kriging algorithm in the geostatistical analyst extension of ArcGIS. The highest incidences of stunting were in the eastern parts of the country, where stunting levels exceeded 40 per cent. Higher levels were also observed in some of the northern provinces and in the southwest. The lowest levels were observed in Ouagadougou, the most urbanized area of the country.

Using multilevel analysis to identify the determinants of childhood stunting

The final stage in the analysis was to use a multilevel approach to analyse the childhood stunting data at both the individual and cluster (community) levels.

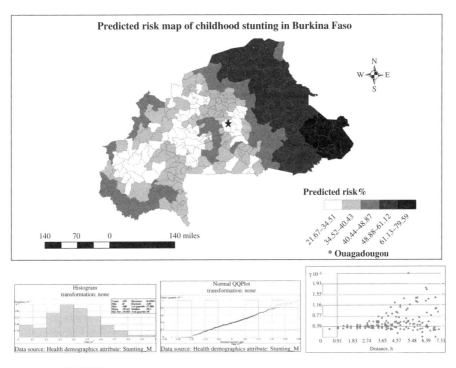

Data source: DHS (2003)

Figure 12.4 *Predictive risk maps of stunting in Burkina Faso*

This approach was deemed the most useful for a number of reasons. First, the technique was ideal because of the inherent structure of the stunting data, with a nesting of children within households, households within clusters, and clusters within regions. This hierarchical structure was most compatible with the conceptual framework proposed earlier consisting of basic, underlying and immediate causes.

A second reason for choosing this approach was to minimize the chances of committing inferential errors. A conventional regression analysis of stunting at the individual level assumes that the cases are independent (meaning that there is no intra-class correlation). Yet we know that many children within the same households or communities are likely to have some commonalities such as ethnicity, socio-economic status (SES), and climatic and physical environments. So, the use of a conventional regression model would have violated this assumption of statistical independence, thus increasing the chances of Type I error. Similarly, by aggregating the individuals and households, and performing the analysis at just the cluster (community) level, one would have increased the chances of Type II inferential errors. Other issues that were imminent in the use of traditional analytical methods were the *small numbers* problem, the loss of individual characteristics, and the likely reduction of power of the statistical test due to a smaller sample size. In light of these potential data issues, a multilevel approach was deemed the most appropriate for the new study. For those wishing to learn more, the analytical benefits and pitfalls of this approach and the applications in public health research are available for further review in many publications including Diez-Roux (2000), Kreft and deLeeuw (1998), Duncan et al (1996) and Bryk and Raudenbush (1992).

In the current study, a two-stage hierarchical model was performed. At the base of the model was Level 1, consisting of the individual children with measures of their stunting outcomes and their immediate and underlying risk factors. Level 2 was based on the residential communities (clusters) of these children and the basic attributes of those communities. These served as the contextual risk factors for childhood nutritional health outcomes. Thus, in the proposed model, stunting of the ith child in the jth cluster was expressed as Y_{ij} where,

$$Y_{ij} = \beta_{0j} + \beta_{ij} + r_{ij}$$

where

$$\beta_{0j} = y_{00} + y_{01}(yes) + y_{02}(cli) + y_{03}(X) + \ldots + u_{0j}$$

$$\beta_{ij} = y_{10} + y_{11}(age) + y_{12}(bweight) + y_{13}(X) + \ldots + \mu_{ij}$$

The outcome in childhood stunting Y_{ij} was a function of β_{0j}, the between groups variance (attributes of the communities such as urbanization, transportation access, agro-climatic conditions); β_{ij}, the within groups variance (attributes of the individual child such as age, birth weight and maternal characteristics), plus r_{ij}, a residual variance, an error term.

Table 12.1 summarizes the sample profiles at the household level, and the maternal and childhood characteristics. Tables 12.2 and 12.3 provide the results

Table 12.1 *Sample profiles of childhood stunting in Burkina Faso*

Household levels
- Urban 16.6%
- Average household size: 9.93
- Wealth index
  - Poorest – 18%; Poor – 20.8%; Middle – 26%
  - Rich – 18.1%; Richest – 16.9%
- Religion: Muslim 56.3%; Christian 27%
- Ethnicity: Mossi (53.7%)
- Household sanitation
  - 84.7% use neither piped nor bottled water
  - 73.4% do not have a toilet facility

Maternal
- Mean age: 29.81 yrs
- Occupation:
  - Agriculture 72.7%
  - Sales 15.7%
- Education
- Health card: 55%

Children
- Mean age: 29 months
- Mean birth wt: 2972kg
- Haemoglobin: 87.96g/dl
- Anaemia level (n = 2746)
  - Severe 13.3%
  - Moderate 60.9%
  - Mild 7.9%

---

derived from the multilevel analysis. Three separate models were produced using stepwise iterations and the model comparisons summarized at the end of the statistical computations (Table 12.4). The first model derived the estimates of fixed effects at the community level. The significant predictors of childhood stunting at this level were ethnicity, wealth index and urbanization. Further review of the ethnic dimension confirmed some variability in the risk of stunting, with two ethnic groups (ETHNIC = 3 and ETHNIC = 4 in the table) in particular experiencing significantly higher risks than counterparts, the

Table 12.2a *Model 1: Results from tests of fixed effects[a]*

Part A: Source	Num df	Den df	F	Sig.
Intercept	1	2717.276	122.9	.000*
ETHNIC	9	941.518	6.391	.000*
WEALTH	4	6011.347	6.531	.000*
URBAN	1	875.359	21.99	.000*
M_AGE5G	6	7392.903	1.079	.372
MSTATUS	5	7155.312	.730	.601
NORTHDRY	1	580.307	3.687	.055*
LAND5%	1	354.815	118.00	.732

[a] Dependent Variable: Stunting.

Table 12.2b *Model 1: Estimates of fixed effects*

Parameter	Estimate	Std. Error	t	Sig.
Intercept	.220699	.089836	2.457	.014**
[ETHNIC=1]	−.033238	.051735	−.642	.521
[ETHNIC=2]	.022833	.043816	.521	.602
[ETHNIC=3]	.101543	.045532	2.230	.026**
[ETHNIC=4]	.213312	.044381	4.806	.000***
[ETHNIC=5]	−.024130	.048384	−.499	.618
[ETHNIC=6]	.033465	.042979	.779	.437
[ETHNIC=7]	.030913	.036244	.853	.394
[ETHNIC=8]	.075661	.045342	1.669	.096*
[ETHNIC=9]	.054354	.071209	.763	.445
[ETHNIC=10]	0[a]	0		
[WEALTH=1]	.121138	.026581	4.557	.000***
[WEALTH=2]	.094018	.025968	3.620	.000***
[WEALTH=3]	.119844	.024673	4.857	.000***
[WEALTH=4]	.090998	.024028	3.787	.000***
[WEALTH=5]	0[a]	0		
[Urban=.00]	.118957	.025367	4.689	.000**
[Urban=1.00]	0[a]	0		
North5dry=.00]	−.077948	.040596	−1.920	.055*
[North5dry=1.00]	0[a]	0		

[a] denotes reference category.

Table 12.2c *Estimates of covariance parameters*

Parameter	Estimate	Std. Error	Wald Z	Sig.
Residual	.221126	.003738	59.161	.000***
Intercept [CLUSTER] Variance	.008391	.001546	5.429	.000***

*p ≤ 0.10   **p ≤ 0.05   ***p ≤ 0.01.

Fulfulde/Puel and Gourmanche groups. Both groups are related to the Fulani, a mostly nomadic people known throughout the West African region.

An analysis of the wealth index confirmed the social gradient hypothesis with children residing in the poorer communities more likely to experience hunger with a greater risk of stunting than those in the wealthier areas. Many of the physical environmental variables were not significant except for

Table 12.3a *Model 2: Adding covariates and random effects*

Estimates of Covariance Parameters[a] Parameter	Estimate	Std. Error	Wald Z	Sig.
Residual	.217470	.003727	58.352	.000
Intercept + CH_AGE + EDUC + meandist [subject = CLUSTER] Variance	9.936722E-6	1.697307E-6	5.854	.000

[a] Dependent Variable: Stunting.
*p ≤ 0.10   **p ≤ 0.05   ***p ≤ 0.01.

Table 12.3b *Model 3: Adding covariates and random effects at the individual level*

Estimates of Covariance Parameters[a] Parameter	Estimate	Std. Error	Wald Z	Sig.
Residual	.192866	.006098	31.629	.000
Intercept + CH_AGE + meandist + EDUC + BWEIGHT + PWATER + NUMKIDS [subject = CLUSTER]				
Variance	8.931327E-10	.294964E-10	2.711	.007

[a] Dependent Variable: Stunting.
*p ≤ 0.10   **p ≤ 0.05   ***p ≤ 0.01.

Table 12.4 *Model comparisons (smaller statistical values imply an improved model fit)*

Model 1 (fixed factors) at community cluster level	Model fit statistics
	AIC: 10116.1
	BIC: 10323.4
Model 2 (fixed and random effects) at community cluster/individual level (maternal attributes)	
	Model fit statistics
	AIC: 10082.8
	BIC: 10290.2
Model 3 (fixed and random effects) at community cluster/individual level (maternal + child attributes)	
	Model fit statistics
	AIC: 2868.3
	BIC: 3046.8

agro-climate where the dry conditions in the North were marginally significant risk sources of stunting ($p < 0.10$).

The second model was based on the fixed and random effects at the community and individual levels. Three variables were added to the list of significant predictors of childhood stunting. These included transportation access (measured as mean distance to primary roads), the educational attainment of the mother and the age of the child. Finally, the third model involved the addition of covariates and random effects at the individual level. The significant variables were the number of children in the household, the birth weight of the child and access to piped water.

A comparison of the model fit statistics derived from the different stages of the analysis confirmed that the third model was comprehensive and also the most predictive of stunting risk among children (Table 12.4). Overall, the analysis showed that at the community level, the nutritional health of young children was dependent on the degree of urbanization of a place, ethnicity and the wealth of the residents. Within the households, the most important determinants were access to main roads, access to piped water conditions, the number of children and better education opportunities for the mothers who are the primary caregivers. At the individual level, the results confirmed the existence of differential susceptibility among the children by age and birth weight. With the exception of the northern areas of the country, variables measuring the physical environmental constraints of food security did not emerge as significant risk factors in this study. A similar finding was noted in the previous study in which stunting levels were comparable across most of the climatic regions (Margai, 2007). These results underscore the earlier recommendations that reactive approaches, used by donor agencies to address food emergencies caused by biophysical conditions, must look beyond these physical/environmental factors to focus instead on social and economic risk factors such as urbanization, transportation access, household, maternal and childhood characteristics of vulnerable communities.

Food deserts and childhood vulnerability to hunger in developed countries

Studies of food insecurity and childhood vulnerability such as the one discussed in the preceding section often focus on poor nations, and rightly so, since statistical forecasts point towards a grim outlook in these regions. But even as we monitor conditions in these low-income countries, it is equally important to keep an eye on the developed countries where child hunger remains a perennial problem for economically and socially disadvantaged groups. In the United States, for example, the recent rise in poverty levels has been accompanied by an upsurge in the proportion of food-insecure households. Estimates released by the United States Department of Agriculture (USDA, 2009) showed a significant rise in hunger prevalence levels in 2008, the highest since the annual survey was first administered in 1995. About 14.6 per cent of all households (or 49.1 million people) are now deemed to be food insecure. Roughly 16.7 million of these residents are children. Further inquiry into these numbers reveals disparities by race, class, household composition and geography (Figure 12.5). About 42 per cent of the food-insecure households earn incomes below poverty levels. Single families with children, particularly those headed by women, experience the most difficulties. Black and Latino households are more impacted than their white or Asian counterparts. When examining the geographical distribution, the prevalence levels are comparatively similar across the census regions; however, residents in the principal cities and metropolitan areas experience the most difficulties in securing healthy meals.

Food deserts and obesogenic environments

In industrialized countries such as the United States, the term that is increasingly used to describe communities where residents encounter geographic and economic hurdles in accessing nutritional foods is 'food desert'. This terminology was reportedly first used by a resident in a public housing development in Scotland in the 1990s (Cummins and Macintyre, 2002). A related terminology is the 'obesogenic' environment. This is used to describe communities that host a high density of food establishments that offer unhealthy diets, large portion sizes and limited opportunities for physical activities. Since the 1990s, several studies have been conducted to validate the existence of these environments and the health impacts among residents, most

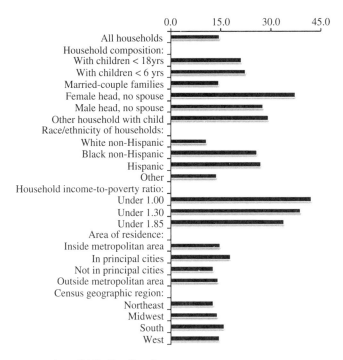

Data source: www.ers.usda.gov/Briefing/FoodSecurity

Figure 12.5 *Hunger prevalence levels by demographic composition in the United States*

notably in metropolitan areas (Swinburn et al, 1999; Smoyer-Tomic et al, 2006; McEntee and Agyeman, 2010).

In a systemic review of food desert studies conducted in the developed countries, Beaulac et al (2009) identified three types of methodological approaches used to delineate vulnerable communities: (i) market-based studies that compare the selection of food items across geographic areas and stores in terms of availability, variety, price and quantity; (ii) geographic-based studies that evaluate the geographic (physical) access to different types of food stores; and (iii) mixed methods that utilize both the market- and geographic-based measures of access. Their research revealed that nearly 70 per cent of the studies on food deserts so far have been completed in the United States, and the rest in the United Kingdom, Canada and Australia. Evidence from US-based studies was found to be compelling enough to support the existence of food deserts while the research from the other developed countries showed mixed results. In the United States, the geographically based studies showed that low-income and African American residents were more likely to be underserved by food retailers than other population groups. Some studies found higher prices in low-income areas and in African American communities, while others reported no differences in prices or, in some instances, lower prices in the disadvantaged areas. Generally however, prices were lower in urban areas than the rural communities. The availability and quality of the food in the disadvantaged communities were also found to be generally lower than other communities.

Causes of food deserts

The existence of food deserts and other obesogenic environments in high-income countries has been attributed to many factors including urbanization and market dynamics that produce systemic inequalities in the food retail environment. With urban sprawl and white flight, food retailers have abandoned the central cities in search of new trade areas and more profitable opportunities in the suburbs and exurbs. Poor residents in these urban areas who lack access to their own transportation are left with limited food options. They are forced to buy food from convenience marts, fast food restaurants and small corner stores that are often stocked with foods that are low in nutritional content but high in fat and calories and often pricier than those sold in other locations.

The challenges facing residents in the inner cities also exist in the rural areas but, surprisingly, few studies have examined the existence of food deserts in these environments. One exception is the recent analysis by McEntee and Agyeman (2010). Using data for Vermont, the researchers identified food deserts in rural areas. They began the research by categorizing food access into three types: (i) informational access which describes the educational, cultural and social constraints that influence how and why people choose to eat certain foods; (ii) economic access which describes the financial factors that impact one's ability to acquire food; and (iii) geographic access which expresses the personal and place accessibility in terms of distance to the food retailer. The study emphasized the geographic aspects of food access, and used the network analyst function in ArcGIS to compute the distance between each residential unit and the closest food retailer. For each census tract, the mean distance was calculated by aggregating the distance between each residential unit and the retailers, and dividing this sum by the number of residential units. Based on the mean distance derived for each census tract, a threshold of ten miles was used to locate the tracts with geographic access to food. Areas exceeding this threshold were identified as food deserts and further characterization of their socio-economic and demographic profiles was performed.

The health status of residents in food deserts

In both the urban and rural environments where food deserts exist, research has shown that there are often poor nutritional health outcomes among the residents in these areas. These residents not only lack geographic access to healthy and affordable food choices, but are also less likely to engage in other health promoting behaviours such as exercise, biking or walking, especially those living in the crime-ridden and stressful urban neighbourhoods. The lack of physical activity coupled with poor diet results in poor health outcomes, most notably obesity, along with other chronic diseases such as hypertension, high cholesterol, type 2 diabetes, stroke, cancer and overall poor health status (Vandegrift and Yoked, 2004).

Obesity, in particular, is a growing epidemic in the United States with alarming rates observed among low-income and minority populations. Prevalence rates among African Americans have been reported at 45 per cent based on the 2003–2004 National Health and Nutrition Examination Survey (NHANES). Kwate et al (2009) observed that blacks were 1.7 times more likely to be obese, and 3.1 times more likely to reside in neighbourhoods with a high proportion of obese residents. They attributed these patterns to not only individual risk factors but also higher levels of isolation, segregation and greater exposure to fast food restaurants. Using data for New York City, the researchers explored the effects of the food environment (or restaurant landscapes) on obesity among African Americans. Fast food restaurants (FFRs) were defined as establishments that do not provide table service, that serve patrons at cash registers or drive-through windows, that require payments before eating, and with primary menu items such as hamburgers, hot dogs and fried chicken (Kwate et al, 2009). Exposure to these establishments was determined by using a GIS grid-based approach to arrive at the total number of FFRs within a 300m radius of the centre of each grid (which was roughly equivalent to half a block in the city). Average exposure for each block group was then calculated by dividing the sum value for all cells in each block group by the number of cells in that block group. Using the FFR exposure index as the dependent variable, a series of statistical models were derived. The researchers found that, when examining exposure in residential areas, the FFR rates were highest in block groups with a high proportion of African Americans. These findings were consistent even in instances where adjustments were made for median household income.

The link between obesity and social and environmental risk factors such as food deserts was also established in an earlier study by Reidpath et al (2002). The environmental determinants were measured by the density of FFRs. Using data from Melbourne, Australia, the researchers found that those living in areas with the lowest individual median weekly incomes were 2.5 times more exposed to fast food chains than those living in areas with the highest individual median weekly incomes. Knowledge of these risk factors and challenges facing residents in these areas is useful in developing health interventive strategies.

Chapter summary and conclusions

The decadal progress made in agricultural productivity and the global fight against hunger has recently been eroded by the world economic downturn, and scandals in the food industry. Alongside these crises have been widening disparities between producers (small farmers versus giant food corporations), and between consumers. The discussions in this chapter have focused largely on consumer issues by exploring the geographies of food injustice by race/ethnicity and class. The global scope of these problems has been illustrated by drawing examples from two vastly different countries, the United States, one of the world's richest countries, and Burkina Faso, one of the world's poorest.

In both countries, we focused on the likely impacts of food deficits on children. While stunting was identified as the primary health outcome of food insecurity among children in Burkina Faso, in the United States, obesity was the primary health concern as children and their families turn to unhealthy food choices to meet their daily consumptive needs. Geographically, the areas lacking access to nutritional foods were also different in these two countries. In Burkina Faso, these were primarily rural environments, in the northern reaches of the country with agro-climatic constraints, and the eastern areas with poor soils and limited access to main access roads. Within the United States, the food deserts were the most urbanized areas (inner cities) with dense transportation networks and fast food establishments. Residents who lacked their own automobiles were limited in geographic access to healthy and affordable foods.

Despite the differences in geography and health outcomes, two commonalities identified in both settings were fairly consistent with the primary themes of this book. Specifically, the socio-economic status of residents, and the racial/ethnic dimensions both emerged as risk factors of food insecurity. In Burkina Faso, the wealth index and ethnic characteristics of the population clusters were significant risk factors of stunting. Similarly, in the United States, hunger prevalence levels were highest among minorities and families below the poverty levels. The maternal characteristics were also important, as evidenced by the educational attainment of mothers in Burkina Faso, and the high risk of hunger among single family households headed by women in the United States.

Finally, geographic methodologies were used successfully to demonstrate the spatial patterning of these disparities in both settings. In Burkina Faso, data were drawn at multiple spatial scales to identify the hotpots for childhood stunting. Using a three-tiered analytical framework, these paediatric nutritional health outcomes were expressed as a function of basic, underlying and immediate causes that are manifested at the regional/community level, the household level and the personal level. In the United States, a review of the literature showed the use of geographic methodologies as prescriptive tools to identify food deserts and obesogenic environments in both urban and rural communities. Though these studies were conducted in vastly different settings, the findings underscore the need for ongoing surveillance of disadvantaged communities in both food-rich and food-poor nations, to assist needy families who are likely to suffer long-term health consequences as a result of chronic food insecurity.

References

Beaulac, J., Kristjansson, E. and Cummins, S. (2009) 'A systematic review of food deserts, 1966–2006', *Preventing Chronic Disease*, vol 6, no 3, pp1–10

Bryk, A. S. and Raudenbush, S. W. (1992) *Hierarchical Linear Models: Applications and Data Analysis Methods*, Sage, Newbury Park, CA

Campbell, C. (1991) 'Food insecurity: A nutritional outcome or a predictor variable', *Journal of Nutrition*, vol 121, pp408–415

Cummins, S. and Macintyre, S. (2002) 'Food deserts: Evidence and assumption in health policy making', *British Medical Journal*, vol 325, no 21, pp436–438

Diez-Roux, A. (2000) 'Multilevel analysis in public health research', *Annual Review of Public Health*, vol 21, pp171–192

Duncan, C., Jones, K. and Moon, G. (1996) 'Health-related behavior in context: A multilevel modeling approach', *Social Science and Medicine*, vol 42, no 6, pp817–830

FAO (2002) *The State of Food Insecurity in the World*, Food and Agriculture Organization of the United Nations, Rome, www.fao.org/docrep/005/y7352e/y7352e00.htm, accessed 28 May 2003

FAO (2009) *The State of Food Insecurity in the World*, Food and Agriculture Organization of the United Nations, Rome, www.fao.org/docrep/012/i0876e/i0876e00.htm, accessed 3 March 2010

Frongillo, E. A. (1999) 'Validation of measures of food insecurity and hunger', *Journal of Nutrition*, vol 129, pp506–509

Garrett, J. L. and Ruel, M. T. (1999) 'Are determinants of rural and urban food security and nutritional status different? Some insights from Mozambique', *World Development*, vol 27, no 11, pp1955–1975

Girma, W. and Genebo, T. (2002) 'Determinants of nutritional status of women and children in Ethiopia', *Demographic Health Survey*, Macro International Inc, Calverton, MD

Goldberg, A. D. and Frongillo, E. A. (2001) 'Cultural perspectives for understanding food security among the Mossi', a Background Paper on Food Security in Burkina Faso, *Food and Nutrition Technical Assistance (FANTA)* Project, Academy for Educational Development, Washington, DC

Kreft, I. and deLeeuw, J. (1998) *Introducing Multilevel Modeling*, Sage, London

Kwate, N. O., Yau, C., Loh, J. and Williams, D. (2009) 'Inequality in obesigenic environments: Fast food density in New York City', *Health and Place*, vol 15, pp364–373

Margai, F. M. (2007) 'Geographic targeting of risk zones for childhood stunting and related outcomes in Burkina Faso', *Journal of World Health and Population*, June, pp1–19

Maxwell, D., Ahiadeke, C., Levin, C., Arman-Klemesu, M., Zakariah, S. and Lamptey, G. M. (1999) 'Alternative food security indicators: Revisiting the frequency and severity of coping strategies', *Food Policy*, vol 24, pp411–429

McEntee, J. and Agyeman, J. (2010) 'Towards the development of a GIS method for identifying rural food deserts: Geographic access in Vermont, USA', *Applied Geography*, vol 30, pp165–176

Millstone, E. and Lang, T. (2008) *The Atlas of Food: Who Eats What, Where and Why*, University of California Press, Berkeley, CA

Nnakwe, N. and Yegammia, C. (2002) 'Prevalence of food insecurity among households with children in Coimbatore, India', *Nutrition Research*, vol 22, pp1009–1016

Olson, C. M. (1999) 'Nutrition and health outcomes associated with food insecurity and hunger', *Journal of Nutrition*, vol 129, pp521–524

Reidpath, D. D., Burns, C., Garrard, J., Mahoney, M. and Townsend, M. (2002) 'An ecological study of the relationships between social and environmental determinants of obesity', *Health and Place*, vol 8, pp141–145

Skalicky, A. M., Frank, D. A., Meyers, A. F., Adams, W. G. and Cook, J. T. (2000) 'Does food security and hunger correlate with lab indices of iron nutrition in young inner city children?', (Abstract 12221), Paper presented at the 128th Annual Meeting of

American Public Health Association, http://apha.confex.com/apha/128am/techpro gram/paper_12221.htm, accessed 7 June 2004

Smith, L. C., El Obeid, A. E. and Jensen, H. H. (2000) 'The geography and causes of food insecurity in developing countries', *Agricultural Economics*, vol 22, pp199–215

Smoyer-Tomic, K., Spence, J. and Amrhein, C. (2006) 'Food deserts in the prairies? Supermarket accessibility and neighborhood need in Edmonton, Canada', *The Professional Geographer*, vol 58, no 3, pp307–326

Swinburn, B., Egger, G. and Raza, F. (1999) 'Dissecting obesogenic environments: The development and application of a framework for identifying and prioritizing environmental interventions for obesity', *Preventive Medicine*, vol 29, pp563–570

UNDP (2003) *Millennium Development Goals: A Compact among Nations to End Human Poverty*, Human Development Report, United Nations Development Programme, United Nations, New York

UNICEF (1990) 'Strategy for improved nutrition of children and women in developing countries', Policy Review Paper, United Nations Children's Fund, United Nations, New York

USDA (2009) *Household Food Security in the United States*, 2008, Economic Research Report # 83, United States Department of Agriculture, Washington, DC

Vandegrift, D. and Yoked, T. (2004) 'Obesity rates, income, and suburban sprawl: An analysis of US states', *Health and Place*, vol 10, pp221–229

Weinreb, L., Wehler, C., Perloff, J., Scott, R., Hosmer, D., Sagor, L. and Gundersen, C. (2002) 'Hunger: Its impact on children's health and mental state', *Pediatrics*, vol 110, no 4, pp1–9

WHO (1995) *Physical Status: The Use and Interpretation of Anthropometry*, Report of a WHO Expert Committee, Technical Report Series No 854, World Health Organization, Geneva, Switzerland

WHO (2006) 'Health profile of Burkina Faso', www.afro.who.int/index.php? option=com_content&view=article&id=1018&Itemid=2045, accessed 25 March 2008

PART III

SOCIAL AND ECONOMIC FACTORS IN POPULATION HEALTH DISPARITIES

13
Poverty, Race and Place: A Triple Whammy Hypothesis for Minority Health Geographies

Introduction

The effect of poverty and class on population health disparities is well recognized in the literature, as noted by the social gradient hypothesis introduced earlier in Chapter 4. In many countries, evidence of these disparities has been linked primarily to class differences among population groups. In the United Kingdom, for example, the most common predictor variable used by scholars to study health disparities is occupation, while in other European countries, education and occupation dominate the literature as the primary predictors (Adler, 2006). Ethnic differences between population groups have also been identified as the root causes of health disparities in other countries (Wu et al, 2003).

Comparatively speaking, the United States represents one of the few countries where health disparities are strongly influenced by not just one, but two or more dimensions, and the intersections between them. Some scholars have appropriately characterized the observed relationships between these multiple dimensions, chiefly race, ethnicity and class, and the related health outcomes as a confluence of risks (Wood, 2003). A related idea is the *double jeopardy hypothesis* which posits that in many communities, those who bear a double burden, such as being poor and being a member of a minority group are more likely to face double health disadvantages than their counterparts (Beal, 1970; Dowd and Bengtson, 1978; King, 1988; Ferraro and Farmer, 1996). Thus, within the context of race and class, one can expect population health disparities to be greater among minority groups who are doubly disadvantaged by their race and class status.

Of greater interest in this book is the geographical context in which these differential health patterns emerge. Many studies have not fully acknowledged the fundamental role of place in explaining these disparities yet there is sufficient evidence that suggests otherwise. As demonstrated in most of the chapters in this book, place critically impacts the living environments of people and their access to all of life's enhancing resources including water, healthy food and a pollution-free environment. The purpose of this chapter therefore is to make the case for the expansion of the double jeopardy hypothesis to a *triple jeopardy*, or *triple whammy hypothesis*, in which the synergistic effects of poverty, race and place are examined as the core drivers of population health disparities. The hypothesis is best proven by evaluating minority health geographies in the United States, a country where a distinct geographical concentration of poverty is evident across racially segregated communities (Massey et al, 2009).

The chapter examines the interconnections between race/ethnicity, class and place and the overall impacts on the health of the nation's largest minority groups: African Americans, Latino Americans, Native Americans and Asian Americans. These issues are addressed within a locational context to bring attention to key geographic themes such as residential segregation, settlement geography, immigration and the socio-spatial experiences of these groups. The first part of the chapter presents the triple whammy hypothesis, and then proceeds to examine the conceptualization of segregation – a process that many scholars would argue is at the root of social and environmental health inequities in the country. This is followed by a separate analysis of the unique health concerns of each minority group. The chapter concludes with a discussion of these emergent themes and pursuable areas for health intervention.

The triple whammy hypothesis

The *triple jeopardy* or *triple whammy hypothesis* proposed in this book is essentially an extension of the double jeopardy hypothesis, in which the fundamental role of place in population health is acknowledged. In addition to the main effects, two-way interactions of poverty and race, poverty and place, and race and place, and the three-way interactions of poverty, race and place, are presented as the core drivers of population health geographies. These dual and triple forces are most evident in the United States where there are distinct geographies of race and class.

A preliminary investigation of the effectiveness of this hypothesis was recently completed by analysing the health effects of poverty on children from different racial and ethnic backgrounds and across different geographic regions in the United States (Margai, 2008). Figure 13.1 presents the conceptual framework of the triple whammy hypothesis that was developed in that study. The hypothesis was tested using 2006 data from the National Health Interview Surveys (NHIS). Among the key indicators used to assess the health outcomes among children were their physical health (birth weight, prevalence of asthma, diabetes), cognitive well-being (learning disability), emotional well-being, behavioural outcomes, self-reported health status, and access and utilization of health care services. Poverty levels were assessed based on two thresholds: family earnings at 100 per cent below the poverty line, and 50 per cent (extreme poverty) levels. A multivariate analysis of the data demonstrated that along with known covariates, the main effects and interactive effects of poverty, race and place were influential determinants in explaining the variability in the four indices of child health. With further analysis of these health indices, the triple whammy hypothesis was most evident among children residing under

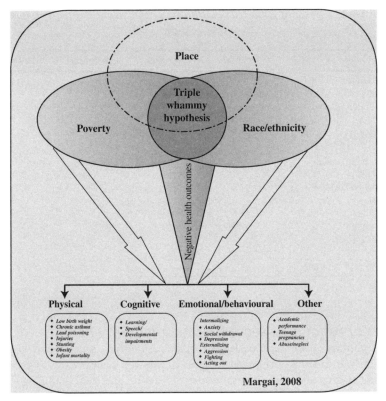

Figure 13.1 *The ecology of poverty, race and place on child health*

conditions of extreme poverty. The combined effects of race, place and poverty were most highly significant in explaining the physical, cognitive health of the children and their access to health care (see Table 13.1).To date, no other study has offered this perspective in which place plays a fundamental role by interacting with race and class to explain population health disparities. Many scholars, however, have commented on the need to study the ongoing evolution of racially distinct landscapes in the United States (Massey et al, 2009), the emergence of sharper economic divisions over economic space, and the so-called balkanization of social and demographic groups (Frey, 1996). Friedman and Lichter (1998) credited these trends to changes in the composition of local industries and labour markets, industrial restructuring and job losses that have been accelerated by globalization and outsourcing of economic activities. The spatial inequalities in poverty are compounded by the racial/ethnic characteristics of the population subgroups such that those who are poor, non-white and live in these areas face triple disadvantages when it comes to their health status. Thus, minorities residing in areas of concentrated poverty such as Appalachia, the southern 'black belt' region, and the inner cities of major metropolitan areas are more likely to face a triple health burden by virtue of their socio-economic status (SES), their race, ethnicity and location.

Table 13.1 *Assessing pediatric health disparities using the triple whammy hypothesis*

Variables	Physical	Cognitive	Emotional	Health access
Race/ethnicity		***	***	***
Place	***	***	***	
Poverty (under 50 per cent)	***	***	***	***
Race × Place		**		**
Race × Poverty	***	***	***	***
Race × Place × Poverty	***	***	*	***
Age	***	***	***	***
Birth weight	***	***	***	
Indigenous households	***	***	**	***
Education				***
Single mother	**	***	*	***
Unemployment	*	*	**	**
Home ownership			**	***
Family size				***
Number of kids in family			***	*

$^{***}p \leq 0.01;\ ^{**}p \leq 0.05;\ ^{*}p \leq 0.10;$

Effects of residential segregation on minority health

Many scholars have acknowledged that residential segregation patterns, particularly in historic urban settlements across the country, say a great deal about the origins of environmental health disparities and their enduring impacts on the nation's minority groups (Lopez, 2002; Gee and Payne-Sturges, 2004; Morello-Frosh and Lopez, 2006). Research efforts to understand these patterns have looked at how segregation is conceptualized and measured in the literature, with applications of these measures in the study of negative health conditions such as poor reproductive health outcomes (Geronimus, 2000; Grady, 2003; Mason et al, 2009), lead poisoning (Oyana and Margai, 2010) and asthma and other forms of air pollution (Morello-Frosh and Lopez, 2006).

The concept of segregation was first introduced by Burgess (1928) and has since being widely used by social scientists to describe and measure the extent to which population subgroups live geographically apart from one another in an urbanized environment. People may willingly or unwillingly reside in different neighbourhoods, census tracts or other areal units because of their racial/ethnic composition (racial/ethnic segregation), their income or class status (economic segregation), or both. Evidence from the literature suggests, however, that residential segregation by race/ethnicity in the United States is stronger than economic segregation.

Historically, studies of racial segregation were based primarily on white and black populations, but more current investigations incorporate Hispanics and Asian Americans, an indication of the increasingly pluralistic nature of the nation's population. Since the 1950s, nearly 20 measurable indices of segregation have been developed for research and policy applications (Iceland et al, 2002). A factor analysis of these measures by Massey and Denton (1988) led to the conclusion that they can all be organized into the five basic geographic dimensions of segregation. These are evenness, exposure, clustering, centralization and concentration. Groups that experience two of more of these attributes are said to be hypersegregated (Osypuk and Acevedo-Garcia, 2008). Below is a brief description of each dimension. Then using data from the US Census in 1980, 1990 and 2000, Figure 13.2a–d shows the different indices obtained for each minority group in metropolitan statistical areas (MSAs) with at least 3 per cent or 20,000 or more of these racial and ethnic minority groups.

1 *Evenness (or unevenness)* is a measure of the disproportionate distribution of racial/ethnic groups across spatial units in a metropolitan area. The measure compares the proportion of a particular racial/ethnic group living in a certain neighbourhood (or census areal units) to the group's relative percentage for the entire urban area. A group is regarded as segregated when the percentages observed in certain areal units are significantly greater than the relative percentage obtained for the city. This implies the need for population redistribution in order to achieve evenness. Traditionally, evenness is calibrated using the dissimilarity index which is expressed in Table 13.2. The derived index, D, varies from 0 to 1, the closer to 0, the lower the segregation. For example, the dissimilarity index for blacks in New York City in 2000 was 0.821 meaning that 82.1 per cent of the blacks and whites would have to be relocated in this city in order to achieve complete integration of the two racial groups. Based on the D index reported in Figure 13.2a–d, the highest levels of residential segregation were observed among the African American and Latino populations.

2 *Exposure* describes the degree to which members of a minority group are exposed only to one another or the likelihood of physical contact with other racial or ethnic groups in the metropolitan area. One measure of exposure is the interaction index, which is calibrated using the formula outlined in Table 13.2. The index, mP_n^*, measures the probability that members of the group m share a neighbourhood with members of another group n. Alternatively, it can be computed as a probability that members of a group m share the same residential areas with each other, mP_m^*. The latter, often called the isolation index, varies from 0 to 1, and the higher this value, the higher the isolation. Again for New York City, the isolation index observed for blacks in 2000 was 0.838 suggesting a high probability that black residents tend to reside next to each other within the same neighbourhoods.

3 *Concentration* measures the relative amount of physical space occupied by specific minority groups within the urbanized area. Proponents of this measure argue that a high level of concentration speaks volumes about the disproportionate impacts of discrimination, poverty, and social and economic constraints among minorities. They are often cramped into small areas relative to the larger urban space resulting in high densities, overcrowding, stressful environments and other social ills. Measures of concentration typically assess the population density of the minority group, relative to the density of other groups. One such measure is the Duncan's delta index outlined in Table 13.2. A value of 0 implies uniform density. A higher value implies residential segregation of the specific minority groups.

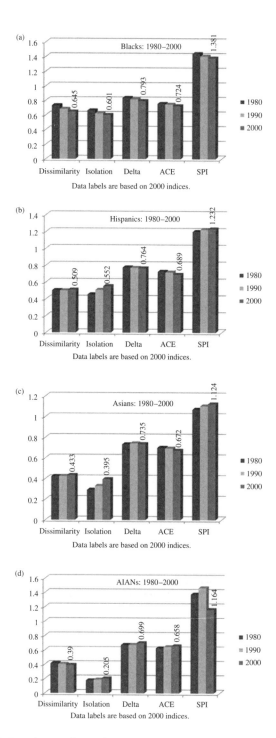

Figure 13.2a–d *Residential segregation trends among US minorities*

Table 13.2 *A summary of the measures used to evaluate the five dimensions of racial/ethnic segregation in US metropolitan areas*

Dimension	Measure	Formula	Spatial	Multi-group
Evenness	Index of dissimilarity	$D = \sum \dfrac{[t_i\lvert p_{im} - P_m\rvert]}{2TP_m - (1 - P_m)}$	Yes	Yes
Exposure	Interaction index	$mP_n^\star = \sum \left[\dfrac{t_i P_{im}/TP_m}{[(P)_{in}]}\right]$	No	No
Concentration	Duncan's Delta index	$\text{DEL} = \sum \dfrac{\left[\left\lvert\left(\frac{t_i p_{im}}{TP_m}\right) - \left(\frac{a_i}{A}\right)\right\rvert\right]}{2}$	No	No
Centralization	Absolute centralization index	$\text{ACE} = \sum[X_{i-1p}A_i] - \sum[X_{ip}A_{i-1}]$ Tracts sorted by land area $X_{ip} = \sum[t_i p_{im}]$, tracts from 0 to i $A_{ip} = \sum[a_i]$, tracts from 0 to i	Yes	No
Clustering	Spatial proximity index	$S_p = \dfrac{TP_m^L P_{mm}^{LL} + TP_n^L P_{nn}^{LL}}{NP_{tt}^{LL}}$ $P_{mn} = \sum\sum\left[\dfrac{t_i P_{im} t_j P_{jn} C_{ij}}{TP_m TP_n}\right]$ $C_{ij} = e^{-d_{ij}}$ $d_{ij} =$ distance between tract I and tract j	Yes	No

Note: T is the number of residents in urban area; t_i is the number of residents in tract I; Pm is the proportion of urban area residents that belong to racial/ethnic group m; P_{im} is the proportion of tract i residents of racial/ethnic group m. A is the land area of the metro area; ai is the land area of tract i.
Source: Modified from Morello-Frosch and Lopez, 2006

For example, in 2000, Abilene, Texas had one of the highest national values for African Americans, with a concentration index of 0.88. Thus, 88 per cent of all blacks would have had to be moved across neighbourhoods in order to achieve a more uniform density in this city.

4   *Centralization* is measured using either the absolute or relative concentration index. Both measures assess the extent to which a population group is located near a central city as opposed to the suburbs of the metropolitan area. The relative centralization index examines the degree of centralization of the minority population relative to the dominant majority group. The value ranges from +1 to 1, with 0 representing a uniform distribution of both groups relative to the city centre. The Absolute Centralization Index (ACE) reported in Table 13.2 focuses only on the spatial distribution of the minority group in relation to the city centre. The value also ranges from +1 to 1. Positive values suggest the tendency for the minority group members to reside close to the inner city whereas the negative values suggest the location of the group in the outskirts of the city. Again, upon review of 2000 housing data for blacks, the ACE measure was mostly positive for the 332 MSAs. Specifically, only the Santa Barbara–Santa Maria–Lompoc Metropolitan area in California had a negative value. Of the remaining locations, 300 of them had values exceeding 0.4 per cent, suggesting very high levels of urban centralization of African Americans throughout the United States.

5 *Clustering* can be measured using the spatial proximity index. This examines the degree to which neighbourhoods that are inhabited by minority groups tend to be contiguous to each other, as opposed to being dispersed across the metropolitan area. A value of 1 represents spatial randomness in the distribution of minorities. Values greater than 1 imply some clustering and less than 1 suggest a tendency for minorities to reside next to non-minorities. For African Americans, the residential clustering index observed in 2000 ranged from 1.002 to 1.907, with Newark, New Jersey having the highest level of clustering of the group.

Overall, these indices have been valuable in the social sciences and research on health disparities in the United States. Concerns about their aspatial characteristics have led to numerous revisions to incorporate a spatial component. Others have developed new variants that accommodate multiple racial and ethnic groups (Wong, 1993; 1998; 2003). In the next section, we shall describe the settlement geographies of the different racial and ethnic groups and how these relate to their health concerns.

The health concerns in racial and ethnic minority communities

A. Black communities

Demographics and settlement geographies
Black Americans make up about 13 per cent of the US population, and are the most urbanized of all racial/ethnic population groups. Nearly 52 per cent of all blacks live in the central city of metropolitan areas (US Census Bureau, 2000). Other than Native Americans, blacks have probably experienced more endemic and lasting levels of discrimination than any of the other minority groups (Polednak, 1996; Acevedo-Garcia et al, 2003). Further, based on the five dimensions of segregation described in the preceding section, blacks are the only racial/ethnic group to have experienced the full impact of hypersegregation in the United States. Figure 13.2a shows that the levels of segregation have declined slightly over the years across all five dimensions though the rates are still high when compared to the other minority groups.

The settlement characteristics of blacks, being urban and hypersegregated in environmentally and socio-economically stressed neighbourhoods, exact a heavy toll on their health status. The long-term impacts were aptly described by Geronimus (1992) in her proposition of the *'weathering hypothesis'*, as a process through which early exposures of blacks to systemic and structural disadvantages such as segregation, poverty, stress, disrupted social networks and polluted landscapes result in cumulative health impacts.

Leading causes of deaths among blacks
When examining the aggregate measures of mortality for blacks, one finds that the top three leading causes of death are similar to the larger white majority: heart disease, cancer and cerebrovascular diseases (Table 13.3). These three health conditions account for about half of all deaths among the two groups

Table 13.3 Leading causes of deaths among the US racial and ethnic groups (both sexes, all ages)

Rank	Whites (non-Hispanic)	Blacks (non-Hispanic)	Latinos	Asian Americans and Pacific Islanders (AAPIs)	American Indians/ Alaskan Natives (AI/Ans)
1	Heart Disease (26.2)	Heart Disease (24.9)	Heart Disease (21.7)	Cancer (26.3)	Heart Disease (19.4)
2	Cancer (23.3)	Cancer (21.7)	Cancer (20.0)	Heart Disease (23.8)	Cancer (17.4)
3	Cerebrovascular Disease/ Stroke (5.6)	Cerebrovascular Disease/ Stroke (5.8)	Unintentional Injuries (9.1)	Cerebrovascular Disease/ Stroke (8.1)	Unintentional Injuries (12.1)
4	Respiratory Disease (5.3)	Unintentional Injuries (4.8)	Cerebrovascular Disease/Stroke (5.3)	Unintentional Injuries (4.7)	Diabetes (5.8)
5	Unintentional Injuries (5.0)	Diabetes (4.4)	Diabetes (4.7)	Diabetes (3.6)	Chronic Liver Disease (4.2)
6	Alzheimer's Disease (3.7)	Homicides (3.1)	Chronic Liver Disease (2.7)	Respiratory Disease (3.0)	Cerebrovascular Disease/ Stroke (3.9)
7	Diabetes (2.7)	Nephritis, Nephrotic Syndrome (2.9)	Homicides (2.6)	Pneumonia and Influenza (3.0)	Respiratory Disease (3.6)
8	Influenza and Pneumonia (2.3)	Respiratory Disease (2.7)	Respiratory Disease (2.5)	Nephritis, Nephrotic Syndrome (1.9)	Suicide (2.8)
9	Nephritis, Nephrotic Syndrome (1.7)	HIV/AIDS (2.4)	Pneumonia and Influenza (2.2)	Suicide (1.8)	Nephritis, Nephrotic Syndrome (2.1)
10	Suicide (1.4)	Septicaemia (2.1)	Birth Defects (2.1)	Alzheimer's Disease (1.6)	Pneumonia and Influenza (1.9)
	All other causes/ Residual (22.9)	All other causes/ Residual (25.1)	All other causes/ Residual (27.0)	All other causes/ Residual (21.8)	All other causes/ Residual (26.6)

Numbers in parenthesis denote percentage of total deaths
Source: Leading Causes of Death for 2006, National Center for Health Statistics

(52 per cent for blacks and 55 per cent for whites). However, further inquiry of these deaths using age-adjusted, cause-specific data shows that far more blacks die of these diseases than whites. For example, the death rate from coronary heart disease among blacks is 280.6 per 100,000, when compared to only 216.3 per 100,000 for whites. Cancer is the second leading cause of death for both groups, but the death rates are 20 per cent higher among blacks than whites. A careful examination of the cause-specific rates shows that certain cancers afflict blacks more than the other groups. Prostate cancer remains a major area of concern among black men. They are one and half times more likely to die from the disease than white men. Breast cancer is prevalent among both African American and white women. The incidence rate is slightly lower for African American women; however, they are more likely to die of the disease than white women. The age-adjusted breast cancer rates are 32 per 100,000 for black women while they are 24 per 100,000 for white women. The disparities between morbidity and mortality risks are apparent for several forms of cancer, with lower survival rates overall for blacks than whites. The health statistics show that five years after cancer diagnosis, the likelihood of survival is significantly lower for blacks (44 per cent) than for whites (60 per cent). The trends in HIV/AIDS within black communities have been particularly disturbing in recent years. Blacks account for half of all new HIV cases that are now diagnosed, of which 72 per cent are black women, and the disease is now the leading cause of deaths among young black women between 25 and 34 years (Dyer, 2004). Blacks also now account for a significant amount (98 per cent) of all cumulative AIDS cases among the incarcerated. Within the context of the urban health penalty alluded to earlier, the scourge of the AIDS pandemic is most evident in the nation's metropolitan areas. In Washington, DC, 3 per cent of the residents are reported to have HIV/AIDs, a level that triples the Centers for Disease Control's (CDC) threshold of 1 per cent for a geographic area to be classified as an epidemic area (Vigilance, 2008). The epidemic rates of AIDs cases in this city have been compared to levels experienced in some African countries. With the exception of those aged 13–19 years, all age groups in the city are experiencing the disease at epidemic levels, the highest being for ages 40–49 years (7.2 per cent). The disease levels are disproportionately higher among blacks, who account for 76.3 per cent of all residents with the disease. A recent study by the city's health department showed racial/ethnic-based differences in the mode of transmission. Male to male sexual contact (MSM) was the leading mode of disease transmission among whites (77.6) and Hispanics (49.1 per cent). Among blacks, the lead mode of transmission was heterosexual contact (32.8), followed closely by MSM and intravenous drug use. The observed transmission mode places black women at significantly higher risk than their counterparts in other racial risk groups.

Other health concerns among blacks

African Americans also face significantly higher risks of infant mortality, diabetes and homicides than other racial and ethnic groups in these communities. Infant mortality rate (IMR) has been, historically, a key indicator of health disparities between blacks and whites. This black–white gap has persisted despite the dramatic reduction in IMR rates over the last several decades. The rate among African Americans (14.1 per cent) continues to be more than twice the rate of whites (5.7 per cent). The consensus among many researchers is that low birth weights (LBW), or babies born weighing less than 2500 grams, account for nearly two-thirds of the observed black/white disparity in IMR. The racial differential in LBW is equally large with prevalence rates of 13 per cent among blacks compared to only 6.5 per cent among whites. Such babies are known to face greater health risks including cognitive and developmental problems, congenital anomalies, respiratory ailments, higher rates of hospitalization and possibly death from health complications prior to their first birthday (McCormick, 1995). Attempts to explain the black–white gap in LBW have yielded complex interactions between risk factors that go beyond personal characteristics of the mother such as age, income, substance abuse or high-risk behaviours. Instead, researchers are now examining neighbourhood and contextual factors such as access to prenatal care, occupational hazards, neighbourhood segregation and exposure to toxic substances. Grady (2003), for example, investigated the risks of LBW among mothers in segregated and non-segregated tracts in Kings County, New York. She concluded, however, that the risks were higher for black mothers regardless of where they lived. Another study reported on environmental quality and the likelihood of poor reproductive outcomes due to exposure to contaminants such as pesticides, industrial solvents, metals and endocrine-disrupting chemicals that lead to adverse reproductive outcomes (Margai, 2003).

Overall, there is a persistent gap in morbidity and mortality rates observed between blacks and whites for many chronic health conditions including heart disease, cancers and diabetes, as well as IMR. The black community has also been hard hit by emerging diseases such as HIV/AIDS. The reasons for these disparities are complex but linked to the triple disadvantages described earlier: poverty, race and place. These determinants play out in many ways including residential segregation, access to quality and affordable health services and utilization of the services, the late diagnoses of diseases, and disparities in treatment and participation in clinical trials.

B. Health concerns in Latino American communities

Latino demographics and settlement geographies

Hispanic Americans are now the largest minority group, comprising 13 per cent of the US population in 2004. Demographic patterns suggest a 58 per cent increase in this population between 1990 and 2000, the largest among all racial/ethnic groups in the country. These increases are due both to the arrival of recent immigrants as well as the high birth rates among the Latino population. Not surprisingly, a key attribute of this population is its relative youthfulness: the median age is 26 years and 35 per cent of the population is less than 18 years. This contrasts with the rest of the US population with a median age of 35 years with only 26 per cent of the population below 18 years of age. These demographic differences are even more revealing in certain states such as California where some experts predict that in the near future, half of all children will be Latinos (Flores et al, 2002).

With the exception of blacks, segregation levels for Hispanics are relatively higher than the other groups. Evidence from the data garnered over the last three decades suggests some modest declines in segregation levels except for the medium sized cities (with 500,000 to 1 million residents). Two areas of concern are the rising levels of isolation and spatial clustering of the group. Using a sample of metropolitan areas with at least ten tracts and 3 per cent or more Hispanics in 1980 and beyond, the data show a positive change in the isolation index and the spatial proximity. Between 1980 and 2000, the index of isolation increased by 22.5 per cent, suggesting increasingly lower exposure of the group to other racial and ethnic groups residing in the city. The spatial proximity index also increased for this group during this period, suggesting further clustering in the urbanized areas.

Given the changing demographic patterns of Hispanics, several studies are now beginning to take a closer look at the health statistics of the population, including those of the children. Previous studies commonly used the term '*epidemiological paradox*', or the Latino paradox, to describe the fact that even though Latinos face the same demographic/economic risk factors and socio-spatial barriers as blacks, their overall health status is more favourable than blacks and, better yet, comparable to those of the dominant white majority (Amaro and De La Torre, 2002; Grady, 2003; Margai, 2003). For most of the health charts depicted in Figure 13.3, this appears to be the case. However, closer scrutiny of the health measures reveals that there are certain conditions that disproportionately impact the group. These disparities are linked to wider systemic problems including their immigration status, occupation, linguistic barriers and the environmental quality of their neighbourhoods.

Leading causes of deaths among Latinos

In comparing the leading causes of deaths between Latinos and whites, one finds that Latinos are disproportionately impacted by unintentional injuries (accidents), which account for the third leading cause of death among the group (see Table 13.3). Latinos, particularly the undocumented migrants, work in low-skilled, menial jobs such as day labourers, meat packing, crop-picking, farming and construction which place them at high risk of occupational injuries. For example, between 1995 and 2000, Mexican foreign-born workers accounted for more than 69 per cent of fatal injuries among foreign-born workers. Further, employers are likely to take advantage of the undocumented status of some of these workers by offering them low wages with no benefits. As a result, 34 per cent of Latinos are uninsured, nearly three times the rate for non-Hispanic whites.

Latino children, especially those from migrant families, also face poorer health outcomes. Of the 1 million children in the United States whose parents are migrant and seasonal workers, about 94 per cent of them are Latinos (Flores et al, 2002). One of the leading causes of deaths among Latinos is from birth defects, the only racial/ethnic group to have this risk category among the ten leading causes of death. These health events are linked to the occupational hazards, specifically to migrant exposure to pesticides and other hazardous substances (Cooper et al, 2001a, 2001b). Additional health problems identified among these children include inadequate preventive care, high rates of infectious diseases, farm injuries, high risk of nutritional disorders and low educational attainment, as well as endocrine, neurological and behavioural disorders that also have potential links to exposure to hazardous substances (Schenker, 1995; Flores et al, 2002).

Other Latino health concerns

As shown in Figure 13.3a–f, the Latino community also faces higher risks of HIV/AIDS along with other health concerns such as obesity/diabetes, homicides, teenage pregnancy and tuberculosis. The severity of these outcomes varies among the different subgroups. In comparing the three major Latino subgroups, Puerto Ricans face more disparate health outcomes than Mexican Americans and Cubans. For example, the age-adjusted death rate for HIV among Puerto Ricans living on mainland United States is 32.7 per 100,000, more than 13 times the rate for non-Hispanic whites. The diabetes rate is 172 per 100,000, when compared to 122 per 100,000 for Mexican Americans, and 47 per 100,000 for Cuban Americans.

The severity of health outcomes among Latinos also depends on nativity and the varying levels of Latino *acculturation* into US society. Acculturation has been evaluated using variables such as place of birth, year of residency in the United States and language use. Most studies have demonstrated negative effects of acculturation on the health of subsequent generations. The foreign-born and less acculturated Latinos have been found to experience fewer health problems but this relative advantage declines with increasing stay in the United States. Second generation Latinos or those who are more acculturated have been shown to face greater health problems such as obesity, illicit drug use, adverse birth outcomes and high rates of teenage pregnancy. Examining the differentials in overweight conditions in the Latino community, Gordon-Larsen et al (2003) noted that there are certain patterns of acculturation and structural factors that placed the Latino youths at risk. Specifically, immigrant adolescents are likely to be influenced by the neighbourhoods in which they reside, and the obesogenic environments described earlier in Chapter 11. These conditions along with existing socio-economic disadvantages result in greater risk factors and more adverse health conditions that impact this rapidly growing population.

C. Health concerns in Asian American communities

Asian demographics and settlement geography

About 4.4 per cent of the US population identify themselves as Asian Americans and Pacific Islanders (AAPI). Like Latinos, this group has undergone explosive growth in recent decades, from just 1 million in the 1960s to 12 million in 2000, and is expected to reach 36.7 million by 2050. Among the factors contributing to this contemporary growth pattern are the relaxation of US immigration laws, the involvement of the US military in Southeast Asia and associated exodus/resettlement of refugees, globalization and the increasing interconnection of US and Asian economies, and the well established migration networks (Zhou and Gatewood, 2000).

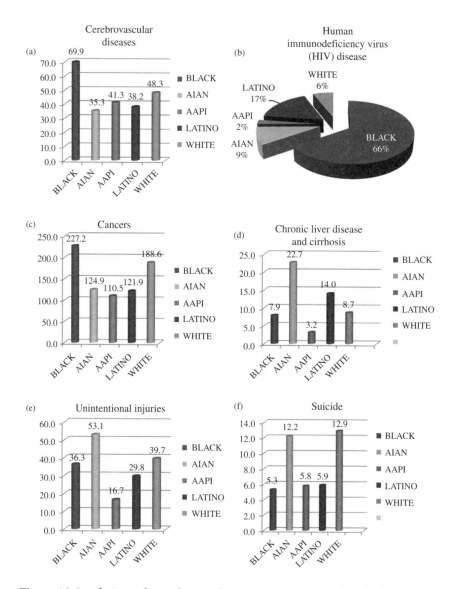

Figure 13.3a–f *Age-adjusted mortality rates among racial and ethnic groups in the United States, 2006*

Asian Americans in the United States today represent a diverse mix of ethnic groups that differ by language, religion, immigration into the United States, and length of stay as well as the degree to which they have acculturated or assimilated into society. Japanese and Chinese Americans, for example, have a longer generational history whereas other groups such as Indians, Koreans, Vietnamese, Cambodians, Laotians and the Hmong people are fairly recent immigrants with more limited levels of assimilation. Despite these notable differences, the public's perception of Asian Americans is still misguided. Asian

Americans are often perceived as foreigners, nerds, high achievers and compliant workers who rarely encounter problems of racism or institutional discrimination. Many are thought to be highly educated and employed as medical doctors, computer programmers, accountants or Wall Street professionals. Further, they are mis-perceived as people who, because of their high earning potential, have no major social, economic or health needs, and are all physically and mentally healthy. Experts warn that these erroneous characterizations, often termed the '*model minority myth*', fail to acknowledge the real health concerns or disparities that exist in the Asian American community. Those who have investigated the SES and health characteristics of this group have identified a line of bifurcation that separates Asian Americans into categories of varying demographic, socio-economic and health status instead of a single homogeneous population (Zhou and Gatewood, 2000; Frazier, 2003). For example, when examining the demographic profile of the group by nativity and age, the Asian American population has a disproportionately large foreign-born component and a disproportionately young native-born component (Zhou and Gatewood, 2000). They also have diverse occupational backgrounds that relate to the unique migration patterns of each subgroup, their national origin and their basis of admission into the United States (family-sponsored, employer-sponsored or refugee resettlement). These range from physicians and nurses, computer programmers, small business entrepreneurs and middle-class professionals to low-skilled workers on farms, in sweat shops and other economic entities. These differential skills translate into varying levels of SES and income by national origin. Immigrants from India, the Philippines and Taiwan reportedly have higher income levels than those from Vietnam, Cambodia or Laos. Similarly, the poverty rates range from 7 per cent for Filipinos, Indians and Japanese Americans to 42 per cent for Cambodians and more than 60 per cent for Laotians (Zhou and Gatewood, 2000).

Asian Americans are historically one of the least segregated groups in the United States, though data garnered in recent years suggest subtle increases in at least three dimensions of segregation – dissimilarity, isolation and the spatial proximity index. Based on the selected sample of metropolitan areas, a comparison of the data collected between 1980 and 2000 shows a 35 per cent increase in the isolation index among the group, along with increasing levels of spatial clustering. A similar pattern has been observed for the Hispanic population, and may reflect the arrival of the more recent migrants.

Leading causes of death among Asian Americans

In examining the health indicators of Asian Americans, the findings are mixed. While the group as a whole experiences a good health status with the lowest rates of deaths from cancer, heart disease and stroke, there are clear indications of high incidence and death rates for certain types of cancers. Unlike the other racial/ethnic groups, cancers (not heart disease) account for the leading cause of death among AAPIs (Table 13.2). Examining the cause-specific cancer rates, one finds that this group experiences the highest incidences of liver cancer (13.8 per 100,000) and stomach cancer (17.3 per 100,000) when compared to those of whites (4.8 per 100,000 for liver cancers and 7.7 per 100,000 for stomach cancers). The group has the highest mortality rates for chronic liver disease and cirrhosis (Figure 13.3). It is also the only racial/ethnic group (along with whites) to have Alzheimer's disease as one of the leading causes of death.

Other health concerns among Asians

Other major health risk factors for Asian American health are smoking, and exposure to tuberculosis and hepatitis, but these vary significantly by population subgroup. For example, a study by Ma et al (2002) concluded that tobacco use was a serious public health problem among Asian Americans but the rates were significantly higher among Southeast Asian men. The authors indicated that smoking rates varied from 33 per cent among Koreans, 55 per cent among Chinese and 56 per cent among Vietnamese to 71 per cent among Laotians and Cambodians. Noting that current smokers were most likely to be foreign born, these authors revealed that the subgroup differences were related to country of birth, immigration status and length of stay in the United States. Similar findings have also been noted for tuberculosis levels among Asian Americans. Even though the overall risk of tuberculosis among Asians (33 per 100,000) in the United States is 15 times the rate of whites, the rates have been shown to vary among the different subgroups, and proven to be highest during the first few years of immigration and then declining gradually to less than 5 per cent after ten years or more of residency in the United States.

Asian Americans have also been disproportionately affected by hepatitis B (HepB), a virus that attacks the liver resulting in chronic infection, scarring, cirrhosis and possibly liver cancer and death. Even though the rates of HepB have been decreasing (due to the increasing availability of the vaccine), the reported rate among Asians is still high (2.95 per 100,000) and twice that of the white population. Yu et al (2004), in their study of health disparities among AAPI children, contend that overall, the health issues facing this community are largely related to issues of citizenship/nativity status and the presence of cultural and linguistic barriers. These factors limit their use of health resources regardless of eligibility. They recommend the use of outreach and promotional programmes to educate the Asian immigrant populations on how to access and navigate the health care system.

D. Health concerns in Native American communities

Demographics and settlement geographies

US citizens who are descendants of the original peoples of the Americas and still maintain tribal affiliation in their communities are classified as American Indians and Alaskan Natives (AIAN). In 2000, there were approximately 560 federally recognized tribes residing in about 35 states (US Census, 2000). Together, these groups comprised roughly 4.1 million or 1.5 per cent of the total US population. Contrary to public perceptions of negative growth and decimation of the group by disease and/or absorption into the larger US population, the trend over the last four decades shows a steady upward increase at an average annual rate of about 4 per cent. Noting that this demographic trend is nearly impossible without immigration, some authors have credited the positive growth to the increasing number of racial self-identifications among people with partial or distant Native American ancestry (Cunningham, 1996). The increase in fertility levels has also played a part. For example, roughly 45 per cent of Native American women have their first child as teenagers when compared to 21 per cent of white women. Another contributory factor has been the improvement in mortality levels that has accompanied the epidemiological transition in the United States as a whole, benefiting all racial/ethnic groups. Infectious diseases that once afflicted more than 90 per cent of the Native American population, killing many and weakening others, have been mostly eradicated. Despite these developments, the AIAN population continues to be disproportionately affected by health conditions that result in significantly higher morbidity and mortality levels. A report in 2004 concluded that Native Americans still bear a greater burden of health risk factors and chronic diseases than any other racial/ethnic minority population (Liao et al, 2004). This group has been previously described as the poorest of the poor in the United States with poverty rates of 26 per cent when compared to 13 per cent for the United States as a whole and only 8 per cent for white Americans. As with the other minority groups, the root causes of these disparities are linked to racial stereotypes, discrimination, geographic isolation, poverty and limited access to health services. Native Americans have been caricatured and stereotyped as lazy, alcoholics, and savages wearing feathers and living in tipis. Until recently, minimal reference was made to the diversity of the group as separate nations with different names, languages, cultures, adaptive behaviours, needs and preferences.

The segregation indices derived for Native Americans suggest very low levels, perhaps obscured by the relatively small population numbers in the metropolitan areas (see Figure 13.2). Almost two-thirds of the population resides in non-metropolitan areas and 31 per cent reside in non-metro areas with very low density (less than ten per square mile). This distribution is in stark contrast to the rest of the US population with 75 per cent in urban areas and only 3 per cent in areas with very low density (Cunningham, 1996). The settlement geography of the group, unlike the other groups, is the result of several treaties and the unique relationship between the various tribal nations and the federal government. They are allowed to exist as sovereign entities but are also entitled to health and educational services provided by the federal government. The Indian Health Service (IHS) was set up in 1955 as the primary agency responsible for providing health care to the Native American population who reside on or near the reservations. Despite these benefits, the Indian reservations remain as relatively isolated pockets of extreme poverty, unemployment and poor health conditions. Nearly 40 per cent of the Native American adults are likely to be unemployed throughout the year and more than two-thirds have family incomes below the poverty line compared to only a third for the general population (Cunningham, 1996). Access to health care is still very limited due to the sparse distribution of those that are eligible for IHS services.

Leading causes of death among Native Americans

Examining the profile of the leading causes of death, heart disease and cancer account for the top leading causes of death among the AIAN population. The good news about cancer among the group is that the aggregate mortality rates have been generally lower (125 per 100,000) than the rates observed for whites and blacks. However, there is some regional variability in these levels with some AIAN communities reporting higher levels of 248 per 100,000 in states such as Alaska and 292 per 100,000 in the Northern Plains (Paisano et al, 2003). Among the cause-specific cancers, the most serious risks are for lung cancer, colorectal cancer, stomach and liver cancer. Incidence rates for stomach and liver cancer among the AIAN population are higher than the overall US rates and potentially related to high levels of alcohol consumption reported earlier.

Another area of concern among Native Americans is the large number of deaths from unintentional injuries (Figure 13.3). Accidents are the leading cause of death for Native Americans aged 1–44 years and the third leading cause of death for the group as a whole (Table 13.2). A study by Wallace et al (2003) showed that injury-related deaths among Native Americans was twice the rate for the United States as a whole and accounted for 75 per cent of all deaths among the children and youth. Unlike Latinos, where accidental deaths are caused by occupational hazards, for Native Americans these deaths are caused by unintentional motor vehicle accidents. Native Americans have the highest deaths from motor vehicle accidents and pedestrian events. These crashes are caused primarily by impaired driving – specifically, alcohol abuse, which is estimated to be as high as 70 per cent in some areas when compared to prevalence rates of 11–32 per cent among whites and blacks. Further, some contend that these accidents occur due to the traffic safety and regulatory codes that are less restrictive in these sovereign nations when compared to the rest of the country (Wallace et al, 2003).

Other health concerns

Other health problems facing Native Americans include diabetes, chronic liver disease, mental illnesses and suicides (Figure 13.3). In a sample of blacks, Hispanics, Asians and Native Americans, the highest prevalence of obesity, current smoking, cardiovascular disease and diabetes was found among Native Americans. Approximately 80 per cent of the AIANs had one or more adverse risk factors or chronic conditions and one-third had three or more of these conditions (Liao et al, 2004). Mental health issues and suicides are particularly problematic in these AIAN communities. Researchers blame these conditions on the depressive state of life on the reservations due to poverty, alienation and relative isolation of these communities.

Emerging geographic themes in minority health geographies

Using the triple-burden perspective in this chapter, minority health geographies in the United States were described as multidimensional, resulting from the synergistic effects of race, class and place. In examining the unique health challenges facing each group, certain geographic themes emerged, many of which underscore the social, economic and place-based dimensions of health disparities: *residential segregation, the urban health penalty, the weathering hypothesis, the epidemiological paradox, nativity, immigration, length of stay, acculturation, geographic isolation and alienation.* Even though these themes were discussed in reference to specific minority groups, they are by no means unique to those groups. For example, the negative effects of acculturation, as described among Latinos, also apply to Asian Americans and immigrants from the African Diaspora. Similarly, the epidemiological paradox, a positive dimension of Latino health, has been documented in the comparison of US-born blacks versus foreign-born blacks, as well as in the comparison of Asian Americans by nativity. Comparing blacks in urbanized communities to Native Americans in the rural areas, one finds that both groups have different settlement geographies, yet face similar problems of relative isolation and alienation from the rest of society. In effect, the weathering hypothesis, as noted earlier to explain the cumulative health impacts on blacks, also applies to Native Americans and possibly other minority groups residing in segregated ethnic enclaves.

A few other countries around the world face situations analogous to those described above; however, the conditions in the United States are unique and inherently challenging for a number of reasons. First, there is ample evidence of an increasingly pluralistic nation that is both multi-ethnic and multi-racial in composition. In 2007, the US Census estimated that nearly a third of the population now belongs to a racial and ethnic minority group, a statistic that they expect to validate during the 2010 census. Demographic projections point towards continuing growth of these minority groups, most likely reaching 50 per cent by 2050. Second, there is a growing sense of urgency among scholars and government officials to do something about these health disparities. As noted in Chapter 3, studies released over the last decade, including a seminal piece produced by the Institute of Medicine (IOM, 2003) affirm the pervasiveness of the disparities in morbidity and mortality, including significant gaps in access and utilization of health services. Concerns about these disparities recently fuelled the health care reform debates. Advocates argue that failure to adequately address these problems will hurt the nation's population health as a whole, as well as its fiscal health. The recent passage of the health care reform bill is a giant step toward addressing these problems and achieving health parity among all groups.

References

Acevedo-Garcia, D., Lochner, K., Osypuk, T. and Subramanian, S. V. (2003) 'Future directions in residential segregation and health research: A multilevel approach', *American Journal of Public Health*, vol 93, no 1, pp215–221

Adler, N. E. (2006) 'Overview of health disparities', in Thomson, G. E., Mitchell, F. and Williams, M. (eds) *Examining the Health Disparities Research Plan of the National Institutes of Health: Unfinished Business*, Committee on the Review and Assessment of the NIH's Strategic Research Plan and Budget to Reduce and Ultimately Eliminate Health Disparities, The National Academies Press, Washington, DC

Amaro, H. and De La Torre, A. (2002) 'Public health needs and scientific opportunities in research on Latinas', *American Journal of Public Health*, vol 92, no 4, pp525–529

Beal, F. M. (1970) 'Double jeopardy: To be black and female', in Cade, T. (ed) *The Black Woman: An Anthology*, Signet, New York, pp90–100

Burgess, E. W. (1928) 'Residential segregation in American cities', *Annals of the American Academy of Political and Social Science*, vol 14, pp105–115

Cooper, S., Burau, K., Sweeney, A., Robison, T., Smith, M. A., Symanski, E., Colt, J. S., Laseter, J. and Zehm, S. H. (2001a) 'Prenatal exposures to pesticides: A feasibility study among migrant and seasonal farmworkers', *American Journal of Industrial Medicine*, vol 40, no 5, pp578–585

Cooper, S., Burau, K., Sweeney, A., Robison, T., Smith, M. A., Symanski, E., Colt, J. S., Laseter, J. and Zehm, S. H. (2001b) 'Ascertainment of pesticide exposures of migrant and seasonal farmworker children: Findings from focus groups', *American Journal of Industrial Medicine*, vol 40, no 5, pp531–537

Cunningham, P. (1996) *Changing Numbers, Changing Needs: American Indian Demography and Public Health*, Commission on Behavioral and Social Sciences and Education, National Academies Press, Washington, DC

Dowd, J. J. and Bengtson, V. L. (1978) 'Aging in minority populations: An examination of the double jeopardy hypothesis', *The Journal of Gerontology*, vol 33, no 3, pp427–436

Dyer, E. (2004) 'The new face of AIDs: Young, black and female', *The Crisis*, November/December, pp29–32

Ferraro, K. F. and Farmer, M. M. (1996) 'Double jeopardy to health hypothesis for African Americans: Analysis and critique', *Journal of Health and Social Behavior*, vol 37, no 1, pp27–43

Flores, G., Fuentes-Afflick, E., Barbot, O., Carter-Pokras, O., Claudio, L., Lara, M., McLaurin, J. A., Pachter, L., Ramos-Gomez, F. J., Mendoza, F., Valdez, R. B., Villarruel, A. M., Zambrana, R. E., Greenberg, R. and Weitzman, M. (2002) 'The health of Latino children: Urgent priorities, unanswered questions, and a research agenda', *Journal of the American Medical Association*, vol 288, no 10, pp82–91

Frazier, J. W. (2003) 'Asians in America: Some historical and contemporary patterns', in Frazier, J. W. and Margai, F. M. (eds) *MultiCultural Geographies: The Changing Racial and Ethnic Patterns of the United States*, Global Academic Publishing, Binghamton, NY

Freidman, S. and Lichter, D. T. (1998) 'Spatial inequality and poverty among American children', *Population Research and Policy Review*, vol 17, no 2, pp91–109

Frey, W. H. (1996) 'Immigration, domestic migration, and demographic Balkanization in America: New evidence for the 1990s', *Population and Development Review*, vol 22, no 4, pp741–763

Gee, G. and Payne-Sturges, D. (2004) 'Environmental health disparities: A framework integrating psychosocial and environmental concepts', *Environmental Health Perspectives*, vol 1123, pp1645–1653

Geronimus, A. T. (1992) 'The weathering hypothesis and the health of the African American women and infants: Evidence and speculations', *Ethnicity and Disease*, vol 2, pp207–221

Geronimus, A. T. (2000) 'To mitigate, resist, or undo: Addressing structural influences on the health of urban populations', *American Journal of Public Health*, vol 90, no 6, pp867–872

Gordon-Larsen, P., Harris, K. M., Ward, D. S. and Popkin, B. M. (2003) 'Acculturation and overweight related behaviors among Hispanic immigrants to the U.S.: The national longitudinal study of adolescent health', *Social Science and Medicine*, vol 57, pp2023–2034

Grady, S. (2003) 'Low birth weight and the contribution of residential segregation: New York City 2000', in Frazier, J. W. and Margai, F. M. (eds) *MultiCultural Geographies: The Changing Racial and Ethnic Patterns of the United States*, Global Academic Publishing, Binghamton, NY

Grady, S. (2006) 'Racial disparities in low birthweight and the contribution of residential segregation: A multi-level analysis', *Social Science and Medicine*, vol 63, pp3013–3029

Iceland, J., Weinberg, D. H. and Steinmetz, E. (2002) 'Racial and ethnic residential segregation in the United States: 1980–2000', Census 2000 special report series no CENSR-3, Bureau of Census, US Department of Commerce, Washington, DC

Institute of Medicine (IOM) (2003) *The Future of the Public's Health in the 21st Century*, The National Academies Press, Washington, DC

King, D. K. (1988) 'Multiple jeopardy, multiple consciousness: The context of black feminist ideology', *Signs*, vol 14, no 1, pp42–72

Liao, Y., Tucker, P., Okoro, C. A., Giles, W. H., Mokdad, A. H. and Harris, V. B. (2004) 'REACH 2010: Surveillance for health status in minority communities: United States, 2001–2002', *MMWR Surveillance Summaries*, 27 August 2004/53 (SS06), pp1–36

Lopez, R. (2002) 'Segregation and black/white differences in exposure to air toxics in 1990', *Environmental Health Perspectives*, vol 110, suppl 2, pp289–295

Ma, G. X., Shive, S., Tan, Y. and Toubbeh, J. (2002) 'Prevalence and predictors of tobacco use among Asian Americans in the Delaware Valley region', *American Journal of Public Health*, vol 92, no 6, pp1013–1020

Margai, F. M. (2003) 'Using geodata techniques to analyze environmental health inequities in minority neighborhoods: The case of toxic exposures and low birth weights', in Frazier, J. W. and Margai, F. M. (eds) *MultiCultural Geographies: The Changing Racial and Ethnic Patterns of the United States*, Global Academic Publishing, Binghamton, NY

Margai, F. M. (2008) 'Disparities in the health effects of childhood poverty by race, ethnicity and place', Paper presented at the Race, Ethnicity and Place Conference, University of Miami, Miami, FL, 5–8 November 2008

Mason, S. M., Messer, L. C., Laraiac, B. A. and Mendolad, P. (2009) 'Segregation and preterm birth: The effects of neighborhood racial composition in North Carolina', *Health and Place*, vol 15, pp1–9

Massey, D. S. and Denton, N. (1988) 'The dimensions of residential segregation', *Social Forces*, vol 67, pp281–315

Massey, D. S., Rothwell, J. and Domina, T. (2009) 'The changing bases of segregation in the United States', *The ANNALS of the American Academy of Political and Social Science*, vol 626, no 1, pp74–90

McCormick, M. (1995) 'The contribution of low birth weight to infant mortality and childhood morbidity', *The New England Journal of Medicine*, vol 312, no 2, pp82–89

Morello-Frosch, R. and Lopez, R. (2006) 'The riskscape and the color line: Examining the role of segregation in environmental health disparities', *Environmental Research*, vol 102, pp181–196

Osypuk, T. L. and Acevedo-Garcia, D. (2008) 'Are racial disparities in pre-term birth larger in hypersegregated areas?', *American Journal of Epidemiology*, vol 167, pp1295–1304

Oyana, T. J. and Margai, F. M. (2010) 'Spatial patterns and health disparities in pediatric lead exposure in Chicago: Characteristics and profiles of high-risk neighborhoods', *The Professional Geographer*, vol 62, no 1, pp46–65

Paisano, R., Cobb, N. and Espey, D. K. (2003) 'Cancer mortality among American Indians and Alaska Natives: United States, 1994–1998', *Morbidity and Mortality Weekly*, August, vol 52, no 30, pp704

Polednak, A. P. (1996) 'Segregation, discrimination and mortality in the U.S. blacks', *Ethnicity and Disease*, vol 6, pp99–108

Schenker, M. B. (1995) 'Farm-related fatalities among children in California, 1980–1989', *American Journal of Public Health*, vol 85, no 1, pp89–92

United States Census Bureau (2000) 'Census of Population and Housing, US Department of Commerce', Economics and Statistics Administration, Washington, DC

United States Census Bureau (2005) 'Racial and Ethnic Segregation in the United States 1980–2000 Census of Population and Housing', US Department of Commerce, Economics and Statistics Administration, Washington, DC

Vigilance, P. N. D. (2008) 'District of Columbia HIV/AIDs Epidemiology, Update 2008', Department of Health, Government of the District of Columbia, p84

Wallace, L. J. D., Patel, R. and Dellinger, A. (2003) 'Injury mortality among American Indian and Alaska Native children and youth: United States, 1989–1998', *Morbidity and Mortality Weekly*, August, vol 52, no 30, pp697

Wong, D. W. (1993) 'Spatial indices of segregation', *Urban Studies*, vol 30, pp559–572

Wong, D. W. (1998) 'Measuring multi-ethnic spatial segregation', *Urban Geography*, vol 19, pp77–87

Wong, D. W. (2003) 'Spatial decomposition of segregation indices: A framework toward measuring segregation at multiple levels', *Geographical Analysis*, vol 35, no 3, pp179–194

Wood, D. (2003) 'Effect of child and family poverty on child health in the United States', *Pediatrics*, vol 44, no 3, pp707–711

Wu, Z., Noh, S., Kaspar, V. and Schimmele, C. M. (2003) 'Race, ethnicity, and depression in Canadian society', *Journal of Health and Social Behavior*, vol 44, no 3, pp426–441

Yu, S. M., Huang, Z. J. and Singh, G. K. (2004) 'Health status and health services utilization among U.S. Chinese, Asian Indian, Filipino and other Asian/Pacific Islander children', *Pediatrics*, vol 113, 1 January, pp101–107

Zhou, M. and Gatewood, J. V. (2000) 'Mapping the terrain: Asian-American diversity and the challenges of the twenty-first century', in Zhou, M. and Gatewood, J. V. (eds) *Contemporary Asian America: A Multi-Disciplinary Reader*, New York University Press, New York

14
Globalization, Population Mobility and Immigrant Health Disparities

Introduction

International migration, the flow of people across political boundaries, is a complex geographical process that is largely driven today by the forces of globalization, transnationalism and cross-cultural interactions. Within the context of rational choice theory, the process may be characterized as an inherent aspect of human behaviour as individuals rationalize and act on their inner quest for better chances in life by relocating to new environments that are deemed to be more lucrative, safer and healthier than their communities of origin. Evidence garnered throughout history, and particularly in the last century, shows that migration has played a central role in the social, economic and demographic transformation of many world regions. Alongside these changes have been the larger societal concerns in the sending and recipient countries on matters relating to brain-drain vs. brain-gain, occupational hazards, worker rights and equity, acculturation, assimilation vs. transnationalism, discrimination and xenophobia, human and drug trafficking, terrorism and homeland security, emergent diseases and migrant health. This chapter examines some of these concerns focusing on the connections between global mobility and immigrant health geographies.

The chapter is divided into three sections. We start with a discussion of the influential role of globalization and the current trends in international migration. Data characterizing these trends are based largely on the US and African immigration flows. In the second section, we explore different models of immigrant health, nativity, acculturation and the larger implications for the morbidity and mortality levels of both the migrants and the host populations in the receiving countries. This discussion will be followed by a case study in the third section that examines the health status of black immigrants in the United States. We offer a comparative analysis of US-born blacks versus African- and Caribbean-born blacks by evaluating the relationships between acculturation and health, the barriers to health access and utilization, and the overall impacts on the chronic health conditions among adults in each population group.

The trends and determinants of international migration

Statistics from the International Organization of Migration (IOM) show that globally there are now more than 300 million migrants around the world (IOM, 2009) and nearly three-quarters of these individuals are foreign-born or international migrants. There has been a 23 per cent rise in immigration rates since the 1990s, and these trends remain largely unabated in the 21st century. Efforts to regulate these movements through immigration laws, passports, visas, border control measures (such as fencing, remote control cameras) and other electronic devices have been barely successful as migrants continue to seek new corridors, underground tunnels and other alternative means to enter these countries.

The key determinants of migration, often called the push and pull factors, remain the primary causes of both voluntary and forced movements. Group inequities within the source areas, political and religious persecution, civil wars, environmental hazards and economic differentials between the source and destination areas all account for these international flows. More recently, these movements have been fuelled by the contemporary forces of globalization (Murray and Smith, 2001; Woodward et al, 2001; Huynen et al, 2005). At least five global forces have been identified as the drivers of population mobility:

The intensification of global governance structures

The reinvigoration and strengthening of regional and global governance structures have contributed to recent immigration flows. The enactment of trade liberalization policies through supranational and regional organizations such as the European Union (EU), North American Free Trade Agreement (NAFTA), or the African Union (AU) have led to increasing economic and trade partnerships, and greater interdependence between countries. The formalization of these relationships, along with ongoing investments by multinational corporations, has created a huge demand for skilled workers in both high- and low-income countries, subsequently leading to labour movements across borders.

The emergence and vulnerability of global economic markets

Globalization has also led to the transformation of global financial infrastructures, expanding global markets and the production of new trading systems (Huynen et al, 2005). These changes have led to strong interdependencies between global corporations and financial markets. They have also revealed the relative vulnerabilities of individual economic systems and the varying abilities of these governments to financially cope or recover from these challenges. Within the EU for example, countries such as Portugal, Italy, Greece and Spain have been recognized as having the most vulnerable economies during the recent global economic crisis. These same countries have witnessed the largest influx of low-income migrants during the last decade, further deepening their economic crises. Globally, persistent differentials in the economic systems within and between these countries continue to serve as one of the strongest determinants of population mobility across borders.

Persistent imbalances in demographic structures across world regions

As with economic differentials, the regional imbalances in population growth patterns and changing demographic structures also contribute to international migration flows. Developed countries continue to face low birth rates and rapidly aging population structures while developing countries struggle with higher growth rates, rapid urbanization and related environmental pressures. These processes exacerbate the population imbalances between the regions, fuelling migration flows outward to the regions where guest workers are needed to meet the labour demands and support other institutions.

Global environmental changes

Historically, floods, droughts and other environmental disasters have produced large numbers of refugees in many world regions. But even more disconcerting are the potential threats from global climate change, including desertification, loss of farmland and other negative environmental impacts that will likely accompany these changes. As noted in Chapter 6, there are varying levels of place vulnerability to these environmental hazards, with developing countries facing greater threats and yet constrained by their ability to cope, adapt or recover from these events. The realization of these global environmental hazards is therefore likely to intensify international migration flows.

The emergence of migrant networks and transnationalism

The increase in population mobility between countries has been enhanced by the existence of migrant networks between the sending and receiving countries. Cross-border activities and transnationalism have also contributed to these flows as more people in host countries choose to closely associate themselves with other countries, preferably their country of origin or those of their ancestors. Collectively, these activities have been the most significant causes of population mobility in recent years, producing a new activity space that is now referred to as the '*transnational migratory space*' (IOM, 2009). This geographical space is populated with individuals that are bilingual or multilingual, with dual citizenship, dual lineages, multiple properties and extended family and social networks. Spatial interaction within this geographic space is enhanced by information flows, international news media and new communication technologies and social media networks. Advanced and cheaper means of transportation have made it easier for people to move people back and forth, in addition to the continuous flow of ethnic foods, products and remittances between the places. Overall, migrant networks and transnational activities have led to greater opportunities for cross-cultural interaction, enabling immigrants to share their experiences, address common problems and assist in the transportation and resettlement process of their fellow migrants, and in so doing contribute to larger population flows.

A look at US immigration flows and the diversification of global source regions

Of the top ten receiving countries in the world, the United States has been the most consistent recipient of immigrants in recent decades. To date, the country has had the highest number of foreign-born migrants, with an observable increase in immigration rates from 23.3 million in 1990 to 38.2 million foreign-born migrants in 2010. A ratio of the foreign-born population relative to the total population shows that the percentage of immigrants is now at its highest levels since the 1930s decennial census.

Among the immigrants in the United States, about 3 per cent are from Africa. Though small in comparison to the other world regions, this number reflects a significant increase in African immigrant flows over the last few decades (US Office of Immigration Statistics, 2004). In 1990, there were only 364,000 documented African-born (AFB) immigrants in the United States. This figure has more than doubled in recent years to more than 1 million documented migrants (Eissa, 2005). A breakdown of the African immigration statistics reveals a diversification of immigrant flows from all parts of the continent (Figure 14.1). Western Africa is now the leading source region of the African immigrants (35 per cent) with Nigeria accounting for at least a third of these immigrants. Eastern Africa is next (26 per cent), with Ethiopians constituting the largest proportion. Immigrants from northern Africa account for 20 per cent, the AFB migrants with Egypt contributing roughly 10 per cent of the flows. Immigrants from southern Africa constitute 7 per cent of the African migrant flows and the majority (6.9 per cent) of these individuals are from South Africa.

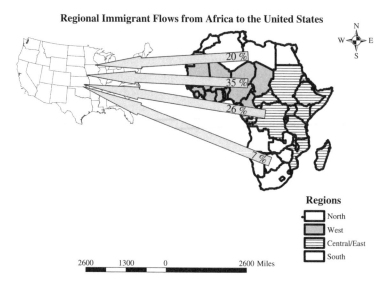

Figure 14.1 *Regional immigrant flows from Africa to the United States*

Contrary to AFB immigrants being a monolithic group in the United States, one finds that these immigrants reflect an eclectic mix of cultures, languages, religions, dress codes, customs, diets and value systems that represent their diverse geographic origins across the continent (Kamya, 1997; Djamba, 1999). Their increase in numbers and diversity also warrant a more detailed examination of the issues that impact them. One such area that needs immediate attention is the health of the immigrants. Specifically, what is the health status of black immigrants upon arrival in the United States? Is it similar to or different from the health outcomes observed among US-born blacks, Caribbean-born blacks or other groups in the United States? How does the health of AFB blacks change or evolve with increasing stay and acculturation in the United States? These questions are addressed in the rest of the chapter. To do so, we first present the models of immigrant health, and then utilize case study data to explain the patterns of health access, acculturation and varying health outcomes within this population subgroup.

Many of the patterns that are described in the ensuing section also apply to other racial/ethnic minority groups. However, the study of the AFB group is important for at least three reasons. First, the study fits in with the general theme of the book which is to engage in a cross-cultural analysis of health challenges facing marginalized populations in both developed and developing countries but with emphasis on the United States and selected countries in Africa. Second, African Americans have been identified in the previous chapter as one of the groups facing significant health disparities in the United States. As more AFB blacks migrate to the country, it will be interesting to see whether the health patterns differ or conform to the patterns observed among the rest of the group. Finally, there is a dearth of research on migration, acculturation and black health, an area that has been researched extensively among Latino and Asian populations. As the black population diversifies, there is a need for such studies to uncover the positive and culturally protective buffers of the group for use in formulating sustainable and culturally acceptable health promotion strategies.

Exploring the models of immigrant health and application to black immigrant populations

Studies of immigrant health suggest that many factors contribute to the overall well-being of these populations: nativity, immigration status, demographic and socio-economic status, linguistic proficiency, cultural background, friendship and kinship networks, and health care access (Leclere et al, 1994; Perez, 2002; Newbold and Danforth, 2003; Gushulak and MacPherson, 2004; Beiser, 2005). Scholars examining these different factors have come up with different models and research paradigms that seek to explain the migrant health status prior to their departure, upon arrival, and on staying in the US environment. Four of these models are introduced in this book: the pre-existing illness paradigm; the healthy immigrant paradigm; resettlement/acculturative stress paradigm; and more recently the racial context of origin paradigm (MacPherson and Gushulak, 2001; Beiser, 2005; Read and Emerson, 2005).

Model I: The pre-existing medical condition

This first paradigm is based on the notion that immigrants typically arrive in their new environment with a pre-existing medical condition. Gushulak and MacPherson (2006) argue that 'migrants and other mobile populations reflect the health characteristics of their place and environment of origin and carry several of these characteristics with them when they move' (p3). For example, if migrants originate from areas with prevalent infectious diseases, coupled with poverty and limited access to health care, upon arrival these individuals are more likely to exhibit these poor health attributes.

The negative health conditions of migrants from challenging environments are compounded further by the migratory process itself. During or after the travel phase, immigrants, particularly refugee populations or those channelled through human trafficking and smuggling operations, are likely to exhibit physical or psychosocial symptoms that reflect the traumatic events they undergo. Hunger, dehydration, rape, violence, injuries and exposure to treacherous conditions are likely to have a lasting impact on the health of these migrants upon arrival in their host community (Gushulak and MacPherson, 2000; Beiser, 2005).

Not surprisingly, the principle underlying the pre-existing illness paradigm is evident in many immigration policies that are formulated by receiving countries. Countries such as the United States, Canada and Australia typically require mandatory health screening of migrants prior to formal admission (Beiser, 2005). In the United States, for example, all potential migrants are required to undergo a rigorous examination to check for diseases such as tuberculosis, HIV/AIDS, leprosy, STDs and other communicable diseases. Those with pre-existing conditions are either denied a permanent residency status in the country, or asked to petition for a waiver to enter the country following which they would undergo medical treatment and disease counselling.

Until recently, many countries did not enforce their health screening policies for incoming migrants; however, with the rise in pandemics and emerging infectious diseases such as drug resistant tuberculosis, SARS and H1N1, these regulations have been reinstated. In the United Kingdom, for example, pre-arrival health screening measures for tuberculosis have been recently implemented for migrants originating from Bangladesh, Sudan, Tanzania and Thailand.

A review of the screening regulations within the United States and other developed countries raises some important health implications. First, the lack of screening for chronic diseases such as hypertension, cardiovascular disease, diabetes and cancers implies that some migrants do indeed arrive with chronic and potentially debilitating illnesses. There are also loopholes that could potentially lead to the entry of individuals with poor health conditions such as those arriving with tourist, student or business visas, and illegal migrants.

On a more positive note, the compulsory health screening policies used by these countries indicate that legal immigrants are *pre-selected* for good health. This selection bias could arguably be used as a possible explanation for the healthy immigrant effect that is widely reported among immigrant populations.

Model II: The healthy immigrant advantage

Unlike the preceding model where immigrants are presumed to have pre-existing illnesses upon arrival in the host country, many scholars have found the opposite outcome, an immigrant health advantage. Specifically, within the US context, findings from various immigrant populations have shown that those who migrate to the United States have excellent health outcomes initially, with low rates of chronic and degenerative diseases, low levels of depression or suicidal tendencies, substance abuse and less adverse reproductive outcomes. These migrants have lower levels of morbidity than their US-born counterparts despite their lower socio-economic status, limited proficiency in the English language, difficulties in accessing the health care system, exposure to racial discrimination and other barriers. This phenomenon, appropriately described as the *epidemiological paradox*, has been widely studied among some Latino and Asian groups (Markides and Coriel, 1986; Scribner and Dwyer, 1989; Gordon-Larsen et al, 2003; McDonald and Kennedy, 2004; Yu et al, 2004). A superior health advantage has also been previously reported among black immigrants. Lucas et al (2003) who examined the health status and health practices of three population subgroups, confirmed that the foreign-born black men reported substantially better health outcomes than the US-born black men and their overall health status was similar to, or slightly better than that of the US-born white men. Their findings also underscored the epidemiological paradox observed among other immigrant families, revealing that, despite the tough circumstances and high-risk factors facing these new residents, they fared better in health than their native-born counterparts.

Some scholars have posited many different perspectives to explain the observed health advantage among new migrants. Some have argued that the mandatory screening process alluded to earlier plays a role in the positive health attributes of migrants. For example, among African immigrants, many recent arrivals were legally admitted on the basis of the diversity lottery programme, professional visas, and similar programmes requiring a stringent health screening process. This process has probably resulted in the selection of healthy African migrants for entry into the United States. At the same time, however, not all migrants enter the country legally. In the United States at least 25 per cent of the immigrants are illegal migrants, and they too have been shown to exhibit some health advantages. So beyond the mandatory health screening programmes, what additional reasons can possibly be offered for the healthy immigrant advantage?

The *self-selectivity* of migrants has been identified as one of the alternative reasons for the superior health status of migrants. Studies have shown that typically the most highly skilled and educated and healthiest individuals are the ones who choose to migrate voluntarily. Such individuals are also likely to have the financial resources to travel to their new destinations, including the support systems and social networks required to survive in the new host societies.

Another possible explanation for the healthy immigrant advantage is the *salmon bias hypothesis*. This originates from the phenomenon in which salmon swim upstream to spawn before their death (Abraido-Lanza et al, 1999; Laveist, 2005). Specifically, immigrants are likened to salmon species such as those from the Pacific Northwest which begin their lives in the rivers in Alaska, British Columbia, Washington, Oregon and California. They swim out into the Pacific Ocean and remain in this ocean for years. When they mature, they ultimately head back home to the same river of origin where they will spawn before their death. The same pattern of behaviour applies to some foreign-born migrants. When they are severely ill and are close to dying, they may choose to return to their home country rather than die in the United States or their host country. What this means is that the recording of their deaths may not necessarily be captured in the US vital statistics database resulting in the underestimation of the death rates among the migrant population.

Laveist (2005) also raises a related issue of *data reliability* that is inherent in the vital statistics database, particularly for Latino populations. Due to the changing classification schemes for recording race and ethnicity in the census and other vital records, there is a greater likelihood to miscode the ethnic status of a patient. These errors also result in the underreporting of health events among the population group, and possibly account for the observed differences in health outcomes between the native and foreign-born populations.

Model III: Resettlement and acculturative stress

The relative health advantage or superior health status observed among migrants does not remain in effect forever. Rather, it declines with increasing stay and acculturation in the host society. Several studies have been conducted particularly among Latinos and Asian Americans (Lee et al, 2000; Gordon-Larsen et al, 2003; Yu et al, 2004) have documented these deteriorating health trends. These health trends, commonly characterized as part of the acculturative, assimilative and convergence health paradigms, show a chronology of health events that start out with positive health outcomes that decline with increasing stay, acculturation and assimilation in the dominant host society. Some contend that the health of the immigrant not only declines with acculturation, it ultimately converges with the health of the native-born residents in the dominant host society.

Both the acculturation and assimilation have been studied extensively as part of a sequential process that results in the partial or complete cultural transformation and integration of immigrants into the mainstream society (Salant and Lauderdale, 2003; Portes et al, 2005). In particular, acculturation, typically viewed as the first step toward assimilation, has been described as a multifactorial process involving behavioural and lifestyle changes as well as structural changes in neighbourhood composition, institutions and social networks. Various terms such as modernization, westernization or American-ization have been used to characterize this complex transformation of migrants through language, behaviour, diet, dress codes, neighbourhood characteristics and social interaction with members of the mainstream society.

It has been noted, however, that most minorities in the United States and other Western countries never fully integrate into the dominant host society. Researchers have argued that because of these trends, emphasis should be placed instead on acculturation and transnationalism, and not on assimilation. Resettlement is now widely believed to be a cross-cultural interactive process between migrants, their host and source countries. This process is bi-directional and more complex than the simple, linear uni-directional pattern that is often portrayed. Not all migrants are likely to follow the same trajectory. The resettlement, acculturative or assimilation process may be segmented, producing a wealth of opportunities for some immigrants but also a host of challenges particularly for those who assimilate downwards into the lower class or more marginalized segments of society (Portes et al, 2005). Upon moving into a new environment, some immigrants may undergo lifestyle and dietary changes that elevate their risk for poorer health outcomes (see Figure 14.2). These changes may include sedentary lifestyles, lack of physical activity, greater exposure to the mass media and heavy advertising and a diet consisting of high-fat, energy-dense foods and large portion sizes. Geographic factors including current residence, duration of stay, citizenship, home ownership and neighbourhood conditions, and contextual factors such as poverty, residential segregation, unemployment and high crime may also be key determinants in explaining the declining health outcomes. There are also post-migration stressors and experiences such as unemployment, racial discrimination and other structural characteristics of the new host society that heighten the risks for chronic diseases.

Model IV: The racial context of origin

This fourth model focuses exclusively on black immigrant families, given their history of enslavement, forced migration and other forms of discrimination in other world regions (Read and Emerson, 2005; Read et al, 2005). This model corroborates the existence of a black immigrant health advantage but notes that the advantage varies by region of birth and health status measure. In the two studies presented by Read and others so far, AFB blacks experienced the best health followed by West Indian and European-born blacks. All of these groups

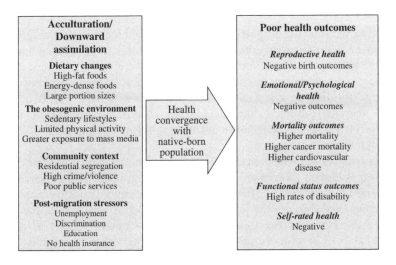

Figure 14.2 *Health effects of downward assimilation, acculturation and resettlement*

fared better than the US-born blacks. In explaining these group differentials and the notable health advantage among AFB blacks, Read and Emerson (2005) confirmed the selectivity hypothesis, specifying, however, that the underlying factors of migrant selectivity were more influential with greater distance between the origin and destination areas of the migrants. More importantly, their study suggested the need for understanding the racial context of origin, specifically the underlying mechanisms of race and class in some societies that worsen the health and well-being of population subgroups such as the native-born black Americans. They argued that cumulative exposure to racism and other systemic problems associated with minority status play an influential role in black health beyond just the lack of exercise and poor diet. Thus, black immigrants from minority white regions in Africa and South America were more likely to have superior health outcomes than their counterparts in majority white regions such as Europe or the United States. These systemic factors, they argued, are also responsible for the deteriorating health conditions of black immigrants with increasing stay in the United States.

Overall these four models reviewed above offer varied perspectives in explaining immigrant health. Three of the four models are applicable to all immigrant populations, while the racial context of origin is exclusive to AFB blacks. Given the strong merits of all of these models, some studies have argued in favour of interactive models of immigrant health. The argument put forth is that the health of all individuals, regardless of nativity or region of birth, is a function of several factors including their personal characteristics (age, income and education), their genetic predisposition, psychological stressors, social sources of strength and the neighbourhood conditions. Following below is a case study that incorporates several of these perspectives in explaining black health disparities and emerging concerns.

A case study of black immigrant health in the United States

As noted earlier, black immigration from other world regions, particularly from Africa, is increasingly relevant in explaining the emergent health care challenges facing the black population in the United States. Recently, a preliminary study was done to compare the health status of the three largest black population subgroups residing in the United States: US-born blacks, Caribbean-born blacks, and African-born blacks (Margai, 2009). The research focused primarily on the adult population using long-term, degenerative or chronic health outcomes.

This analysis was based on the 2003 national survey data collected through the National Health Interview Survey (NHIS) programme (US Department of Health and Human Services 2003). The NHIS is an annual multipurpose survey that is conducted through the joint auspices of the National Center for Health Statistics (NCHS) and the Centers for Disease Control (CDC) in Atlanta, Georgia. Trained personnel conduct face-to-face interviews among members of the non-institutionalized civilian population. Using a complex methodological design that includes stratification, clustering and multistage sampling procedures, the data collected are nationally representative. Further, a series of post-adjustment strategies are often applied to account for the variability in the age, sex and race/ethnicity of the population.

This analysis utilized the combined adult core sample data obtained from the 2002 and 2003 surveys. These records included data gathered on 93,386 persons in 2002 and 92,148 persons in 2003, resulting in an aggregated dataset of 185,534 persons. Variables included subject identification and geography (nativity, region of current residence, housing tenure, US citizenship), health status and behaviours, health care access and utilization, and socio-demographic information. The data were preprocessed, following which a statistical query by race was performed to extract only the individuals characterized as blacks/African Americans. A total of 26,334 cases were retained. A second query by age of the respondents led to the extraction of 17,348 adults in the sample (those aged 18 years and over). A third query was completed using the geographic region by birth to focus on the three subregions of interest in the study. Approximately 88 per cent of the respondents were United States-born blacks (denoted from here on as USB), 8.8 per cent originated from the Caribbean Islands and neighbouring countries (denoted as CRB), and 2.3 per cent were African-born blacks (denoted as AFB). To avoid oversampling from one region, a randomized subsample of 400 cases was selected from each of the three subregions for further statistical analyses. All subsequent statistical analyses were based on the comparison of residents from these three subregions: USB, CRB and AFB. Following is a brief overview of the sample profiles based on the major variable sets utilized in the study.

Resettlement and acculturative attributes

Table 14.1 provides a profile of the current residential patterns of the three population subgroups. The results underscore what is generally known about the geography of these groups, especially USB and CRB. The USB are still highly concentrated in the south, a pattern that is reflective of the historical geography of the group but also the more recent reverse migration shifts to the south. CRB predominate in the northeast, with an almost equal representation in the south. AFB are the most widely dispersed group, although they also appear to favour the northeastern and southern regions of the United States.

Three variables – duration of residence in the United States, citizenship and home ownership – were used as proxies for characterizing the acculturative attributes of the residents. A cross-tabulation of the variables that measure duration and citizenship against geographic region of birth confirms the newcomer status of African immigrants in the United States. Roughly 26 per cent have lived in the United States for less than five years and another 23 per cent for less than ten years (Table 14.1). On the contrary, nearly three-quarters of the CRB respondents have been in the United States for more than ten years, with half of the group indicating over 15 years of residency. Further evidence is provided by their citizenship status, with half of the CRB being US citizens when compared to only a third of all AFB respondents. Home ownership patterns also tend to favour those who were born in (USB) and/or resided in the United States for a longer time period (CRB). Nearly two-thirds of the AFB are renters, though an increasing number of them are now purchasing homes.

Table 14.1 *Settlement, acculturative and socio-economic characteristics of blacks groups*

Variable	Nativity: Geographic region of birth		
	US born $n_1 = 400$	Caribbean born $n_2 = 400$	African born $n_3 = 400$
Settlement and acculturative attributes			
Current residence (%)			*** $\Phi = 0.35$
Northeast	14.3	46.5	32.5
Midwest	19.5	2.5	18.8
South	60.5	45.5	39.3
West	5.8	5.8	9.5
US citizenship (%)			*** $\Phi = 0.56$
	–	54.3	35.1
Duration of stay in US			*** $\Phi = 0.51$
Under 5 (yrs)	–	10.3	26.3
5–10	–	13.3	23.8
10–15	–	19.5	16.8
Over 15	–	57.0	33.3
Housing tenure (%)			*** $\Phi = 0.21$
Own	54	58	30
Socio-demographic attributes			
Mean age (yrs)***	44.3	42.6	38.0
Males (%)			*** $\Phi = 0.11$
	37.8	41.5	50.2
Education (%)			*** $\Phi = 0.29$
< High school	25.8	24.1	9.7
High school/GED Dip.	31.5	28.3	19.6
Some college	28.4	30.7	34.2
Bachelor's degree	11.2	10.8	24.0
Master's/PhD	3.1	6.0	12.5
Unemployed (%)			*** $\Phi = 0.13$
	33.2	22.4	20.5
Family income (%)			ns
Under $20,000	28.7	23.3	26.5

Note: Significance based on contingency analysis using chi-square statistics; ***$p < 0.01$; Φ = phi coefficient representing strength of the observed relationship.

Socio-demographic characteristics

A comparison of the socio-economic profiles of the three subgroups shows that the African blacks are relatively younger (mean age of 38 years) when compared to the 42.6 years for Caribbean-born blacks and 44.3 years for the resident US-born population ($p < 0.01$). This is in concert with the typical age structures of immigrants being relatively younger than their native-born counterparts. The sex ratios differ within the subsamples, with slightly more females in the USB and CRB samples while both sexes were equally represented in the AFB sample. A comparison of the educational attributes of the respondents also indicates marked differences among the three population groups. AFB are more highly educated than their US-born or Caribbean counterparts (see Figure 14.2). A detailed comparison of the groups based on educational attainment revealed that only 14 per cent of the USB and 16 per cent of the CRB had completed four-year bachelor's or advanced degrees, whereas among the AFB, more than twice as many respondents (36.8 per cent) had four-year or advanced college degrees.

The high educational attainment of AFB was also reflected in their employment status. Despite their shorter duration of residency in the United States, only 20 per cent of AFB respondents were unemployed last year. CRB also fared better with only 22 per cent unemployed when compared to 33 per cent of the USB adults. The high human capital in this foreign-born population was not, however, reflected in the annual earnings. All groups reported comparable levels of household earnings (see Figure 14.3). Family income levels across the three groups were fairly consistent, with approximately 30 per cent of the households earning below the poverty level ($20,000).

Health status
The health assessment of the three population subgroups was based on three sets of measures: health insurance coverage, self-reported health status and a

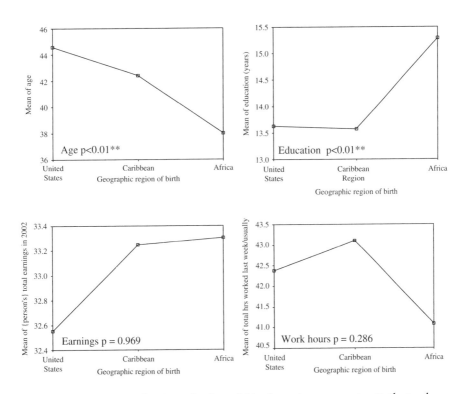

Figure 14.3 *Distribution of selected black socio-economic attributes by nativity*

Table 14.2 *Health care access and differentials in health status among black groups*

Variable	Nativity: Geographic region of birth		
	US born $n_1 = 400$	Caribbean born $n_2 = 400$	African born $n_3 = 400$
Health insurance			*** $\Phi = 0.158$
Uninsured (%)	16.8	30.3	32.5
Reported health status			*** $\Phi = 0.27$
Excellent health (%)	22.0	39.5	45.8
Very good health	30.3	24.0	29.0
Good health	27.0	27.3	18.3
Fair health	15.0	6.8	5.8
Poor health	5.5	2.3	1.0

Note: Significance based on contingency analysis using chi-square statistics; ***$p < 0.01$; $\Phi =$ phi coefficient representing strength of the observed relationship.

chronic health index (CHI). Health insurance coverage was a binary measure based on whether or not the respondents had access to health insurance. As reported in Table 14.2, the analysis showed statistically significant group disparities in health care access ($p < 0.01$). AFB faced the greatest disadvantage with 32.5 per cent having no health insurance, followed closely by the CRB. On the contrary, only about 16 per cent of USB were uninsured, the numbers being fairly consistent with previous studies (Margai, 2006). These findings confirm that AFB and CRB share similar patterns to the Hispanic Americans, with more than 30 per cent lacking insurance.

The documentation of self-reported health status also showed major differentials among the groups. Despite the higher portion of uninsured persons, nearly half of the AFB respondents reported excellent health outcomes when compared to 39.5 per cent of CRB and 22 per cent of the USB respondents. Overall, there were significantly more USB in fair or poor health, nearly three times greater, than the AFB respondents ($p < 0.01$).

Not surprisingly, the results obtained from the self-reported health status were congruent with the chronic health index computed in the study. This index was created using 12 well documented measures of chronic health conditions and known risk factors: heart disease, stroke, hypertension, diabetes mellitus, lung/respiratory disease, cancer, depression/anxiety, obesity, nervous system disorders, digestive system disorders, urinary system disorders and physical limitation. A reliability analysis of the index showed that it was acceptable with strong inter-item correlations (Cronbach's $\alpha = 0.81$). A descriptive analysis of this measure by population subgroup showed group differences, with native-born blacks scoring slightly higher on the index when compared to their foreign-born counterparts (see Figure 14.4a). The index also showed a statistically significant increase with increasing duration of stay in the United States (see Figure 14.4b).

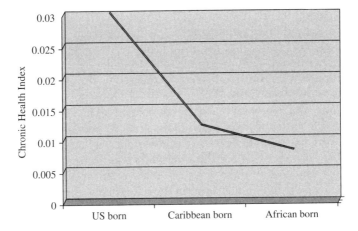

Figure 14.4a *Mean chronic health index by nativity*

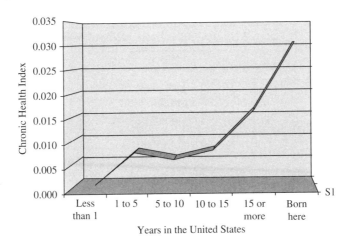

Figure 14.4b *Chronic health index by length of stay in the United States*

Evaluating the risk factors for chronic health conditions among black immigrants

A final step in this study was to conduct a logistic regression analysis to identify the existing risk factors among the different black subgroups in the United States. Two models were developed. The first model assessed whether the health status of the adult black population can be correctly explained by nativity, citizenship and duration of residency in the United States. The second model examined the preceding relationships while controlling for the socio-economic and demographic characteristics of these individuals. To carry out these two analytical objectives, the CHI was used to stratify the respondents into two groups. Those with a CHI above the mean were classified as having poor (or negative) health outcomes. Those with a CHI below the mean were placed in the second group, characterized as having positive health outcomes. Approximately 90.3 per cent of the respondents fell into the latter group. Next, using the dichotomized CHI measure as the dependent variable, two separate regression models were run. The first model focused on the origin and settlement geographies of the respondents. The second model incorporated all of the other socio-economic and demographic factors as contextual factors in explaining the observed health status of these individuals. Prior to both analyses, a series of tests were run to evaluate levels of multicollinearity among the predictor variables. The tolerance of all of these variables was above 0.10, indicating the statistical independence of these variables in the multivariate analysis.

Results from the first model confirm the relevance of the geographic region of birth (nativity) in explaining the observed differences in health (Table 14.3). Using USB as the reference category, the results show that the likelihood of a poor health status was significantly lower among the Caribbean-born, and even

Table 14.3 *Odds ratios derived from logistic regression analysis*

	Chronic health index	
	Model 1	*Model 2*
Nativity		
US born (Ref)		
CR born	0.30(0.18, 0.52)***	0.26(0.12, 0.52)***
AF born	0.21(0.11, 0.40)***	0.15(0.07, 0.35)***
Current residence		
Northeast	0.54(0.28, 1.0)*	0.22(0.10, 0.48)***
Midwest	0.55(0.28, 1.1)*	0.30(0.13, 0.69)***
South	0.61(0.35, 1.1)*	0.28(0.14, 0.54)***
West (Ref)		
Duration of stay in US		
Under 5 years	0.36(0.15, 0.94)**	0.27(0.1, 0.75)**
5–10	0.23(0.08, 0.70)***	0.25(0.07, 0.83)**
10–15	0.40(0.16, 0.99)**	0.44(0.16, 1.21)ns
Over 15 (ref)		
US citizenship	0.36(0.22, 0.59)***	0.14(0.07, 0.27)***
Age (years)		1.02(1.0, 1.03)**
Family income		
Percentage < $20,000		1.51(0.89, 2.59)ns
Marital status		
Married		1.20(0.69, 2.10)ns
Employment		
Unemployed		4.75(2.82, 7.9)***
Home ownership		
Renter		1.1(0.68, 1.8)ns
Educational attainment		
Without high school Dip		2.0(1.2, 3.4)***
Health insurance		
With coverage		0.36(0.18, 0.71)***

Note: ***denotes significance at $p < 0.01$; **at $p < 0.05$; *at $p < 0.10$; and ns is not significant; numbers in parentheses: 95% confidence bands derived from the analysis.

lower among the African-born counterparts. The analysis of the duration of residency showed that those who had lived in the United States for less than five years had the greatest health advantage. Consistent with other findings, this health advantage was less apparent among those who had stayed longer in the United States. The citizenship status in the United States, noted earlier as a proxy for acculturation, also appeared to have a negative impact on the chronic health status of the black adult population. The analysis by settlement region showed marginal differences. Using the Western states as the reference category, the results showed slightly higher but marginally significant risks for those in the Northeast, Midwest and the South, the latter being the most at-risk region for poor health. Overall, the fit of the model was good, with a Nagelkerke R^2 of 0.731.

In the second logistic regression model, the same variables were analysed while controlling for the socio-economic and other contextual factors such as age, income, marital status, employment status, housing and availability of health insurance. Among these variables, age was positively related to the health status of the black residents ($p < 0.01$). Poverty was not statistically significant; however, those who were unemployed were nearly five times more likely to have a negative health condition. The latter relationship might be bi-directional, with the negative health status possibly accounting for the unemployment status of the individual and vice versa. The risks of poor health conditions were also greater among renters than homeowners and nearly three times higher among those without a high school diploma. Not surprising also was the fact that those without health insurance were statistically three times more likely to suffer from a chronic health condition.

The statistical findings in the second model revealed that all but two of the geographic/settlement indicators remained key determinants of health status, while adjusting for these socio-economic factors. The geographic region of birth was still a significant predictor of health status, with even greater health advantage among the AFB. This implies that, when the socio-economic attributes are taken into account, the observed differentials between the groups widen, with foreign-born blacks enjoying even better health outcomes. The duration of residency in the United States also remained a strong predictor in the analysis, with the lowest risks among those who had lived between five and ten years in the United States. When controlling for socio-economic factors, US citizenship and geographic region of current residence were no longer significant in explaining health status. Overall, the addition of the socio-economic and contextual factors led to a slight improvement in the fit of the model. Model 2 had a Nagelkerke R^2 of 0.80, indicating that nearly 80 per cent of the observed differentials in the chronic health status of adult black residents in the United States had been explained by the variables included in the analysis.

Chapter summary and implications

As the world becomes ever more connected through cultural, economic, environmental, political and social processes, people will continue to move across political borders to take advantage of new opportunities that are offered through these global interactions. Not surprisingly, international immigration remains a hot button topic in many developed countries. The United States, being the top receiving country and the top choice for prospective migrants, remains at the centre of this debate as it grapples with a range of issues that extend beyond jobs to national security and health. In this chapter, our review of the immigration data shows that the percentage of foreign-born residents in this country is now at its highest since the 1930s, and the origin of these migrants has expanded beyond the European borders to include all world regions. AFB still constitute a tiny fraction of the US immigrants; however, their numbers have grown significantly in recent decades. Given the increasing heterogeneity of the US black population, the analysis of the settlement/ acculturative attributes of these immigrants and the health differentials between the population subgroups was deemed essential for health policy formulation to address existing and emergent health disparities. Along these lines, we reviewed four paradigms on immigrant health in this chapter: pre-existing illness; healthy immigrant advantage; acculturative stress; and racial context of origin paradigm. Then, using the national health survey data, the chronic health status of three black subgroups in the United States was analysed as a function of nativity, acculturation and socio-economic characteristics of the residents.

The black immigrant case study confirmed the existence of a healthy immigrant advantage among foreign-born blacks in the United States. AFB and CRB fared better than native-born blacks, based on the self-reported health measures as well as the chronic health index. Patterns of migrant selectivity were also evident from the age and educational characteristics of the migrant population.

The case study also provided evidence of an epidemiological paradox among AFB and CRB. These two groups had better health outcomes, despite the low levels of health insurance coverage that limit their access to health care services in the United States. The positive health outcomes observed among the foreign-born blacks, particularly Africans, were most evident among those who had lived in the United States for less than ten years. Age and education were found to be strong predictors of these chronic health outcomes; however, these variables were not the only factors responsible for the observed differentials among the groups. These results showed that upon controlling for these socio-demographic factors, AFB showed even greater health advantages than their US-born counterparts. Collectively, the results from the case study provide strong evidence in favour of the healthy immigrant effect and acculturative models in explaining US black health outcomes. As noted earlier, several processes may be at work, including the self-selectivity of the migrants, the mandatory health screening programmes, the 'salmon bias' hypothesis, and the underutilization and under-reporting of health incidences due to the lack of health insurance among the immigrants. The relative contribution of these factors in explaining the observed group disparities is largely unknown, and will require a more detailed health assessment and longitudinal study of foreign-born blacks. Such information would be highly beneficial in developing health protective strategies aimed at reducing the prevalence gaps in chronic diseases between the native-born and foreign-born blacks, with more far-reaching goals of expanding health access among all groups and eliminating black/white health disparities.

References

Abraido-Lanza, A. F., Dohrenwend, B. P., Ng-Mak, D. S. and Turner, J. B. (1999) 'The Latino mortality paradox: A test of the "salmon bias" and healthy migrant hypotheses', *American Journal of Public Health*, vol 89, pp1543–1548

Beiser, M. (2005) 'The health of immigrants and refugees in Canada', *Canadian Journal of Public Health*, vol 96, supplement 2, pps30–s40

Djamba, Y. K. (1999) 'African immigrants in the United States: A socio-demographic profile in comparison to native blacks', *Journal of Asian and African Studies*, vol 34, no 2, pp210–215

Eissa, S. O. (2005) 'Diversity and transformation: African Americans and African immigration to the United States', Immigration Policy Brief, www.ailf.org/ipc/diversityandtransformationprint.asp, accessed 31 March 2006

Gordon-Larsen, P., Harris, K. M., Ward, D. S. and Popkin, B. M. (2003) 'Acculturation and overweight related behaviors among Hispanic immigrants to the US: The national longitudinal study of adolescent health', *Social Science and Medicine*, vol 57, pp2023–2034

Gushulak, B. D. and MacPherson, D. W. (2000) 'Health issues associated with the smuggling and trafficking of migrants', *Journal of Immigrant Health*, vol 2, pp67–78

Gushulak, B. D. and MacPherson, D. W. (2004) 'Population mobility and health: An overview of the relationships between movement and population health', *Journal of Travel Medicine*, vol 11, pp171–178

Gushulak, B. D. and MacPherson, D. W. (2006) 'The basic principles of migration health: Population mobility and gaps in disease prevalence', *Emerging Themes in Epidemiology*, vol 3, no 3, pp1–11

Huynen, M., Martens, P. and Hilderrink, H. (2005) 'The health impacts of globalization: A conceptual framework', *Globalization and Health*, vol 1, no 14, pp1–12

IOM (2009) 'International Migration Report: A Global Assessment', Department of Economic and Social Affairs Population Division, International Organization of Migration, United Nations, New York

Kamya, H. A. (1997) 'African immigrants in the United States: The challenge for research and practice', *Social Work*, vol 42, no 2, pp154–165

Laveist, T. A. (2005) *Minority Populations and Health: An Introduction to Health Disparities in the United States*, Jossey-Bass, Wiley Imprint, San Francisco, CA

Leclere, F. B., Jensen, L. and Biddlecom, A. E. (1994) 'Health care utilization, family context, and adaptation among immigrants to the United States', *Journal of Health and Social Behavior*, vol 35, no 4, pp370–384

Lee, S. K., Sobal, J. and Frongillo, E. (2000) 'Acculturation and health in Korean Americans', *Social Science and Medicine*, vol 51, pp159–173

Lucas, J. D., Barr-Anderson, J. and Kington, R. S. (2003) 'Health status, health insurance and health care utilization patterns among immigrant black men', *American Journal of Public Health*, vol 93, no 10, pp1740–1747

MacPherson, D. W. and Gushulak, B. D. (2001) 'Human mobility and population health: New approaches in a globalizing world', *Perspectives in Biology and Medicine*, vol 44, no 3, pp390–401

Margai, F. M. (2009) 'Acculturation and the health of black immigrant families', in Okpewho, I. and Nzegwu, N. (eds) *The New African Diaspora*, Indiana University Press, Bloomington, IN, pp164–182

Markides, K. S. and Coreil, J. (1986) 'The health of Hispanics in the Southwestern United States: An epidemiological paradox', *Public Health Reports*, vol 101, pp253–265

McDonald, J. T. and Kennedy, S. (2004) 'Insights into the "healthy immigrant effect": Health status and health service use of immigrants to Canada', *Social Science and Medicine*, vol 59, pp1613–1627

Murray, C. J. L. and Smith, R. (2001) *Diseases of Globalisation*, Earthscan, London

Newbold, K. B. and Danforth, J. (2003) 'Health status and Canada's immigrant populations', *Social Science and Medicine*, vol 57, no 10, pp1981–1995

Perez, C. (2002) 'Health status and health behavior among immigrants', *Health Reports*, (Supplement), vol 13, Statistics Canada Catalog 82-003, Ottawa

Portes, A., Fernández-Kelly, P. and Haller, W. (2005) 'Segmented assimilation on the ground: The new second generation in early adulthood', *Ethnic and Racial Studies*, vol 28, no 6, pp1000–1040

Read, J. G. and Emerson, M. O. (2005) 'Racial context, black immigration and the US black/white health disparity', *Social Forces*, vol 84, no 1, pp181–199

Read, J. G., Emerson, M. O. and Tarlov, A. (2005) 'Implications of black immigrant health for US racial disparities in health', *Journal of Immigrant Health*, vol 7, no 3, pp205–212

Rennen, W. and Martens, P. (2003) 'The globalisation timeline', *Integrated Assessment*, vol 4, no 3, pp137–144

Salant, T. and Lauderdale, D. S. (2003) 'Measuring culture: A critical review of acculturation and health in Asian immigrant populations', *Social Science and Medicine*, vol 57, pp71–90

Scribner, R. and Dwyer, J. H. (1989) 'Acculturation and low birthweight among Latinos in the Hispanic HANES', *American Journal of Public Health*, vol 79, pp1263–1267

US Department of Health and Human Services (2003) 'National Health Interview Survey Description, National Center for Health Statistics: Division of Health Interview Statistics, and Centers for Disease Control and Prevention, December 2004'

US Office of Immigration Statistics (2004) *2004 Yearbook of Immigration Statistics*, Department of Homeland Security, Washington, DC

Woodward, D., Drager, N., Beaglehole, R. and Lipson, D. (2001) 'Globalization and health: A framework for analysis and action', *Bulletin of the World Health Organization*, vol 79, no 9, pp875–881

Yu, S. M., Huang, Z. J. and Singh, G. K. (2004) 'Health status and health services utilization among US Chinese, Asian Indian, Filipino and other Asian/Pacific Islander children', *Pediatrics*, vol 113, pp101–107

15
Group Disparities in Access, Quality and Utilization of Health Resources

Introduction

A topic that has come up repeatedly in the preceding chapters has been the unevenness in the distribution of poor health outcomes among population groups and the varying patterns of access, quality and utilization of health services to address these problems. This chapter examines these parameters of health care access, focusing on the types of health resources that are available, the increasingly pluralistic nature of these resources, and the efforts to develop measurable and mappable indicators to monitor progress in health access, affordability and quality. The topics are addressed in tandem with the various conceptualizations that have been presented in the literature. Examples are drawn from the United States, a country that has recently passed a new health care legislation to expand coverage across all population groups. We use data from the Census and National Center for Health Statistics to map out the distribution of the uninsured in America. This is followed by a statistical analysis to identify the social and economic attributes that best describe these uninsured Americans. These findings are used to generate new ideas and strategies for promoting health equity and the broader objectives of social justice

Health resources: Emerging trends in medical pluralism and syncretism

Under the umbrella of social justice, all individuals and groups, regardless of race, class and place, are entitled to equitable access to health resources and the highest attainable standards of health. This broad statement underlies the core principles of both the Universal Declaration of Human Rights (1948) as well as the International Declaration of Health Rights (1992). Understanding and promoting these principles of health equity requires the development of baseline indicators for evaluating and mapping existing health resources, visualizing inequities in access, and using the derived information to track progress over time. By health resources, we are referring to the complete realm of services that are available for use in disease prevention, diagnosis and treatment of individuals. Using this description, health resources may be grouped into five categories: (i) the health personnel such as primary care and specialized care physicians, nurses, aides, traditional birth attendants and other traditional healers; (ii) the physical structures and facilities such as the hospitals, clinics, group homes, nursing homes, assisted living centres, wellness centres and drug rehabilitation centres; (iii) equipment including the monitors, scanners, lasers, X-ray machines and other diagnostic tools and surgical technologies; (iv) materials covering the various medications, including prescriptions, over-the-counter drugs and other therapies available to the patient; and (v) the financial support systems consisting of private insurance and health maintenance organizations, government funded programmes, foundations and other charitable organizations that assist with the coordination of health care delivery. While emphasis is often placed on the caregivers and insurance agencies, all of these five types of health resources collectively serve to improve the quality of life and well-being of individuals in a given environment (Meade and Earickson, 2000).

Beyond the different health resources noted above, it is important also to acknowledge other modalities of health care and the increasingly pluralistic nature of these systems. Conventional therapies that are rooted in Western medicine are dominant in many developed countries, but there are other valuable health care systems and products. Homeopathic and naturopathic therapies are popular particularly in Europe and increasingly so in the United States. Many of the other systems are rooted in non-Western approaches such as traditional Chinese medicine (TCM) and Ayurvedic medicine. In the United States, efforts are currently underway at the National Institutes of Health (NIH) to evaluate the efficacy of these complementary and alternative medicines (CAM) and gauge their use within the general population.

CAM therapies include biological-based medicines, energy-based, manipulative therapies, body-based and mind–body medicinal systems. A recent study in the United States showed that these therapies are growing in popularity with almost 40 per cent of the adult population claiming to use them. The study also found notable differences by race and ethnicity in the use of these CAM therapies. The use of CAM was greatest among the Native Americans (50.3 per cent) and surprisingly high among whites (43.1 per cent) as well. Asians followed next with 39.9 per cent and only about one out of every four Blacks (25.5 per cent) or Latinos (23.7 per cent) reported using these alternative therapies (Barnes et al, 2008).

Two concepts in the geographic and public health literature that describe the diffusion and use of these alternative therapeutic systems are *medical pluralism* and *medical syncretism*. Medical pluralism reflects the existence of multiple sources of medical care and the diverse range of health systems and options that are available for the treatment of illnesses among patients. A related term, medical syncretism, refers to the blending of more than one medical system and the simultaneous use of both conventional and CAM therapies by patients to address their health care needs. Wade et al (2008) examined this phenomenon among American women aged 18 years and older. Using a survey of 808 respondents, the researchers examined the use of different CAM therapies among the women with varying health conditions, their reasons for use and disclosure of use to conventional physicians. About half of the women were found to use these therapies particularly when diagnosed with chronic pain. Biologically based therapies such as natural supplements and herbs were the most commonly cited therapies and most of the women were likely to divulge this information during clinical encounters with their providers. These findings contrasted with another study in which about 65 per cent of Americans aged 50 and older were found to use CAM therapies, yet less than a third were inclined to disclose this information to their doctors (Chao et al, 2008). The researchers concluded that given the increasing adoption and use of these different medical systems, it is incumbent on health care professionals to learn more about these options and determine whether or not their patients are utilizing them. The lack of full disclosure limits the ability to coordinate treatment and more importantly increases the likelihood of harm from potential drug interactions (Chao et al, 2008; Wade et al, 2008). Both the health risks and benefits of polypharmacy must therefore be recognized at all levels of the health care system.

Developing measurable and mappable dimensions of health access

The health policy literature is replete with many descriptions and operational frameworks of access to health care. Over the years, several conceptualizations have been offered to better understand and measure health access, and evaluate the role of environmental and social factors in promoting or inhibiting the use of these health services. From a geographic perspective, the most valuable frameworks have been those that offer indicators that are not only measurable, but also mappable to identify the areas that are medically underserved.

Earlier, in Chapter 9, we introduced the framework by Penchansky and Thomas (1981), which successfully described access as a multidimensional construct with five dimensions: availability, accessibility, accommodation, affordability and acceptability. Though this framework was discussed within the context of water access, it is equally applicable to the study of health access (Cromley and McLafferty, 2002). Of greater interest in this chapter is the Behavioural Model of Health Service and Utilization, a model that has been widely applied in public health studies of access. Andersen first presented his description of health access in 1968 and later, with assistance from Aday, offered a conceptual and operational framework of access and utilization (Aday and Andersen, 1974). The framework was subsequently updated by Andersen (1995) and more recently by others (Phillips et al,1998; Litaker et al, 2005; Hall et al, 2008). In its current form, access to health care services is defined as the ability of individuals to use health services when and where they are needed (Andersen, 1995). The interrelationships between access and utilization of health services, and the resulting health outcomes are dependent on three defining constructs in a community: (i) the environment; (ii) population characteristics; (iii) health behaviour (see Figure 15.1).

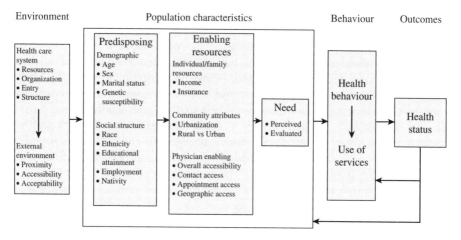

Source: Modified after Phillips et al (1998)

Figure 15.1 *Behavioural model of health service utilization*

The environmental construct

As shown in Figure 15.1, the environment is an exogenous construct consisting of all of the health resources described earlier along with the organizational attributes of the health care delivery system. The availability of these resources, the distributional networks, the health policies, and manner in which the health services are coordinated and delivered within the local environment are important drivers of health access and use. Other items for consideration are the relevant attributes of the external environment such as geographic proximity to health services, the accessibility of the providers and waiting times in the reception areas. More recently, the cultural acceptability of service has also been added as a valuable dimension of access. An environment in which patients have many options within their community and are satisfied with the way in which they are treated when they seek help would likely promote greater use of its health facilities.

The population construct

Population characteristics form the core of the behavioural model. When the model was initially proposed, three major components of the population were identified: the predisposing component, the enabling component and need. The *predisposing component* consists of measurable attributes that are present before the onset of the disease. These attributes also describe the likelihood or propensity of individuals to use the health services. The first set of predisposing factors includes demographic variables such as gender, age and genetic susceptibility. A second group consists of the social structure or characteristics that reflect the status of individuals in the larger society, in terms of occupational status, power and their ability to garner resources to address their health challenges. Thus, variables such as race, ethnicity, education, employment and occupational status can be integrated into the model to evaluate the role of these attributes.

Predisposing factors also include the health beliefs of individuals, their awareness, attitudes, values, knowledge and other belief systems about health and the existing services. Andersen (1995) noted that health beliefs were perhaps the least conceptualized and measured in the study of access yet these play an important role in influencing the subsequent perceptions of need and use of health services. He argued for ongoing efforts to measure and specify ways in which health beliefs might influence the use of different types of services. In an increasingly pluralistic society, people are likely to have different beliefs about the benefits and efficacy of different health systems. Such differences in health beliefs may help explain the varying patterns of health services use, particularly among Native Americans and Asian American subgroups who, as noted before, believe in other health modalities.

The enabling component is another feature of the population that impacts health access. This component is best captured by personal as well as community measures that allow people to use these health facilities. The personal enabling resources may include measures such as income level, access to health insurance, transportation, time constraints and a regular source of care. The community enabling resources are the health personnel and facilities that must be present in the person's local environment for them to access and utilize those resources. These attributes are partly dependent on the degree of urbanization of the area.

In the United States and other countries where health care has been market driven, the placement of health services has followed the classic central place theory (Christaller, 1966). Health facilities are strategically placed in urbanized areas to maximize the number of patients required to support and maintain the facility. There is a tendency therefore for most health services to aggregate in the urbanized centres to take advantage of the larger population sizes and patients needed to maintain their operations. Mapping of the distribution of health facilities shows that rural populations are more likely to be the medically underserved areas. Figure 15.2 illustrates this pattern in Erie County, New York with most of the health services located in the most urbanized areas in the county, the city of Buffalo. This distribution is highly representative of other regions where urban centres serve as the functional node or hub of health services rendered to residents within the city and those residing in the immediate vicinity. This produces disparities in access for residents in the small rural communities.

Hall et al (2008) recently suggested the addition of a new component in the enabling domain, namely the *physician-enabling component*. This new component can be measured and mapped at either the individual or community level. It consists of four indicators of access to providers. The first is the *overall accessibility of the physicians*. The relevant variables to include here are the percentage of primary care providers (PCPs) or specialized care providers (SCPs) that accept new patients, and the accessibility rate to these physicians based on the type of insurance coverage of the patient. The authors contend that though a community, on record, may have an adequate number of physicians, the accessibility rate may not be the same for individuals wishing to see these providers. In their study for example, they found that 86 per cent of the PCPs were accepting new patients. Similarly, high acceptance rates of 84.15 per cent

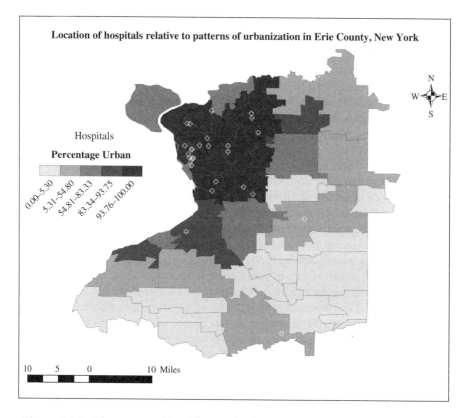

Figure 15.2 *Placement of health care facilities relative to urbanization in Erie County*

were observed among the obstetricians/gynaecologists (OBGYNs), and 89 per cent among paediatricians. However, when asked about accepting new Medicaid patients, the overall accessibility rates declined by about 10 per cent or more for each of these groups of providers.

A second index is *contact accessibility*, and for this domain, Hall et al (2008) suggest the use of variables that measure the frequency of unanswered phone calls to physicians' offices, the proportion of patients that encounter a phone tree or automated answering system, and how long patients are placed on hold before talking to a receptionist. In their study, they found that on average 20 per cent of the calls were unanswered on the first attempt, anywhere from 15 to 32 per cent of the calls were transferred once answered, and about 18 to 30 per cent involved an automated system. The average minutes on hold also varied from 4.07 minutes for PCPs, 4.7 minutes for paediatricians and lower for the OBGYNs (2.3 minutes).

The third index, *appointment accessibility*, captures the degree to which the health providers accommodate the needs of the patients based on appointment scheduling and waiting times prior to and during their visit. Hall et al (2008) suggest variables that measure how long patients wait before they get their first appointment when they need care; the percentage of providers that offer same-day, weekend or evening appointments; and how long patients wait in the reception area before seeing the physician. In their study, they found that at least 65 per cent of the patients could see a PCP or pediatrician within a week; however, the rates were significantly lower for the OBGYNs. Those offering evening or weekend appointments were also greater for pediatricians (43.6 per cent) and PCPs (34 per cent) and significantly lower for the OBGYNs (25.6 per cent)

The fourth index of the physician enabling component is *geographic accessibility*. This measure has been universally applied in all frameworks of health access and utilization, demonstrating the importance of distance as a major constraint or enabler in health assessment. The geographic proximity of providers to patients can be measured using distance in miles, travel time and the mode and cost of transportation. A related concept is *distance decay*, a derivative of the gravity model which predicts an exponential decline in health service utilization with increasing distance away from the health care providers. The principle applies to many spatial interactive processes where consumer activities are likely to decline as a result of the friction of distance. Figure 15.3 demonstrates this principle using the same data set described earlier for Erie County, New York. There is an inverse relationship between the location of the providers and consumers' use of services such that the frequency of trips to the health facilities declines dramatically with distance. Of note here is nature of the health episode. There are observable differences in the friction of distance

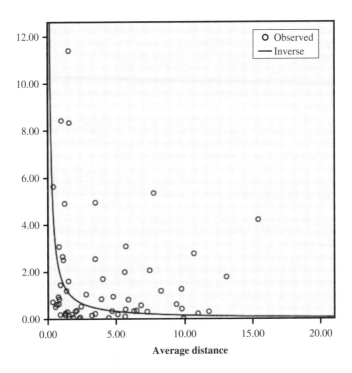

Figure 15.3 *Distance decay effect on health care utilization in Erie County*

between emergency and non-emergency visits, and the attending physician's affiliation with a facility, all of which may override the patient's choice and use of the health facility. Generally, however, for non-emergency visits, the factors that contribute to the distance decay phenomenon in health care utilization are many of the enabling characteristics of the population, such as the person's income, which in turn influences their means of transportation and willingness to travel to seek health care (Haynes et al, 1999). Also relevant is the need for the service which constitutes the final component of the population construct.

The *need component* as described by Aday and Andersen (1974), can be perceived or evaluated. Perceived need is based on the patient's own assessment of their health condition. It contributes to the treatment-seeking patterns of individuals and their likelihood to adhere to medical advice. The evaluated need is based on the provider's assessment using a battery of diagnostic tests, and contributes directly to the kind and amount of treatment that a patient will receive following a visit to the provider.

Health behaviour and utilization of services

The last component of the model is the utilization of the health service. As shown in Figure 15.1, use is directly impacted by all of the factors noted above, and this in turn influences the health status and overall well-being of the individual.

Overall, the Aday and Anderson model is ideal for evaluating the role of the external environment, and the social, economic and behavioural risk factors that shape health access and utilization patterns within communities. The model uses an integrative approach to incorporate these factors as either constraints or enablers of access and use of health services. All of the indicators noted above are measurable and mappable if the geographically referenced information on the patients is included. The use of geographic information systems (GIS) provides the platform for integrating these different risk factors, enabling the visualization of the distributional patterns (Graves, 2009). The relationships between these factors can also be assessed statistically, enabling one to discern the inequities within and between communities and population groups. These findings then become useful for the formulation of health strategies to ensure a more equitable distribution of resources to meet the needs of the disadvantaged and underserved populations.

Disparities in health care affordability: A geographic profile of the uninsured

Of all of the health access components described above, the one that typically receives the most attention in the media is health care affordability, particularly in countries lacking national health coverage for their citizens. Health affordability can be evaluated by using either the prices of health services or people's ability to pay for these services. Both attributes are dependent on many factors including the median household income, the occupational status of individuals and the type of health insurance coverage they receive from either public or private sources. Until the recent passage of the health care reform bill in the United States, health care affordability was one of the major indicators of health disparities among the various population groups. Based on data from the 2007 Current Population Survey, there are approximately 46 million people who are uninsured in the United States, representing approximately 15 per cent of the population. This figure represents an upward trend in the uninsured over a ten-year period, from about 32 million in 1987. Among those who are insured, nearly 60 per cent were covered by an insurance plan affiliated with their place of employment. Another 9 per cent purchased their insurance directly, and approximately 28 per cent of the insured were covered through government sponsored plans. Two of the major plans administered by the government are Medicare and Medicaid. Medicare is offered to approximately 41 million Americans (or 14 per cent of the insured populace). These are mostly individuals who are aged 65 years and older, or those under 65 years with certain disabilities and end-stage renal disease. Medicaid, which covers about 39.6 million people or 13 per cent of the insured, is a state administered programme that is offered to low-income individuals and families. Eligibility guidelines vary from state to state but generally depend on the financial resources of the individual, age, disability status and citizenship. Other government sponsored programmes include the military health care system administered by the Veteran's Administration, and the State Children's Health Insurance Program (SCHIP). The latter was recently expanded by the Children Health Insurance Reauthorization Act of 2009 (CHIPRA), and now provides financial assistance to all states to support uninsured children.

Mapping the distribution of the uninsured reveals geographical differences across the country with states in the south, southwest, and west having significantly higher levels than the national average. States with the highest percentage of people lacking insurance were Louisiana, Texas, New Mexico, California, Florida, Arizona (and Washington, DC), with observable levels exceeding 16 per cent. Using the Getis-Ord (GO) statistic, a hotspot analysis was performed in ArcGIS to confirm these patterns. As shown in Figure 15.4, the results revealed the geographic clustering of counties with large numbers of the uninsured across the United States. More than 80 per cent of the counties in California, Texas, New Mexico, Louisiana and Florida fell within the hotspots of the uninsured. Not surprisingly, these are mostly the border states with immigrant gateway cities. As one progresses inward to states such as Nebraska, Iowa, Illinois, Wyoming and Pennsylvania, the number of uninsured population declines. Other states such as Colorado, Alabama, Mississippi, Arizona and, surprisingly, Maine and Montana also have a few of their counties identified as hotspots.

In an effort to explain these geographic inequities and identify the defining characteristics of the at-risk populations, the results of the hotspot analysis were exported into the SPSS software. The goal here was identify the characteristics that best explain the differences between the hotspots and coldspots for the uninsured in America. Specifically, do these counties vary in terms of race, ethnicity, socio-economic attributes, urbanization and access to providers and health care facilities? To address this question, the GO statistic obtained for each county was recoded into one of three classes: those with values less

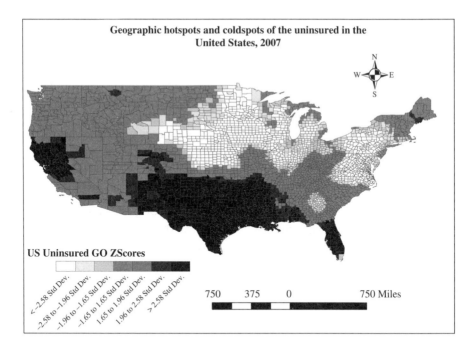

Figure 15.4 *Geographic patterns of hotspots and coldspots for the uninsured*

than − 1.96 standard deviations were classified as the *coldspots*; those with GO values between − 1.96 and + 1.96 standard deviations were classified as *normal* areas; and those with values greater than 1.96 standard deviations were coded as the *hotspots* with above normal levels of the uninsured. Of the 3111 counties in the analysis, 36 per cent (or 1119) were coldspots, 41 per cent (1274) were normal areas and the remaining 23 per cent (718) were hotspots.

A discriminant analysis was performed to explain the variability in demographic and socio-economic characteristics and health access characteristics across these three sets of US counties. Twelve variables were included: the percentage of whites, blacks, Asians, Native Americans and Latinos; the percentage of foreign-born populations; the degree of urbanization of the counties; the percentages of poor and unemployed; the percentage without a high school diploma; the ratio of medical doctors per 10,000 people; and the number of hospitals. To avoid the problem of collinearity, correlation analysis was first performed. The highest observed correlation was for blacks and whites (r = −.820); given the importance of both variables in the analysis, they were retained. Other than these two demographic variables, all of the other variables were fairly independent with absolute correlations below .60. Therefore no action was necessary prior to the discriminant analysis. Further, the use of the stepwise approach was deemed to be a great way to selectively choose the variables that matter most in explaining the observed differences between the counties. The preliminary assessment using univariate analysis of variance showed that surprisingly, all of these variables were statistically significant indicators, except for the two measures of health access: MD ratio and hospitals. These two variables appear to be equitably distributed across the three groups of counties. For example, there are on average five to six hospitals in each county. The MD ratio observed in coldspot and normal counties is slightly higher than hotspot counties; however, this observed difference is not statistically significant. Table 15.1 summarizes the group means observed for variables that were significantly different across the three groups of counties.

Subsequent analysis using stepwise discriminant analysis enabled the identification of the most relevant characteristics of the uninsured. Since the analysis was based on three types of counties, the model derived two linear functions (see Table 15.2). The first function, explaining the difference between the coldspots and the rest of the US counties, has a canonical correlation score of 0.594 meaning that nearly 60 per cent of the variability between these counties was accounted for by the demographic and socio-economic variables included in the model. The second function, explaining the difference between the normal areas and the hotspots, produced a canonical correlation score of 0.302 suggesting that an additional 30 per cent of the variance was explained. Collectively both functions produced a highly significant model explaining the spatial differences in the uninsured across America. Using the structure matrix, one is able to identify the variables that best explain these differences. The first function depicts the population characteristics of the coldspots. Only two of the variables are positively linked to this function – the percentage of whites and the MD ratio (the latter not being significant). Using the strength and direction of function coefficients, one finds that the coldspots are most strongly characterized by a lower percentage of Hispanics, and fewer residents that live below poverty levels. These coldspots also have moderately lower levels of blacks, the unemployed, female headed households, residents without high school education and lower levels of urbanization.

Table 15.1 *Group means observed in different geographic clusters across the United States*

Variable	Coldspot	Normal	Hotspot	Wilk's Lambda
% Latino	2.66	4.01	15.51	.816***
% Poor	12.47	17.11	21.6	.698***
% < High school	12.04	15.32	16.02	.672***
% Blacks	6.89	7.97	13.38	.659***
% Female households	11.27	13.47	14.78	.639***
Per capita income	18,352	17,648	17,154	.629***
% Urban	33.29	33.40	41.7	.623***
% Unemployed	4.7	6.35	6.81	.618***
% Native Americans	1.06	1.89	1.95	616***
% Whites	88.9	86.13	75.52	.606***
% Asian Americans	0.81	0.65	0.89	.604***

Note: Variables are ordered based on the their entry into the stepwise analysis; ***$p < 0.01$
Canonical correlations: Function 1 (0.585); Function 2 (0.285)
Wilk's Lambda: Function 1 (0.604); $X2 = 1562$ df. 22; $p < 0.01$
Wilk's Lambda: Function 2 (0.919); $X2 = 263$ df.10; $p < 0.01$

Table 15.2 *Structure matrix obtained from the discriminant analysis of geographic clusters of the uninsured across the United States*

Variables	Function 1	Function 2
% Latino	−0.651*	0.234
% Poor	−0.610*	−0.561
% White	0.465*	−0.026
% Blacks	−0.245*	0.045
% Urban	−0.163*	0.100
% Unemployed	−0.316	−0.622*
% less than high school	−0.244	−0.528*
% Female-headed households	−0.313	−0.425*
% Asian Americans	−0.044	0.180*
% Native Americans	−0.061	−0.161*
Per capita income	0.122	0.148*

Note: Correlations between the variables and the derived functions: variables are ordered by absolute size of correlation with the functions; *denotes the largest absolute correlation for each variable on the functions.

The second function separates the more "normal" counties from the hotspots. Here the defining characteristics of race and ethnicity are less evident. Rather, one finds that the strongest disparities are linked to the socio-economic characteristics of the population. The normal counties are significantly less likely to have residents that are unemployed, poor, with lower educational attainment and female-headed households.

Overall, the results are fairly consistent with the aspatial analyses of the uninsured in America (DHHS, 2005). These studies confirm a strong correlation between the uninsured and low-income residents. These individuals are less likely to be employed, or work only part time and are therefore ineligible for insurance. Though not included in the preceding analysis, disparities have also been noted among different age groups, particularly younger adults (aged 25–34) who are too old to remain under their parents' insurance and yet do not earn enough to purchase their own. The recent health care reform policy has eliminated this disparity allowing young adults to remain eligible under their family insurance until age 27.

When examining the insurance status by race and ethnicity, the spatial analysis conducted above confirms the disproportionately high levels of Hispanics who lack coverage. The latter are negatively impacted because of their occupational niches, such as construction, agriculture and domestic jobs, which typically do not offer health insurance. Hispanics are also overly represented among non-citizens. They constitute 13 per cent of the general population and yet account for 59 per cent of the non-citizens in the country (DHHS, 2005). Non-citizens have been shown to have significantly lower incomes and to work for firms with fewer than 100 employees. Thus, counties with significantly greater numbers of non-citizens, such as those in the border regions, are likely to emerge as hotspots of the uninsured. The 2010 health reform bill does not provide coverage for non-citizens or illegal immigrants; therefore some of the geographic differences observed in the preceding analysis are likely to persist.

Measurable dimensions of quality of health services

Though several aspects of health quality are embedded in the preceding discussions, this concept deserves separate attention in this chapter. Health quality reflects the degree to which health services for individuals and populations increase the likelihood of desired health outcomes and are consistent with current professional knowledge (TOM, 1991, p21). In assessing the quality of health services in the United States, a research project directed by Donaldson (1999) identified three major issues, and these challenges remain nearly a decade later. The first has to do with the *overutilization* of health services. This involves the excessive or unnecessary use of certain health resources such as diagnostic tests involving magnetic resonance imaging (MRI), X-ray machines and other devices, unnecessary surgical procedures and over-prescription of drugs. Donaldson and others (1999) argued then that such practices not only led to wasteful use of valuable resources, they were also likely to produce harmful side effects in patients.

A second challenge impacting health quality in the United States is linked to the underutilization of health services that are considered to be necessary, effective and clinically appropriate. This problem, often known as the *quality chasm*, is the gap between what is known to be effective care, and what patients actually receive from their providers. Examples of such services include the underuse of preventive services such as mammography, immunizations and treatable mental health conditions such as depression.

A third area of concern has to do with the overall *performance* of the health professionals who may lack the expertise and mastery in clinical practice, or lack the skills necessary to communicate effectively with the patients. These limitations often may result in medical errors that are otherwise preventable, such as drug interactions, surgical mishaps, failure to follow-up on abnormal test results, lack of coordination of care, and cultural incompetence.

The question that often arises is how best to monitor the problems noted above. Guidelines offered are built around the Donabedian (1980) framework which requires data collection on structural indicators, process indicators and outcome indicators. The structural measures focus on many of the health resources described earlier. Health quality can be calibrated, for example, by tracking the accreditation of the health facilities, the providers, the institutional policies and procedures, along with their track record of safety. The process measures examine the clinical aspects of care, specifically the diagnosis and management of diseases in the health care environment. Measures such as the timeliness, accuracy of diagnosis, the appropriateness of the recommended therapies, the likelihood of complications or mishaps, misuse of medications and the overall adequacy of care plans are integrated in the process measures. Also included are the sanitary conditions of the environment, and the quality and nutritional value of food offered to patients within the health facility. The third set of measures is based on the health outcomes. Traditional indicators of morbidity and mortality rates can be used here, including the survival rates and recovery rates of patients. Also relevant is the self-report from the patients and their overall level of satisfaction with the quality of care received.

Finally, researchers are beginning to pay attention to the patient's evaluation of health services, notably the non-clinical aspects of health quality. This new area of research is called 'health systems' responsiveness. It examines individual experiences in health care settings and the likely impacts on health utilization (WHO, 2002). Studies conducted in the United States and around the world have shown instances where patients have failed to utilize health care services because of the treatment received in a previous visit. In one such study conducted in Seattle, Kings County, Washington, researchers found that about 32 per cent of African Americans felt that they had been discriminated against in a previous visit to one of the county's health care facilities (Smyser and Ciske, 2001). As a follow-up, a more detailed study was set up to better understand the experiences of this group. Through interviews conducted, many respondents described more than one incident of racial discrimination. The incidents were geographically widespread, occurring in public and private facilities around the county. The experiences ranged from rude behaviours and racial slurs, to the lack of racial sensitivity of the health personnel. As a result of these experiences respondents were likely to modify their health seeking behaviours. Some indicated avoiding the facilities where the incidents took place, delaying treatments, or not knowing where else to go for treatment. The findings from this study underscored the need for including both clinical and non-clinical attributes of the health care delivery environment when evaluating access and utilizing of these services.

At a global level, the health systems approach has been expanded into a more formal structure for evaluating health quality and comparing these levels across countries. The approach is based on eight domains that are grouped into two areas:

1   Respect for persons (dignity, autonomy, confidentiality and communication);
2   Client orientation (choice, prompt attention, quality of basic amenities, access to social support networks during inpatient care).

Each of these attributes is believed to be universally important to all people, regardless of culture, sex, age, income or other group differences. Using a multi-country framework, data are now collected in different countries to examine the geographical variations in the importance of these domains. For example, Valentine et al (2008) used data consisting of 105,806 respondents in 41 countries to evaluate the differences in patient rankings by country of residence. The researchers concluded that the respondents' views on these issues both within and across countries were more convergent than divergent. Most people selected *prompt attention* in a health care setting as the most important element of health quality. This was followed closely by *dignity* and then *communication*. Integrating such findings in the reformulation of health policies will significantly improve the quality of care that people receive and subsequently improve the utilization of services.

Chapter summary

Addressing health disparities requires the investigation of not only the etiological circumstances of the health challenges facing individuals but also the enabling factors and constraints that impact access, use and quality of the health services received. In this chapter, our emphasis has been on the parameters that are measurable and mappable for use in tracking these disparities. Using the behavioural model of health service utilization, we have discussed the different types of health resources in a given environment, and the population characteristics and behaviours that contribute to the observable health outcomes. Separate attention was also given to the issue of health care affordability for which we documented the demographic and geographic profiles of the uninsured using case data from the United States. We then concluded our discussion with the national and global efforts to assess health quality using both clinical and non-clinical measures.

References

Aday, L. A. and Andersen, R. (1974) 'A framework for the study of access to medical care', *Health Services Research*, vol 9, no 3, pp208–220

Andersen, R. M. (1995) 'Revisiting the behavioral model and access to medical care: Does it matter?', *Journal of Health and Social Behavior*, vol 36, no 1, pp1–10

Andersen, R. M., McCutcheon, A. and Aday, L. A. (1983) 'Exploring dimensions of access to medical care', *Health Service Research*, vol 18, no 1, pp49–74

Barnes, P. M., Bloom, B. and Nahin, R. L. (2008) 'Complementary and alternative medicine use among adults and children: United States, 2007', *National Health Statistics Reports*, no 12, pp1–24, www.cdc.gov/nchs/data/nhsr/nhsr012.pdf, accessed 12 February 2010

Chao, M. T., Wade, C. and Kronenberg, F. (2008) 'Disclosure of complementary and alternative medicine to conventional medical providers: Variation by race/ethnicity and type of CAM', *Journal of the National Medical Association*, vol 100, no 11, pp1341–1349

Christaller, W. (1966) *Central Places in Southern Germany*, Prentice Hall, Englewood Cliffs, NJ

Cromley, E. K. and McLafferty, S. L. (2002) *GIS and Public Health*, The Guilford Press, New York

DHHS (2005) 'Overview of the Uninsured in the United States: Analysis of the 2005 Current Population Survey', Assistant Secretary for Planning and Evaluation (ASPE), US Department of Health and Human Social Services, Washington, DC, http://aspe.hhs.gov/health/reports/05/uninsured-cps, accessed 5 January 2010

Donabedian, A. (1980) *Explorations in Quality Assessment and Monitoring: The definition of quality and approaches to assessment*, Health Administration Press, Ann Arbor, MI

Donaldson, M. S. (ed) (1999) 'Measuring the quality of health care', The National Roundtable on Health Care Quality, Institute of Medicine, www.nap.edu/catalog/6418.html

Graves, A. (2009) 'A model for assessment of potential geographical accessibility: A case for GIS', *Journal of Rural Nursing and Health Care*, 22 March 2009

Hall, A. G., Lemak, C. H., Steingraber, H. and Schaffer, S. (2008) 'Expanding the definition of access. It isn't just about health insurance', *Journal of Health Care for the Poor and Underserved*, vol 19, pp625–638

Haynes, R., Bentham, G., Lovett, A. and Gale, S. (1999) 'Effects of distances, hospitals and GP surgery on hospital inpatient episode, controlling for needs and provision', *Social Science and Medicine*, vol 49, pp425–433

Litaker, D., Koroukian, S. M. and Love, T. E. (2005) 'Context and healthcare access: Looking beyond the individual', *Medical Care*, vol 43, no 6, pp531–540

Meade, M. S. and Earickson, R. J. (2000) *Medical Geography*, The Guilford Press, New York

Penchansky, R. and Thomas, J. W. (1981) 'The concept of access: Definition and relationship to consumer satisfaction', *Medical Care*, vol 19, no 2, pp127–140

Phillips, K. A., Morrison, K. R. and Andersen, R. (1998) 'Understanding the context of healthcare utilization: Assessing environmental and provider-related variables in the behavioral model of utilization', *Health Service Research*, vol 33, no 3, pt 1, pp571–596

Smyser, M. and Ciske, S. (2001) 'Racial and Ethnic Discrimination in Health Care Settings', *Public Health Special Reports*, www.kingcounty.gov/healthservices/health/-news/2001/01012401.aspx, accessed 10 April 2006

Valentine, N., Darby, C. and Bonsel, G. J. (2008) 'Which aspects of non-clinical quality of care are most important? Results from WHO's general population surveys of "health systems responsiveness" in 41 countries', *Social Science and Medicine*, vol 66, pp1939–1950

Wade, C., Chao, M., Kronenberg, F., Cushman, L. and Kalmuss, D. (2008) 'Medical pluralism among American women: Results of a national survey', *Journal of Women's Health*, vol 17, no 5, pp829–840

WHO (2002) *Health Systems: Improving Performance*, The World Health Report 2000, World Health Organization, Geneva, Switzerland

16
Exploring Pathways to Environmental, Health and Social Equity

Introduction

The preceding chapters of this book have provided ample coverage of the kinds of environmental health hazards that impact people around the world and how these interact with various social and behavioural risk factors to produce negative health outcomes. A review of the scientific literature along with case studies drawn primarily from the United States and African countries have demonstrated the complexity of these problems, their manifestation at multiple spatial scales, and the challenges facing governments to come up with sustainable strategies that ensure environmental health equity and social justice among all groups. Disparities have been noted across many different geographic entities, from wealthy industrialized countries, to egalitarian societies such as Sweden, transitional and emerging economies in Eastern Europe, Asia, and the rest of the Global South.

As we move forward in the 21st century, a key question that remains is how best to tackle these challenges individually within each country, and collectively at the international level. Specifically, what pathways can we adopt as global citizens to promote equity in health? What steps can we take to ensure that all people regardless of race, ethnicity, class, region or other social and spatial dimensions will have adequate resources to maintain their health? Many scholars have contemplated similar questions in the past and offered some suggestions (Roby, 1997, 1998; Schoenhals and Behar, 2000; Krieger, 2006) yet the pathways remain fuzzy particularly for residents in the developing regions. In this chapter, we offer four of these strategies that are deemed valuable in promoting environmental and health equity as part of the broader mission of social justice. These are discussed below.

Maintaining an active research agenda

The first path to health equity requires ongoing research to continue to uncover the root causes, complex processes and detrimental impacts of social and environmental injustices within marginalized communities. Maintaining an active research agenda that addresses group inequities through data collection, monitoring, analysis, mapping and visualization of environmental hazards, socio-demographic correlates and health outcomes is critical, and adds greater credibility to the environmental and social justice movement. As illustrated in this text, the work must be theoretically grounded, guided by epidemiological principles and geographical perspectives in the literature, and the use of robust tools and methodologies to validate the claims of residents. Research findings emanating from such investigations would allow health care policy and decision makers to figure out ways to assist in environmental health remediation, and to reallocate resources to prevent future inequities. In making the case for more research on social justice and health disparities, Krieger (2006) recently noted, and rightly so, that the

> *facts never speak for themselves. Rather, the research findings must be critically evaluated in relation to i) the theoretical frameworks that researchers use; and ii) the rigor with which we conceptualize, operationalize, analyze and interpret the relevant constructs; and iii) the intellectual honesty that we must muster to address thoughtfully the likely limitations of any given study and the implications for the conclusions reached. (p461)*

The approaches used in this book have followed these principles. For nearly all health issues introduced in the text, we have presented the theoretical underpinnings and conceptualizations that frame the discussion in the literature. The research has also entailed the compilation of health statistics along with geographically referenced data from communities selected as case studies to evaluate the hypotheses and research questions. Data analysis has also required the use of rigorous methodologies, mostly from geographical and statistical approaches, enabling the computation and visualization of these issues at different spatial scales. These analytical strategies allow the public and decision makers to see for themselves where the risks are, identify the groups that are most vulnerable to those risks, and in so doing take the right steps to minimize those disparities.

Educating and promulgating a social justice mindset for future health professionals

The success of health equity and the social justice movement lies in the hands of future health professionals who must not only be cognizant of the social and environmental injustices that produce health disparities, but must also take an active step in addressing the health needs of these disadvantaged population groups. As we have learned in the preceding chapters of this book, some of the key indicators of health quality and health utilization among patients are linked directly to the cultural competence of the workforce, cultural sensitivity and cultural acceptability, otherwise known as health systems responsiveness. These are all the non-clinical aspects of health quality yet they are the important attributes that patients look for when they visit health care facilities. Patients need health care providers who are culturally aware of their socio-spatial experiences, can communicate effectively and treat them with dignity and respect regardless of their race, ethnicity or class status. Promulgating this social justice mindset among health professionals requires a revision of the core curriculum, integrating courses that include multiculturalism, medical pluralism, environmental injustices and health disparities by race, ethnicity and class, these being the most perennial sources of disparities around the world.

Advocacy for disadvantaged populations

Reducing social and environmental injustices and the concomitant health problems also requires advocacy on the part of the groups that are most affected by these issues. Within all countries and internationally, there are many advocacy groups that try to bring attention to environmental and social injustices and the plight of vulnerable populations, and advocate the protection of the fundamental rights of these people. These groups function through public and private international agencies, foundations, charitable organizations and civil society organizations within various countries. Nationally, tactics such as letter writing campaigns, demonstrations, voter mobilization campaigns and corresponding with government and elected officials are all valuable ways to shine the media spotlight on these issues. Some of these efforts do translate into success stories such as the case of the environmental justice movement in Warren County. However, success in one locality often implies that violators will relocate elsewhere, introducing the same set of negative externalities in other areas. Advocacy groups must therefore be vigilant, and form coalitions to keep polluters away from compounding the problems of the poor and disadvantaged, and work to promote greener and healthier environments for all people.

Promoting sustainable human development through individual and community participation

The fourth pathway to health equity involves the promotion of sustainable human development with individuals and their local communities occupying the centre of these development efforts. Specifically, individuals and communities must be given equitable access to life-enhancing opportunities. These should include the provision of relevant information, materials and resources required to maximize control over their own lives, and make the decisions that will impact their own community, environment and health. Many experts in field of development and scholars have taken a similar position in the past (Roby, 1998; Aronson et al, 2006; Jolly, 2006). For example, Jolly (2006) argues for the empowerment of individuals to take charge of their own lives and consequently their own health. To do so, governments must provide the ideal environments for people to learn, and provide opportunities for them to work and earn a living to support themselves and their families. Strengthening human capabilities also requires access to safe water and sanitation in the living environments of the poor and marginalized groups to minimize the risks of infectious diseases. As we learned in the previous chapters, water-related hazards account for many deaths globally, therefore the path to social and health equity must address such challenges. The formulation of the Millennium Development Goals (MDGs) and the implementation of the related strategies especially in developing countries represent giant steps towards these efforts.

Local community and neighbourhood empowerment also provide avenues to environmental, health and social equity. Aronson et al (2006) suggest several advantages that come with the integration of neighbourhoods and communities in this effort. Such strategies incorporate social networks, social support systems, social capital and their capacity to identify and resolve their own unique problems. Further, as reported in the previous chapters of this book, the value of these social networks and social capital on health outcomes has been widely illustrated in the health literature. In some of the case studies presented in this text, the local context also offers valuable insights into the root causes and processes that produce health disparities. Efforts to address these challenges must therefore build on the experiences of the individuals residing within these communities, engaging them and working with them collaboratively in order to bring a long lasting solution to the problem.

In conclusion, environmental hazards and health disparities are complex, unwieldy and originate from a host of factors. In this book, we started out by offering a very broad view of the environment and this allowed us to undertake a comprehensive examination of a wide array of hazards and risk factors that produce disproportionate outcomes among people. Achieving health equity among these populations is a gargantuan but not necessarily impossible task. It will require a multi-tiered effort with full support and cooperation from the individuals, their communities, governments and international agencies. Interdisciplinary efforts that require input from geographers, spatial epidemiologists and public health professionals will contribute significantly to the targeting of at-risk groups, particularly those that have a limited voice in resource allocation and decision making.

References

Aronson, R. E., Lovelace, K., Hatch, J. W. and Whitehead, T. L. (2006) 'Strengthening communities and roles of individuals in community life', in Levy, B. S. and Sidel, V. W. (eds) *Social Justice and Public Health*, Oxford University Press, New York

Jolly, R. (2006) 'Promoting equitable and sustainable human development', in Levy, B. S. and Sidel, V. W. (eds) *Social Justice and Public Health*, Oxford University Press, New York

Krieger, N. (2006) 'Researching critical questions on social justice and public health: An ecosocial perspective', in Levy, B. S. and Sidel, V. W. (eds) *Social Justice and Public Health*, Oxford University Press, New York

Roby, P. A. (1997) *Working Toward a Just World: Visions, Experiences and Challenge*, The Society for the Study of Social Problems, Knoxville, TN
Roby, P. A. (1998) 'Creating a just world: Leadership for the twenty-first century', *Social Problems*, vol 45, no 1, pp1–20
Schoenhals, M. and Behar, J. E. (2000) *Visions of the 21st Century: Social Research for the New Millennium*, Global Publications, Binghamton, NY

Index

Page numbers in *italic* refer to Figures and Tables.